PROSTATE CANCER
UNDERSTANDING THE PATHOPHYSIOLOGY AND RE-DESIGNING A THERAPEUTIC APPROACH

Editors

Fernand Labrie, *MD, Ph.D, Quebec, Canada*

Michael Koutsilieris, *MD, Ph.D., Athens, Greece*

PMP

PASCHALIDIS MEDICAL PUBLICATIONS

PMP

PASCHALIDIS MEDICAL PUBLICATIONS

PMP (Paschalidis Medical Publications, Ltd.).
14th, Tetrapoleos str., Athens, 115 27, Greece
Tel.: 003-210-7789125, 003-210-7793012, Fax: 003-210-7759421,
e-mail:
orders: Paschalidis@Medical-Books.gr
© information: GP@Medical-Books.gr, CP@Medical-Books.gr

Notice

Medicine is an ever-changing science. As new research and clinical experiences broaden our knowledge, changes in treatment and drug therapy are required. The editor and the publisher of this work have checked with sources believed to be reliable in their efforts to provide information that is complete and generally in accord with the standards accepted at the time of publication. However, in view of the possibility of human error or changes in medical sciences, neither the editor nor the publisher nor any other party who has been involved in the preparation of publication of this work warrants that the information contained herein is in every respect accurate or complete, and they disclaim all responsibility for any errors or omissions or for the results obtained from use of the information contained in this work. Readers are encouraged to confirm the information contained herein with other sources. For example and in particular, readers are advised to check the product information sheet included in the package of each drug they plan to administer to be certain that the information contained in this work is accurate and that changes have not been made in the recommended dose or in the contraindications for administration. This recommendation is of particular importance in connection with new or infrequently used drugs.

ISBN: 960-399-195-3

Copyright © 2004 by PMP (Paschalidis Medical Publications, Ltd.). All rights reserved. Printed in Greece. Except as permitted under the Greek Laws, no part of this publication may be reproduced or distributed in any form or by any means, or stored in a data base or retrieval system, without the prior written permission of the publisher.

*Dedicated
to our families*

Fernand Labrie & Michael Koutsilieris

Contributors/Author's & Affiliations

Bennett, Charles
The Chicago VA Healthcare System/Lakeside Division, the Robert H. Lurie Comprehensive Cancer Center, The Division of Hematology/Oncology of the Department of Medicine, and the Institute for Health Services Research and Policy Studies of Northwestern University, Chicago, Ill

Berman, Craig
University of Colorado Health Sciences Center, Department of Urologic Oncology, Denver Colorado, USA

Bogdanos, John
Department of Experimental Physiology, Medical School, University of Athens, Goudi, 115 27 Athens, Greece
Urology Clinic, METAXA Anticancer Hospital, Pireaus, Greece

Brousseau, George
Oncology and Molecular Endocrinology Research Center, CHUL Research Center and Laval University, Quebec City, G1V 4G2, Canada

Candas, Bernard
Oncology and Molecular Endocrinology Research Center, CHUL Research Center and Laval University, Quebec City, G1V 4G2, Canada

Chevrette, Éric
DSP, Radiology, Centre Hospitalier de l' Université Laval, Québec City, G1V 4G2, Canada

Crawford, E. David
University of Colorado Health Sciences Center, Department of Urologic Oncology, Denver, Colorado, USA

Cusan, Leonello
Oncology and Molecular Endocrinology Research Center, CHUL Research Center and Laval University, Quebec City, G1V 4G2, Canada

Dardoufas, Constantine
Department of Radiology & Radiotherapy, Medical School, University of Athens, ARETAIEION University Hospital, Athens, Greece

Diamandis, Eleftherios P.
Department of Pathology and Laboratory Medicine, Mount Sinai Hospital, University of Toronto, Toronto, Canada

Dimopoulos, Theodoros
Urology Clinic, PANAGIA General Hospital, Thessaloniki, Greece

Dumont, Martine
Oncology and Molecular Endocrinology Research Center, CHUL Research Center and Laval University, Quebec City, G1V 4G2, Canada

Gomez, José Luis
Oncology and Molecular Endocrinology Research Center, CHUL Research Center and Laval University, Quebec City, G1V 4G2, Canada

Highley, Howard R.
NCI, Division of Cancer Treatment and Diagnosis, Rockville, MD, USA

Jung, Klaus
Humboldt University Berlin, Berlin, Germany

Karamanolakis, Dimitrios
Department of Experimental Physiology, Medical School, University of Athens, Goudi, 115 27 Athens, Greece
Urology Clinic, METAXA Anticancer Hospital, Pireaus, Greece

Kelloff, Gary J.
NCI, Division of Cancer Treatment and Diagnosis, Rockville, MD, USA

Koutsilieris, Michael
Department of Experimental Physiology, Medical School, University of Athens, Goudi, 115 27 Athens, Greece

Kurhanewicz, John
Magnetic Resonance Science Center, Department of Radiology, University of California, San Francisco

Labrie, Fernand
Oncology and Molecular Endocrinology Research Center, CHUL Research Center and Laval University, Quebec City, G1V 4G2, Canada

Contributors/Author's & Affiliations

Lembessis, Peter
Department of Experimental Physiology, Medical School, University of Athens, Goudi, 115 27 Athens, Greece
Endo-OncoResearch Laboratories, Athens, Greece

Lévesque, Jacques
DSP, Imagery and Physiology, Centre Hospitalier de l' Université Laval, Québec City, G1V 4G2, Canada

Milathianakis, Constantine
Department of Experimental Physiology, Medical School, University of Athens, Goudi, Athens, Greece
Urology Clinic, METAXA Anticancer Hospital, Pireaus, Greece

Mitsiades, Constantine
Department of Experimental Physiology, Medical School, University of Athens, Goudi, 115 27 Athens, Greece
Department of Medical Oncology, Dana Farber Cancer Institute and Department of Medicine, Harvard Medical School, Boston MA USA

Nathan, Derek
The Chicago VA Healthcare System/Lakeside Division, the Robert H. Lurie Comprehensive Cancer Center, The Division of Hematology/Oncology of the Department of Medicine, and the Institute for Health Services Research and Policy Studies of Northwestern University, Chicago, Ill

Sigman, Caroline C.
CSS Associates, Mountain View, CA, USA

Simard, Jacques
Oncology and Molecular Endocrinology Research Center, CHUL Research Center and Laval University, Quebec City, G1V 4G2, Canada
Canada Research Chair in Oncogenetics & Cancer Genomics Laboratory, CHVL Research Center and Laval University, Quebec City, GIV 4G2, Canada

Soucy, Penny
Oncology and Molecular Endocrinology Research Center, CHUL Research Center and Laval University, Quebec City, G1V 4G2, Canada

Sourla, Antigone
Endo-OncoResearch Laboratories, 115 27 Athens, Greece

Stephan, Carsten
Humboldt University Berlin, Berlin, Germany

Swanson, Mark G.
Magnetic Resonance Science Center, Department of Radiology, University of California, San Francisco

Tavtigian, Sean V.
International Agency for Research on Cancer, 69372, Lyon Cedex 08, France

Têtu, Bernard
Department of Pathology, Centre Hospitalier Universitaire de Québec, l'Hôtel-Dieu-de-Québec, Québec, Canada.

Tsintavis, Athanassios
Urology Clinic, METAXA Anticancer Hospital, Pireaus, Greece

Van der Kwast, Theodorus
Department of Pathology, Erasmus University, Rotterdam, The Netherlands, (TvdK)

Vigneron, Daniel B.
Magnetic Resonance Science Center, Department of Radiology, University of California, San Francisco

Yousef, George M.
Humboldt University Berlin, Berlin, Germany

Zagaras, Evangelos
Urology Clinic, PANAGIA General Hospital, Thessaloniki, Greece

Contents

1. PROSTATE CANCER SUSCEPTIBILITY GENES 1
2. INTRODUCTION AND HISTORY OF PSA SCREENING 39
3. PROSTATE SPECIFIC ANTIGEN AND OTHER KALLIKREINS IN PROSTATE CANCER 53
4. PROSTATE CANCER SCREENING AND EARLY TREATMENT: THE ONLY POSSIBILITY FOR A MAJOR IMPACT ON SURVIVAL IN PROSTATE CANCER. 67
5. MAGNETIC RESONANCE IMAGING AND SPECTROSCOPIC IMAGING OF PROSTATE CANCER: IMPROVED THERAPEUTIC SELECTION AND ASSESSMENT. 79
6. MOLECULAR STAGING IN CLINICALLY LOCALIZED AND ADVANCED PROSTATE CANCER. 97
7. BONE MICROENVIRONMENT PARTICIPATION IN THE DEVELOPMENT OF ANDROGEN ABLATION REFRACTORINESS IN PROSTATE CANCER PATIENTS WITH BONE METASTASES: CLINICAL APPLICATION OF AN ANTI-SURVIVAL FACTOR THERAPY. 109
8. COMBINED ANDROGEN BLOCKADE WITH NON-STEROIDAL ANTI-ANDROGENS FOR ADVANCED PROSTATE CANCER: A REVIEW OF THE EVIDENCE ON EFFICACY AND TOXICITY. 135
9. PATHOLOGIC CHANGES INDUCED BY HORMONE THERAPY IN NORMAL PROSTATE CARCINOMA 145
10. STATUS OF ANDROGEN BLOCKADE IN PROSTATE CANCER IN 2003 157
11. STRATEGIES FOR PROSTATE CANCER PREVENTION. 171

REFERENCES 185

PREFACE

Prostate cancer is the most frequently diagnosed cancer and the second cause of cancer death in men in North America and Western Europe. In fact, one out of eight men will be diagnosed with prostate during his life time. Prostate cancer is thus a major challenge in urgent need of significant improvements in diagnosis and treatment. Fortunately, the death rate from prostate cancer has dropped by 17% in the United States between 1994 and 2003, this decrease coinciding with the routine use of the prostatic specific antigen (PSA) test. In fact, as presented in this book, PSA and the other available diagnostic procedures permit the diagnosis of prostate cancer at the localized stage in 99% of cases, thus permitting treatments having the possibility of a cure, namely surgery, radiotherapy, brachytherapy and/or androgen blockade.

It is most timely to mention a recent metaanalysis presented at the ECCO Meeting in September 2003 showing a one-third decrease in deaths from prostate cancer in patients with localized disease who received androgen blockage (usually an LHRH agonist) immediately at diagnosis versus those who were treated later at time of clinical progression. In fact, until recently, any treatment of early disease was controversial, due to the absence of studies on the subject. The situation has changed since 1997 with the publication on six randomized clinical trials showing a decrease in deaths from prostate cancer ranging from 37% to 81% at five years of follow-up. These results obtained with monotherapy are quite remarkable and demonstrate that androgen blockade is highly efficient in localized prostate cancer, its success being comparable or even better than that achieved with tamoxifen which has become the standard therapy in breast cancer.

An important advance in our understanding of the endocrinology of the prostate and prostate cancer is that about 50% of androgens are left in the prostate following castration. In fact, 50% of androgens are made locally in the prostate from adrenal precursors. This finding has led to the development of combined androgen blockade (CAB) or the addition of a pure antiandrogen to medical (LHRH agonist) or surgical castration. When CAB was used in patients with advanced disease and bone metastases, all the metaanalyses of all the studies performed have shown a decrease in the risk of prostate cancer death death ranging from 10 to 20%. When the same combined androgen blockade was used in patients with localized disease, long-term control or even probably a cure of the cancer could be achieved in 90% of patients.

It is important to identify the genes involved in the development and growth of prostate cancer. Accordingly, you can read in this book a review on the genes already found as being linked to an increased susceptibility to prostate cancer. It is also the important to identify the genes which are involved in the unique environment of the bones where resistance to endocrine therapy is the major issue. Clearly, while localized prostate cancer is highly sensitive to androgens and resistance does not develop to combined androgen blockade, the local factors specific to the bones are a major limitation to the success of any hormonal therapy. It is also of great interest to provide a description of the histopathological changes which accompany androgen blockade and to discuss the potential strategies for prostate cancer prevention. All these aspects of prostate cancer diagnosis, treatment and pathogenesis are presented as well as a look into the future. In fact, an important part of our hope lies with further development of more efficient androgen blockade in parallel with early diagnosis at a time when the cancer is most sensitive to the blockade of androgens. It is clear that androgen blockade has not been used at its optimal level of efficacy in the past and that major progress can be accomplished in this area. On the other hand, the answer to a series of remaining issues should come from the current studies in genomics and proteomics which look at the pathogenesis of prostate cancer at the level of the whole genome.

Fernard Labrie, MD, PhD
Department of Physiology, Faculty of Medicine, Laval University and Endocrine - Oncology Laboratory Research Center CHUL - CHVQ, Quebec City, P.Q. Canada

Michael Koutsilieris, MD, PhD
Department of Experimental Physiology, Medical School, University of Athens, Goudi, Athens, Greece

PROSTATE CANCER SUSCEPTIBILITY GENES

*By Jacques Simard, Martine Dumont,
Penny Soucy, Fernand Labrie, Sean V. Tavtigian*

SUMMARY

In most developed countries, prostate cancer is the most frequently diagnosed malignancy in men. The extent to which the marked racial/ethnic difference in its incidence rate is attributable to screening methods, environmental, hormonal and/or genetic factors remains unknown. A positive family history is among the strongest epidemiological risk factors for prostate cancer. It is now well recognized that the role of candidate genetic markers to this multifactorial malignancy is more difficult to identify than the identification of susceptibility genes for breast, ovary and colon cancer. Several reasons may explain such a difficulty: 1) prostate cancer is diagnosed at a late age, thus often making it impossible to obtain DNA samples from living men of more than one generation; 2) the presence within high-risk pedigrees of phenocopies, associated with the lack of distinguishing features between hereditary and sporadic forms and 3) the genetic heterogeneity of this complex disease with the accompanying difficulty of developing appropriate statistical transmission models which simultaneously take into account these multiple susceptibility genes which, individually, confer only moderate or modest risk. Despite the localization of several susceptibility loci, there has been limited success in identifying high-risk susceptibility genes analogous to BRCA1 or BRCA2 for breast and ovarian cancer. Nonetheless, three strong candidate susceptibility genes have been described, namely *ELAC2* (chromosome 17p11/ *HPC2* region), 2'-5'-oligoadenylate–dependent ribonuclease L *(RNASEL)*, a gene in the *HPC1* region, and Macrophage Scavenger Receptor 1 *(MSR1)*, a gene within a region of linkage on chromosome 8p. Additional studies using larger cohorts are needed to fully evaluate the role of these susceptibility genes in prostate cancer risk. Although initial segregation analyses supported the hypothesis that a number of rare highly penetrant loci contribute to the Mendelian inheritance of prostate cancer, current experimental evidence better supports the hypothesis that some of the familial risks may be due to inheritance of multiple moderate-risk genetic variants. In this regard, it is not surprising that analyses of genes encoding key proteins involved in androgen biosynthesis and action led to the observation of a significant association between a susceptibility to prostate cancer and common genetic variants, such as those found in type 2 5a-reductase, type 2 3b-hydroxysteroid dehydrogenase/isomerase and androgen receptor genes.

1. INTRODUCTION

In most developed countries, prostate cancer is the most frequently diagnosed non-cutaneous malignancy among men. In the United States, one in eight men will develop prostate cancer during his life. The incidence of prostate cancer varies markedly throughout the world, with United States, Canada, Sweden, Australia and France having the highest rates (ranging from 48.1 to 137.0 cases per 100,000 person-years as estimated between the 1988-1992 period), whereas most European countries have intermediate rates (23.9 to 31.0 cases per 100,000 person-years). The lowest prevalence is observed in Asian populations (2.3 to 9.8 cases per 100,000 person-years)[1]. The extent to which this racial/ethnic difference is attributable to screening methods, environmental, hormonal and/or genetic factors is unknown. Although early detection using prostate-specific antigen (PSA) and improved treatment have emerged as the most critical strategies to decrease prostate-cancer mortality[2], the potential of early detection through genetic indicators is also particularly relevant. Nevertheless, scientists involved in cancer genomics acknowledge that obvious heterogeneity exits, making the association of candidate genetic markers to this multifactorial malignancy more difficult than the identification of susceptibility genes for some common cancers such as breast, ovary and colon cancer.

A positive family history is among the strongest epidemiological risk factors for prostate cancer. Familial clustering of prostate cancer was first reported by Morganti et al.[3]. Thereafter, various case-control and cohort studies have investigated the role of family history as a risk factor for prostate cancer (see for recent reviews[4-7]). Much evidence comes from the study of pedigrees having a large number of cases, as those observed in the Utah population[8,9]. The relative risk of prostate cancer increases markedly when the age of the index case decreases or when the number of affected individuals in a cluster increases, thus suggesting that this increased risk has a genetic component. For example, the brother of a proband diagnosed at age 50 has a 1.9-fold relative risk of developing prostate cancer compared to the brother of a case diagnosed at age 70[10]. Moreover, having one, two or three affected first-degree relatives increases the relative risk by 2.2-, 4.9- and 10.9-folds, respectively[11]. It should be noted that family studies offer the opportunity to estimate risks of siblings and parent-offspring pairs, but cannot distinguish between genetic and non-genetic causes of familial aggregations of cancer. In contrast, comparisons of the concordance of cancer between monozygotic and dizygotic pairs of twins provide valuable information on whether the familial clustering is due to hereditary or environmental influences. Thus, the importance of inherited predisposition to prostate cancer is also supported by the finding that monozygotic twins have a four-fold increased concordance rate of prostate cancer compared to dizygotic twins[10]. In support of this latter observation, it has recently been estimated, using the combined data from 44,788 pairs of twins listed in Swedish, Danish and Finnish twin registries, that 42% (95% CI = 29%-50%) of all prostate-cancer risk may be explained by inheritable factors[12].

The first segregation analysis, which included 691 families affected by prostate cancer ascertained through 740 consecutive probands undergoing radical prostatectomy, suggested that inherited predisposition was due to a rare, highly penetrant autosomal dominant allele(s) with a population frequency of 0.003, and with carriers having an 88% cumulative risk of disease by 85 years of age compared to only 5% in non-carriers[10]. The gene accounted for approximately 43% of prostate cancer cases diagnosed before age 55 and 9% of cases diagnosed through age 85. In two other segregation analyses, similar transmission models were proposed[13,14], however, the Grönberg model proposed a more common allele (1.67%) and a lower life span penetrance (63%). All these studies thus supported the presence of at least one highly penetrant autosomal dominant prostate cancer predisposition gene. However, consistently higher risks observed in brothers of prostate cancer affected relatives compared to sons of affected individuals have led to hypotheses of an X-linked, recessive, and/or imprinted component to the genetics of prostate cancer susceptibility[15, 16]. Finally, Cui et al.[17] recently suggested a model of a dominantly inherited increased risk that was greater at younger ages, whereas a recessive or X-linked-risk that was greater at older ages.

2. MAPPING PUTATIVE LOCI FOR PROSTATE CANCER SUSCEPTIBILITY GENES

Several factors may contribute to the difficulty of identifying prostate cancer susceptibility genes[4-8]. Prostate cancer is typically diagnosed at a late age, thus often making it difficult to obtain DNA samples from living affected men for more than one generation. Another significant problem is the lack of clear distinguishing features between hereditary and sporadic forms of the disease, making it difficult to distinguish, within high-risk pedigrees, men who have developed a cancer that is sporadic rather than due to an inherited germline mutation (phenocopies). Indeed, the presence within a pedigree of a sporadic case who harbors a meiotic recombinant within a *bona fide* region of linkage that is not actually relevant to his disease can push a peak of LOD score away from the true location of an underlying susceptibility gene or lead a positional cloning team to incorrectly narrow a putative region of linkage, thus misleading scientists to focus their analysis of candidate genes in the wrong chromosomal region. A particularly difficult problem is the apparent genetic heterogeneity of the trait; appropriate analysis would require development of statistical transmission models that can take into account multiple susceptibility genes, many of which are apparently of moderate or modest penetrance[4-7].

To date, chromosome by chromosome results of genome scans for prostate cancer susceptibility loci have been published by four independent groups. Three additional independent groups have published focused results derived from at least nearly complete genome scans. Because most of the subsequent replication studies are based on the family sets assembled for these genome scans, we will identify most of the study sets either by the acronym for the underlying family study or by the name of the research center most clearly associated with ascertainment of the family set. Sources of the four genome scans that have been, to date, well described are: a Johns-Hopkins/ Sweden collaboration "Johns-Hopkins set"[18]; the Seattle based Prostate Cancer Genetic Research Study "PROGRESS set"[19, 20]; a family collection ascertained largely through staff urologists at the Washington University School of Medicine and consisting mostly of affected sib pairs "WUSM set"[21-23] and a family collection that developed out of a multiethnic case-control study ascertained in Hawaii, California, British Columbia, and Ontario "Stanford/ USC set"[24]. Sources of three additional genome scans that have both identified candidate loci and contributed to replication studies are: a collection of large Utah pedigrees ascertained through a genealogy/cancer diagnosis resource for an excess of closely and distantly related prostate cancer cases among the descendants of a single ancestor "Utah set"[25, 26]; a family collection ascertained through the Mayo Clinic radical prostatectomy database "Mayo set"[27]; and a set of French and German prostate cancer pedigrees "Progene set"[28].

Largely as a result of analysis of these seven collections of prostate cancer pedigrees, hints of linkage have been described on every autosome as well as the X chromosome. Many of the stronger hints have either been cross-referenced between genome scans, reevaluated on one or more of the independent family sets used in one of the other genome scans, or further evaluated on an extended version of the family set from which the hint of linkage was originally derived. Recognizing that strength of evidence in support of these various hints of linkage exists on a continuum complicated by different ascertainment criteria for the underlying family collections as well as differences in analytic methods, it seems useful to discuss two groups of linkages.

The first group (5 linkages) are supported by at least one analysis with LOD >3.0 and nominal support from at least two or more independent analyses. In chronological order by when the hypothesis-generating linkage was first described, these are: *HPC1* at 1q23-25 (Johns-Hopkins set)[18,29], *PCAP* at 1q41-43 (Progene set)[28], *HPCX* at Xq27-28 (Johns-Hopkins set)[30], *CAPB* at 1p36-35 (PROGRESS set)[19], and *HPC20* at 20q11-13 (Mayo set)[27] (Figure 1).

The second group (5 linkages) are supported by at least one analysis with LOD >2.5 and nominal support from at least one independent study, but without reaching the group one criteria. This time ordered by chromosomal location with reference given here to the report presenting strongest evidence of linkage to the locus, these are: a hint of linkage at Chr 4q24-25 (WUSM set)[22], a hint of linkage at Chr 8p23-22 (Johns-Hopkins set)[29], a hint of linkage at Chr 16p13 (WUSM set)[22], a hint of linkage at 17p11 *(HPC2/ELAC2)* (Utah set)[26], and a hint of linkage to tumor aggressiveness at Chr 19q (WUSM set)[23] (Fig. 1).

As one considers the evidence relevant to each of these linkages, it is important to recognize that the multiple testing inherent in executing a complete genome scan for disease susceptibility will generate false-posi-

1. Prostate Cancer Susceptibility Genes

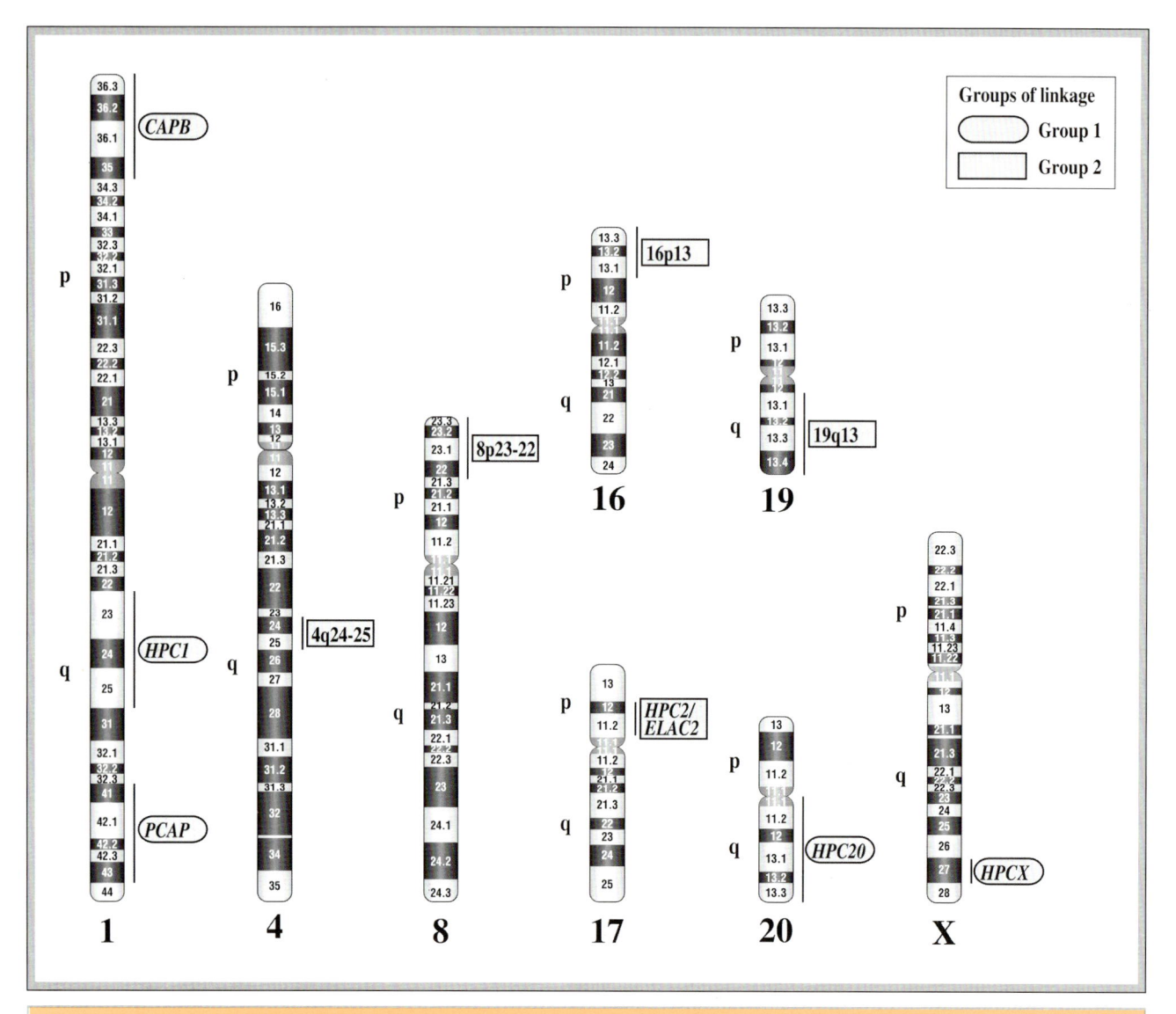

FIGURE 1. Localization of prostate cancer susceptibility loci reported in the literature. The first group of linkages identified by circles, are supported by at least one analysis with LOD > 3.0 and nominal support from at least two or more independant analyses. *HPC1* at 1q23-25[18, 46], *PCAP* at 1q41-43[28], *HPCX* at Xq27-28 [30], *CAPB* at 1p36-35[19, 29], *HPC20* at 20q11-13[39]. The second group of linkages identified by boxes, are supported by at least one analysis with LOD > 2.5 and nominal support from at least one independant study. 4q24-25[22], 8p23-22[46], 16p13[47], HPC2/ELAC2 at 17p11[26] and 19q[23].

tive hints of linkage. Even without error in genotyping or analysis, it is very common to generate false positives with LOD scores between 2.0 and 3.0. Indeed common problems such as miss-specifying allele frequencies contribute to an appreciable level of false positives with LOD scores between

3.0 and 4.0. Until an underlying susceptibility gene has been found, the best evidence in support of a candidate linkage is concordance with independent genome scans or independent targeted analyses of the region with evidence of linkage. Given the number of independent genome scans for prostate cancer susceptibility gene(s) that have been reported to date along with the multiple testing burden created by the analysis of those data with many different models, it would not be surprising to find examples of false-positive results that have been independently corroborated by other false positive results. However, it is very clear from segregation studies that sequence variants that confer risk of prostate cancer do exist which implies that some of the reported hints of linkage, and most likely those with stronger independent support, almost certainly reflect the presence of an underlying prostate cancer susceptibility gene.

2.1 Group 1 linkages

2.1.1 HPC1

Linkage at HPC1 (1q23-25) was first described in 1996 from an analysis of the Johns-Hopkins pedigree resource[18], which was largely ascertained on the basis of early onset familial prostate cancer. In that study, a multipoint LOD score of 5.43 was obtained, and heterogeneity analysis suggested that *HPC1* accounts for up to 34% of prostate cancer families with four or more cases[18]. While several of the initial studies to reexamine this locus found little or no evidence for existence of a linkage at HPC1[28, 31, 32], later studies, often using specific stratifications of their pedigree resources, were much more supportive. Linkage was confirmed through analysis of a set of 41 large (average of 10.7 cases per pedigree) Utah high risk pedigrees[25], with 3-point LOD scores of 2.43 and 2.82 obtained from the full set of pedigrees and youngest quartile (average age at diagnosis) of pedigrees, respectively. Further confirmation came through reanalysis of the PROGRESS pedigree resource[33]. In that study, there was little evidence of linkage at *HPC1* from the overall data set, consistent with earlier analyses from their group. However, when the set of pedigrees was stratified by evidence of linkage at any of the other three loci considered in the analysis (*CAPB*, *PCAP*, and *HPCX*) and further stratified by disease aggressiveness within each pedigree, a NPL score of 2.55 was obtained from the pedigrees displaying a pattern of more aggressive disease but little evidence of linkage to the other loci. When the pedigrees were further stratified by average age at diagnosis, an NPL score of 3.47 was obtained from the pedigrees with age at diagnosis ≥65. One must note that this last stratification gave a result opposite from that obtained from the Utah pedigrees[25] and contrary to the set of criteria used to ascertain the set of pedigrees from which the linkage was first described[18]. Significant support from several studies entirely independent of the original hypothesis generating study make it quite likely that Chr 1q23-25 indeed harbors one or more significant prostate cancer susceptibility genes, although these analyses have not progressed towards a tight localization of the underlying gene(s).

While the fraction of families initially estimated to be linked to *HPC1* was quite high[18], a subsequent pooled analysis of 772 families[34] was more consistent with the actual proportion being much lower, in the vicinity of 6%. In that meta-analysis, a disproportionate amount of linkage was derived from families characterized by male-to-male disease transmission, early age at diagnosis (≤65 years) and having five or more affected members. Interestingly, a large scale, high resolution reanalysis of Chr 1 using an extended version of the Johns-Hopkins pedigree resource[29] provided some evidence for two independent peaks of LOD score within the region, a proximal peak characterized by larger families with higher average age at diagnosis, and a distal peak characterized by smaller clusters with earlier average age at diagnosis. Finally, reanalysis of the WUSM group's genome scan, which did not initially find evidence for *HPC1*[22], found strong evidence in support of the proximal *HPC1* peak just described when Gleason score was used as a covariable[21].

2.1.2 PCAP

A second putative Chr 1 locus, PCAP, located near the 1q telomere, was detected following a genome scan of the Progene pedigree resource and reported to be responsible for 40 to 50% of French and German families[28]. Families with age of onset before 65 years contributed significantly to initial evidence for this linkage. A subsequent study used an extended version of the Progene pedigree resource to determine the contribution of several susceptibility loci, including *HPC1, PCAP, CABP* and *HPCX,* to prostate cancer in the southern and western European population. In that study, the authors found that *PCAP* was the only region showing evidence of linkage in the 64 HPC families studied[35]. Independent groups have also seen some evidence of linkage to 1q41-43. In the initial genome scan of the Johns-Hopkins pedigree resource, a 2-point LOD score of ~1.4 was revealed at D1S235, the third highest peak in that analysis [18]. When the same group conducted a high resolution scan of Chr 1 on an extended version of their pedigree resource, weak evidence at D1S235 did remain[29]. Overall evidence from the genome scan of the WUSM family resource did not show evidence of linkage to the distal segment of 1q. However, when the pedigrees were stratified on the basis of family history, those with greater family history showed modest evidence of linkage in the region, with Z-scores of 2.10 and 1.84 at two closely spaced markers in the region (P = 0.018 and P = 0.034, respectively)[22]. When the data from this genome scan was later reanalyzed with various covariates, weak evidence remained, with a maximum LOD score of 1.90 (P = 0.007)[21]. Analysis of the Progress pedigree resource also provided some supportive evidence. Specifically, a 2-point LOD score of 1.99 was observed at D1S1656 under a recessive analysis model. When this pedigree resource was divided by average age at diagnosis, most of the evidence was found in the earlier onset group[20]. In contrast, there was no evidence for linkage to the distal segment of 1q from the genome scan of the Stanford/ USC pedigree resource[24].

Given that the *PCAP* linkage is not very far from the *HPC1* locus and that linkage studies conducted over family sets that contain phenocopies, sporadics, and false-positive recombinants tend to maximize at some distance away from the actual underlying susceptibility gene, it is not entirely clear that *PCAP* and *HPC1* are independent loci. On the other hand, the linkage data are also consistent with two or even three independent susceptibility loci present on the distal half of chromosome 1q. In this scenario, each locus would have some tendency to interfere with both evidence for and localization of the neighboring loci, creating a complicated and particularly difficult problem of linkage analysis.

2.1.3 HPCX

Linkage at *HPCX* was first described in 1998[30]. Evidence of linkage was quite strong, with a 2-point LOD score of 4.6 and a multipoint LOD of 3.85. The analysis was comprised of prostate cancer pedigrees from 4 centers: Johns Hopkins, the Mayo Clinic, Tampere, and Umea. It should be noted that the Johns Hopkins set of families overlaps strongly with the set that was used to obtain the initial linkage at *HPC1,* and in fact there was suggestive evidence for linkage at Xq in that genome scan[18]. In a heterogeneity analysis, linkage to *HPCX* was estimated to account for 16% of prostate cancers in the data set of 360 families, and the proportion of linked families from each of the four centers was similar. Further analysis of the Finnish families that contributed to the initial study suggested that most of the evidence for *HPCX* comes from families with no evidence of male-to-male transmission[36].

As at *HPC1,* many independent tests for evidence of linkage at *HPCX* have been at best neutral. For instance, genome scans of neither the WUSM pedigree resource nor the PROGRESS pedigree resource observed any evidence of linkage at Xq27-28[20-22]. On the other hand, other independent groups have reported supportive evidence for the linkage. For instance, analysis of a set of 153 prostate cancer pedigrees ascertained though the University of Michigan and the Ann Arbor Veterans Hospital revealed positive LOD scores over a 30 cM region containing *HPCX,* again with the greatest evidence for linkage in the male-to-male transmission pedigrees (peak NPL Z-score of 1.20), and especially those pedigrees with early average age at diagnosis (<65 years of age)[37]. Analysis of genotyping data from the genome scan of the Stanford/ USC pedigree resource revealed a 1-point Z-score of 2.57 at DXS2390. Again, a disproportionate amount of the linkage evidence came from the male-to-male transmission families in that sample set[24]. Finally, analysis of a set of 104 German prostate cancer families gave a maximum NPL Z-score of 1.20, and stratification of the families by average age at diagnosis gave a Z-score of 2.32 in the earlier onset families[38]. Overall, independent analyses are consistent with a susceptibility gene at Xq27-28 contributing to a fraction of hereditary prostate cancer pedigrees, but not to the extent predicted by the hypothesis generating linkage study.

2.1.4 HPC20

Results from a prostate cancer susceptibility genome scan performed on 162 families with ≥3 cases (Mayo pedigree resource) gave strongest evidence for a locus at 20q11-13, *HPC20*[27]. Across the whole set of families, the highest 2-point LOD score was 2.69 while after increasing marker density in the region of interest, the maximum multipoint NPL score was 3.02. In a more detailed analysis, the pedigree set was subdivided on 3 variables: < 5 vs ≥ 5 cases per pedigree, average age at diagnosis < 66 vs ≥ 66 yrs, or +/- male-to-male transmission. Both multipoint NPL and multipoint hetLODs were higher in families with < 5 cases, families with ≥ 66 years at diagnosis (average), and families without male-to-male transmission. The highest multipoint NPL and multipoint hetLODs, 3.94 and 3.61, were observed in the families without male-to-male transmission

In their primary analyses, none of the other three completely reported genome scans observed supportive evidence for this locus[18,22,39]. In a replication analysis, data generated from the Progene pedigree resource also was not supportive[28,35]. On the other hand, analysis of an extended version of the Johns-Hopkins pedigree resource revealed supportive evidence of linkage to *HPC20* when the families were stratified according to the same criteria defined by Berry et al.[40] In that analysis, the subset of Johns Hopkins families with average age at diagnosis ≥65 gave a NPL score of 1.94, and those with < 5 cases gave an NPL score of 1.74. In addition, some evidence supportive of *HPC20* was generated from an analysis of 172 HPC families ascertained through the University of Michigan Prostate Cancer Genetics Project[41]. While this study generated essentially no evidence of linkage from the complete set of families, nor when the families were stratified by average age at diagnosis, number of cases, or +/- male to male transmission, the subset of 16 African-American families in the study gave a Z-score of 1.99 (P = 0.023) at D20S893, just 4 cM from the original *HPC20* peak of LOD score.

2.1.5 CAPB

Analyzing early data from a genome scan of the PROGRESS prostate pedigree resource, Gibbs et al. observed evidence of linkage to Chr 1p36-35, especially in the subset of prostate cancer pedigrees that also reported one or more cases of primary brain cancer. After adding additional families and increasing marker density in the region, they observed a LOD score of 3.22 in the 12-pedigree subset in which both prostate cancer and primary brain cancer were present[19]. Several groups have analyzed their independent pedigree resources for evidence of linkage to this locus. There was no evidence for linkage at 1p in the original genome scan of the Johns-Hopkins pedigree resource[18], nor was there evidence from the total (expanded) set of Johns-Hopkins families used in the subsequent high-resolution scan of chromosome 1 resource[29]. However, a very slight positive LOD score (LOD = 0.61, P = 0.09) was observed in the small subset of prostate families that had a history of primary brain cancer. In contrast, when the Mayo pedigree resource was specifically examined for linkage evidence at each of the 3 published Chr 1 loci, there was no evidence for linkage at CAPB in either the complete pedigree resource or the small subset (12 pedigrees) that was positive for both prostate and brain cancer[27].

On the other hand, one might argue that there is slightly better evidence for a prostate cancer susceptibility gene on 1p slightly proximal to the localization suggested for *CAPB*. In the initial genome scan of the WUSM pedigree resource, there was some evidence of linkage around D1S1622 (57 cM), especially in the subset of prostate cancer pedigrees that reported a family history of breast cancer. The Z-score in this subset of the pedigrees was 3.78 (P < 0.001)[22]. When the genotyping data from that genome scan was reanalyzed under a model that was sensitive to heritability of tumor aggressiveness (Gleason score)[23], evidence for the same locus was again observed (P = 0.003). A 207 pedigree prostate cancer genetics resource assembled by an Anglo/ Canadian/ Texas/ Australian/ Norwegian/ EU Biomed consortium (ACTANE) has also been analyzed for evidence of linkage in the *CAPB* region[42]. While there was no evidence for linkage in any two-tumor type combination (for instance brain and prostate), the earliest average age at diagnosis subset of pedigrees in the resource did show evidence of linkage in the region. Finally, such an interpretation would be more consistent with the 1p localization of slight positive linkage evidence observed under several linkage models in the high resolution analysis of the expanded Johns-Hopkins pedigree set resource[29].

2.2 Group 2 linkages

2.2.1 Chromosome 4q

In the initial genome scan of the Johns-Hopkins pedigree resource, the second-highest 2-pt LOD score, ~1.6, was on chromosome 4q at D4S430[18]. In the initial data from the genome scan of the WUSM pedigree resource, the 2-point Z-score in this region was about 1.3. However, when the pedigrees were bifurcated by average age at diagnosis, essentially all of the linkage evidence was in the older average age at diagnosis pedigrees resulting in a maximum Z-score of 2.85 ($P = 0.002$) at a marker 12 cM from the linkage hint observed in the Johns-Hopkins data[22]. After reanalysis of data generated from the WUSM set using covariates, evidence at 4q remained. Evidence was strongest when number of affecteds was the covariate, resulting in a maximum Z-score of 2.80 ($P = 0.0038$)[21]. Very modest support of linkage in this region was also observed in the Stanford/ USC data set, where there was a cluster of 2-point Z-scores between 1.8 and 2.0 just distal to the region detected by the Johns-Hopkins and WUSM groups, though multipoint evidence was even weaker than 2-point evidence[24]. The genome scan of the PROGRESS pedigree resource did not reveal any evidence of linkage to 4q[20].

2.2.2 Chromosome 8p

Several lines of evidence have implicated the short arm of chromosome 8 as harboring genes important for prostate cancer initiation and/ or progression (for a recent review, see ref. 43). The initial genome scans of the Johns-Hopkins and PROGRESS pedigree resources both detected modest hints of linkage at 8p. In the PROGRESS pedigrees, evidence for linkage was stronger in the later age at diagnosis subset[18, 20]. When number of affected cases was used as covariate in reanalysis of linkage data from the genome scan of the WUSM pedigree collection, there was also a modest hint of linkage at 8p[21]. Accordingly, a high marker density reanalysis of 8p was carried out on an expanded version of the Johns-Hopkins pedigree resource[44]. In this last analysis, a peak hetLOD of 1.84 ($P = 0.004$) was obtained from complete pedigree set. When the pedigrees were stratified by average age at diagnosis, essentially all of the evidence for linkage came from the older age at diagnosis pedigrees (≥65), where the maximum NPL allele sharing LOD was 2.64 (P = 0.0005). As multiple groups have detected at least modest evidence of linkage at 8p and there is clear evidence for one or more genes involved in prostate tumor biology in the region, more detailed analysis is clearly warranted.

2.2.3 Chromosome 16p

Two groups have reported some evidence of linkage to chromosome 16p. In the genome scan of the WUSM set of prostate cancer pedigrees, which consisted mostly of affected sib pairs, the most consistent evidence of linkage was on chromosome 16, with a Z-score of 2.8 on the p-arm, 3.1 on the q-arm, and some separation between the two hints of linkage[22]. When the WUSM data were reanalyzed using covariates, evidence at 16p was stronger than at 16q where the best LOD score (2.68) was obtained when number of cases in the pedigree was the covariate[21]. Analysis of the genome scan of the PROGRESS family collection also revealed a hint of linkage at 16p. The best evidence was under a recessive model, where the 2-point LOD score was 1.58, whereas evidence in the younger age at diagnosis pedigrees was stronger than in the older pedigrees[20]. In contrast, there was absolutely no evidence for linkage to chromosome 16 from initial genome scans of either the Johns-Hopkins or the Stanford/USC pedigree resources[18, 24].

2.2.4 Chromosome 17p (HPC2/ELAC2)

In an almost complete genome scan of 33 large Utah high-risk prostate cancer pedigrees, Lisa Cannon-Albright and Susan Neuhausen found best evidence of linkage at chromosome 17p11[26]. In the initial set of 33 pedigrees (average of 10.2 cases per pedigree with an average age at diagnosis of 68.3 years), the maximum 2-point LOD score was 4.5 at D17S1289, and the maximum 3-point LOD score, using D17S1289 and D17S921, was 4.3. An additional set of 94 Utah prostate cancer pedigrees added only very weak evidence for this linkage, with a maximum multipoint tLOD[45] of 0.44 at 17-MYR0110, a microsatellite marker within the minimal region defined by recombinants on apparently linked haplotypes[26]. Evidence for linkage at this locus was reanalyzed on two of the other available collections of prostate cancer pedigrees, the Johns-Hopkins set[46] and the WUSM set[47]. Neither of these two studies observed supportive evidence. On the other hand, in the genome scan of the Stanford/USC set[24], a 2 point Z-score of 2.44 was observed at D17S1303, a marker within the *HPC2/ELAC2* region.

2.2.5 Chromosome 19q

Genotype data from the genome scan of the WUSM family set has been reanalyzed under a variety of phenotype-specific linkage models. In one of these analyses, Gleason score was used as a quantitative trait measure of prostate tumor aggressiveness, and the mean corrected cross-product between brother's Gleason scores was used as a measure of the heritability of that trait[23]. In that analysis, evidence for prostate cancer aggressiveness genes was observed at chromosomes 5q, 7q, and 19q. Very recently, genotype data from the Mayo clinic set of prostate cancer pedigrees was analyzed under a very similar model. Significant evidence for an aggressiveness locus was found at D19S902 (P = 0.0001)[48], within the region suggested by Witte et al.[23]. Such a concordant result from the first two such analyses would seem quite promising.

3. GENES CONTRIBUTING TO FAMILIAL PROSTATE CANCER

It is one thing to have a hint of linkage, or better yet a well supported linkage, for a disease susceptibility locus. It is quite another thing to identify the underlying susceptibility gene and risk conferring sequence variants in that gene. From the point of view of the positional cloner, every gene within reasonably well defined bounds of a genetic linkage is a candidate gene for the linked trait. When a research group finds sequence variants in such a gene that appear to explain an appreciable fraction of the apparently linked families and appear to confer increased risk of the trait in question, the gene is then properly recognized as a "strong" candidate gene. However, one must recognize that as mutation screening/gene resequencing technology has improved, positional cloners have been able to thoroughly screen more and more genes within regions of linkage. This is a form of multiple testing, so consequently, as the number of candidate genes screened within any given region or for any given trait increases, so does the likelihood of observing a false positive. Therefore, when the discovery of a strong candidate susceptibility gene is published, the publication should be regarded as a hypothesis-generating study and then judged both on the basis of how well the initial hypotheses (or new closely related hypotheses) stand up to independent reanalysis and on the basis of how well the data indicating that the gene is in fact a susceptibility gene explain the genetic linkage from which the gene was localized.

To date, three strong candidate familial prostate cancer susceptibility genes have been described, one each from three of the linkages described in the proceeding section. These are in chronological order *ELAC2* (chromosome 17p11/ *HPC2/ELAC2* region)[26], *RNASEL* (chromosome 1q23-25/ HPC1 region)[49], and *MSR1* (chromosome 8p region)[50].

3.1 ELAC2 (chromosome 17p11/ HPC2/ELAC2 region)

The discovery of the first prostate cancer susceptibility gene characterized by positional cloning was achieved through a long-standing collaboration between Myriad Genetics and several academic groups, taking advantage of the Utah Family Resource which has proven to be an invaluable asset for cloning of cancer susceptibility genes in the past[9, 51-53]. A genome-wide search for prostate cancer predisposition loci using a small set of Utah high risk prostate cancer pedigrees and a set of 300 polymorphic markers done by Cannon-Albright's group provided evidence for linkage to a locus on chromosome 17p (Figure 2)[26]. These pedigrees were

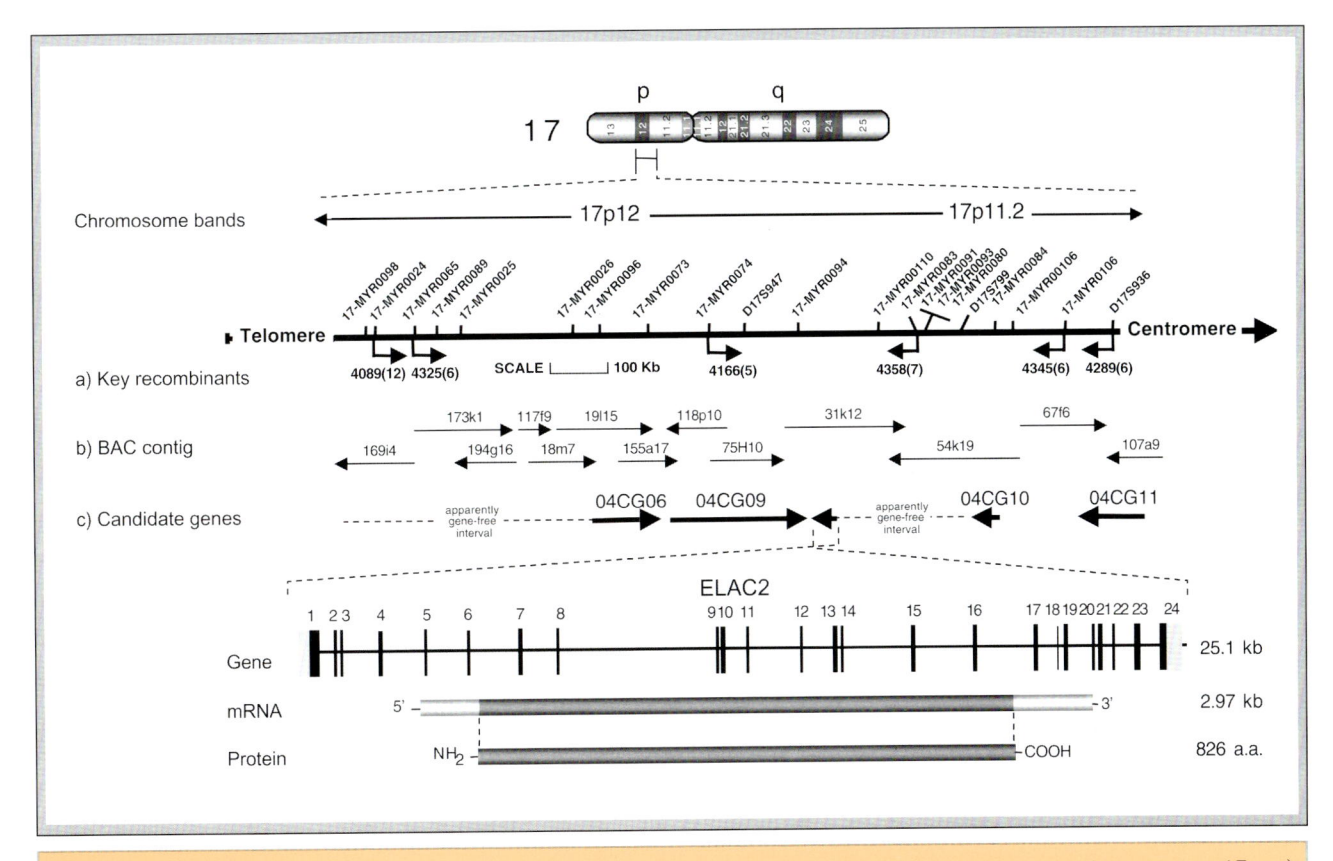

FIGURE 2. Recombinant, physical and transcript map centered at the human *ELAC2* locus on chromosome 17p. a) Key recombinants. Under the arrows, which represent meiotic recombinants, are indicated the number of the kindred in which the recombinant occurred and, in parentheses, the number of cases carrying the haplotype on which the recombinant occurred. b) BAC contig tilling path across the interval. The T7 end of each BAC is denoted with an arrowhead. c) Candidate genes are identified in the interval and below an expanded view of the structure of the *ELAC2* gene[26].

not selected for early age of cancer onset, but consisted of a subset of families ascertained using the Utah Population Database.

Positional cloning and mutation screening within the refined interval identified a gene *ELAC2*, harboring a frameshift mutation, 1641insG, that segregated with prostate cancer in the high-risk pedigree kindred 4102. Three out of four male carriers of the frameshift of age > 45 years had been diagnosed with prostate cancer, and the fourth had a PSA of 5.7 at age 71. The frameshift, which occurred within the most highly conserved segment of the protein and eliminated one-third of the protein, including several other conserved segments, was predicted to be highly disruptive to the gene product's function. A second high-risk Utah pedigree was found to segregate an allele of *ELAC2* that carried 3 missense changes: Ser217Leu (q = 0.30), Ala541Thr (q = 0.04) and Arg781His (very rare or pedigree specific). Of 14 prostate cancer cases in the pedigree, 6 carried the triple missense allele, 6 did not carry, and 2 were unknown. Of 8 male carriers of the triple missense allele who were over age 45 and within the generations of the pedigree for which phenotype information is known, 6 were prostate cancer cases, 1 died of heart disease at age 62 but had two sons and a grandson who carried the allele and were cases, and the remaining one had a PSA of 0.6 at age 60. Another interesting point about the pedigree is that the youngest age at diagnosis carrier of the triple missense allele (diagnosed at age 50) was homozygous for the Leu217 and Thr541 variants. In addition, an ovarian cancer case in the pedigree, diagnosed at age 43, also carried the triple missense allele. The 17p11 tLOD[45] for this pedigree, which peaks at a microsatellite marker within *ELAC2* and is almost entirely accounted for by the triple missense allele, was 1.3[26].

At the time of its cloning, the function of *ELAC2* was unclear. Sequence analysis predicted the gene to encode a metal-dependent hydrolase domain conserved among eukaryotes, archaebacteria, and eubacteria, and bearing striking sequence similarity to domains present in two better understood protein families, namely the PSO2 (SNM1) DNA interstrand crosslink repair proteins and the 73 kDa subunit of mRNA 3'end cleavage and polyadenylation specificity factor (CPSF73). This gene was designated *ELAC2* because it is the larger of two human genes that were found to be homologues of *E. coli* elaC (Figure 3)[26]. From analysis of the complete genome sequences available to date, it appears that all prokaryote and archaebacterial genomes encode one or two genes that are orthologous to *E. coli* elaC, whereas all eukaryotes encode one or two genes that are orthologous to *ELAC2*, which is actually comprised of homologous amino and carboxy halves and appears to have arisen as a direct repeat-duplication of an ancestral elaC-like gene. The first amino half of ELAC2s has suffered considerable sequence divergence, but the carboxy

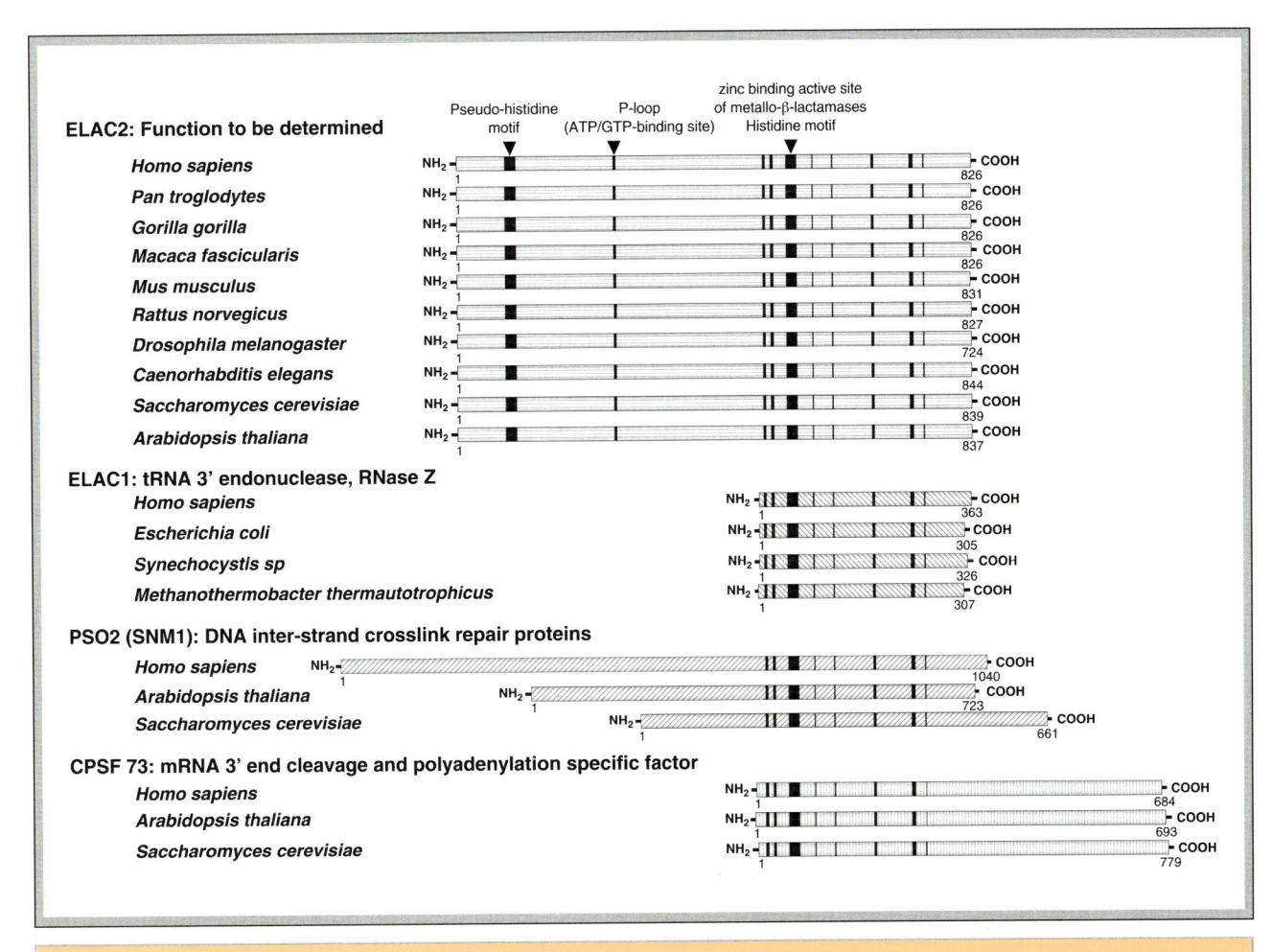

FIGURE 3. A schematic multiple protein alignment of ELAC superfamily members including the ELAC1, PSO2 and CPSF73 families and the ELAC2 orthologs. The conserved motifs are indicated by black boxes. Localization of known motifs are outlined by an arrow.

half is very similar to prokaryotic elaCs. Many eukaryotes, including the so-far sequenced vertebrates and plants, but not the protostomate invertebrates, encode one or two copies of another member of the gene family, *ELAC1*. This gene is of similar size and structure to the prokaryotic elaCs. Recently, *in vitro* analyses have clearly demonstrated that the prokaryotic elaCs encode binuclear zinc-dependant phosphodiesterases[54]. In addition, both archaebacterial elaCs and plant *ELAC1s* have been demonstrated to have a tRNA 3' endonuclease activity, RNase Z, that is required for tRNA maturation[55]. Given that the closely related CPSF73 genes play a role in mRNA 3' end cleavage and polyadenylation, this later result in not at all surprising. An interesting remaining question, though, is whether ELAC2s also encode RNase Z and what sort of functional specialization has occurred during the divergence between *ELAC1* and *ELAC2*.

In the original analysis, both of the common missense changes in *ELAC2* were tested for association with familial prostate cancer[26]. The results from this analysis suggested that both Leu217 and Thr541 conferred increase risk of disease, and allowed us to postulate 5 hypotheses: (1) There is very strong linkage disequilibrium between the two variants, such that virtually all instances of Thr541 (q = 0.04) occur on an allele that also carries Leu217 (q = 0.30). (2) Both sequence variants confer modestly increased risk of disease. (3) The odds ratio measured for that risk of disease depends on the nature of the case-control comparison conducted. For instance, when we compared Leu217 carrier frequencies between familial cases and male controls who were cancer free and had little family history of cancer, we found an odds ratio for Leu217 homozygotes of 2.4 (P = 0.026), but when we compared those same cases to unaffecteds from the prostate cancer pedigrees, the odds ratio dropped to 1.5 (P = 0.014). Similarly, when we compared Thr541 carrier frequencies between familial cases and male controls who were cancer free and had little family history of cancer, we found an odds ratio for carriage of Thr541 of 3.1 (P = 0.022), but when we compared those same cases to unaffecteds from the prostate cancer pedigrees, there was very little evidence for increased risk of disease. (4) In our data, most of the increased risk appeared to be in the earlier age of onset cases. As essentially all segregation analyses that have examined the familiality of prostate cancer have concluded that early onset cases are disproportionately likely to have a genetic basis, it would seem likely that the missense changes in *ELAC2* confer relatively higher risk in early onset rather than later onset prostate cancer cases. (5) Finally, we predicted that the order of risk conferred by the three common missense alleles was Ser217/Ala541 < Leu217/Ala541 < Leu217/Thr541[26] (Figure 4).

To confirm our observation in a cohort unselected for family history, Rebbeck et al.[56] studied 359 incident prostate cancer case subjects and 266 male control individuals that were frequency matched for age and race and were identified from a large health-system population. Among control individuals, the Leu217 frequency was 31.6%, whereas the Thr541 frequency was 2.9%. They observed that the relative risk of having prostate cancer is increased in men carrying the Leu217/Thr541 allele (odds ratio = 2.37; 95% CI = 1.06-55.29). This risk did not differ significantly by family history or race.

Since that time, seven additional analyses of *ELAC2* have been published[46, 47, 57-61]. Results have varied from significantly higher carrier frequencies of the Leu217/Thr541 allele in familial cases compared to low risk controls (OR = 2.83, P = 0.008), but without evidence of increased risk when familial cases were compared to unaffected men from those same pedigrees[47], to essentially no evidence of any increased risk at all[57,61].

Heterogeneity in the association study results led us to prepare a met-analysis of the data published through July, 2002. From that analysis and excluding the data from our hypothesis generating study, there was strong evidence that carriage of the Leu217/Thr541 allele is significantly associated with risk of prostate cancer. However, that risk varied depending on the nature of the case-control comparison made. In very discordant sets (familial cases vs low risk controls, based on familial cases from the Johns-Hopkins and WUSM pedigree resources[46,47]), the OR was relatively higher and the evidence stronger (OR = 1.96, P = 0.008), whereas in a comparison of all cases vs all controls, which is numerically dominated by sporadic cases and population controls, the OR was reduced and not quite significant (OR = 1.25, P = 0.081). Results with Leu217 followed a similar trend, but with lower odds ratios and less significant P-values. For instance, in the comparison of familial cases to low risk controls, the result for Leu 217 dominant was OR = 1.37, P = 0.017 (again, based on familial cases from the Johns-Hopkins and WUSM pedigree resources[46,47,62]). As the case control comparisons made by the Johns-Hopkins and WUSM groups, most closely match the format of our original case-control analysis[26] and actually corroborate four of the five hypotheses generated from our data, although there was no evidence for relatively higher risk in early onset cases, this would seem very strong evidence in support of risk conferred by the Leu217 and Thr541 variants, albeit at slightly lower odds ratios than we originally described.

Subsequent to the preparation of our metanalysis, two more ELAC2 association studies were published[60,61]. Analysis of a series of British prostate cancer cases, many of them diagnosed before the age of 55, and population controls[60] found a trend towards elevated risk in Leu217/Thr541 carriers, though the effect was not significant. Stratification by age at diagnosis demonstrated that most of the risk was present in the earlier onset cases (diagnosis ≤ age 55)(OR = 1.50, 95% CI 0.79 – 2.85). In addition, very slightly increased risk was seen in Leu217 carriers, though this was not nearly significant. Still, as the overall trend matches that observed in the metanalysis, the result can be viewed as supportive. In contrast, a case control comparison of Afro-Caribbeans from Tobago resulted in odds ratios of 1.0[61]. In fact, Thr541 was not even observed in this population, which has relatively little admixture from the European gene pool, suggesting that the Leu217/Thr541 allele is either European or Eurasian in origin.

Overall, mutation screening results indicate that inactivating mutations in *ELAC2*, and even pedigree specific missense changes, are exceedingly rare[26, 46, 47, 58, 59]. Consequently, it will be very difficult to determine whether, or to what extent, such variants confer increased risk of prostate cancer. In fact, there is little evidence that *ELAC2* is a tumor suppressor. Knowing that knockout of the *ELAC2* ortholog in *S. cerevisiae* is lethal, one might hypothesize that at least one functioning allele is required for cellular viability. On the other hand, the Leu217 and Thr541 missense changes are quite common and will eventually be used to tightly constrain the role that this gene plays in prostate cancer genetics. Finally, it must be noted that while the open reading frame of *ELAC2* has been thoroughly screened for sequence variants, the promoter and upstream transcriptional regulatory sequences have not. Thus the possibility remains that some of the inconsistency in current results is due to varying levels of linkage disequilibrium with as yet unknown sequence variants.

3.2 RNASEL (HPC1 region)

The best supported linkage to prostate cancer susceptibility is the *HPC1* locus at chromosome 1q23-25. One of the candidate genes within the broadly-defined *HPC1* region is 2'-5'-oligoadenylate–dependent ribonuclease L *(RNASEL)*. The gene encodes a constitutively expressed latent endoribonuclease that mediates the antiviral and proapoptotic activities of the interferon-inducible 2-5A system.

Mutation screening of *RNASEL* from the germline DNA of one index case from each of 26 pedigrees selected from the Johns-Hopkins pedigree resource, including 8 pedigrees that showed linkage to the *HPC1* locus and that had at least four affected individuals sharing an *HPC1* haplotype, revealed two particularly interesting mutations: the nonsense mutation Glu265X and the initiation codon mutation Met1Ile[49] (Figure 4). The nonsense mutation Glu265X was found in an index case from a pedigree of European ancestry. There were 5 prostate cancer cases in the pedigree and their average age at diagnosis was 67.6 years. DNA was available from four of the five cases, all brothers, and they all carried this mutation. It is not known whether the fifth case, the father, was a carrier. This, however, may not be relevant because the mother was diagnosed with breast cancer at age 59. The Met1Ile mutation was found in the African-American pedigree 097 and is either very rare or pedigree-specific. The six prostate cancer cases in pedigree 097 had an average age at diagnosis of 59. The four out of six cases who carried the mutation had an average age at diagnosis of 57.8 years while the two non carriers were diagnosed at ages 59 and 64. An interesting datum in support of a role for these mutations in their carrier's prostate tumors was that tumor material was available from several

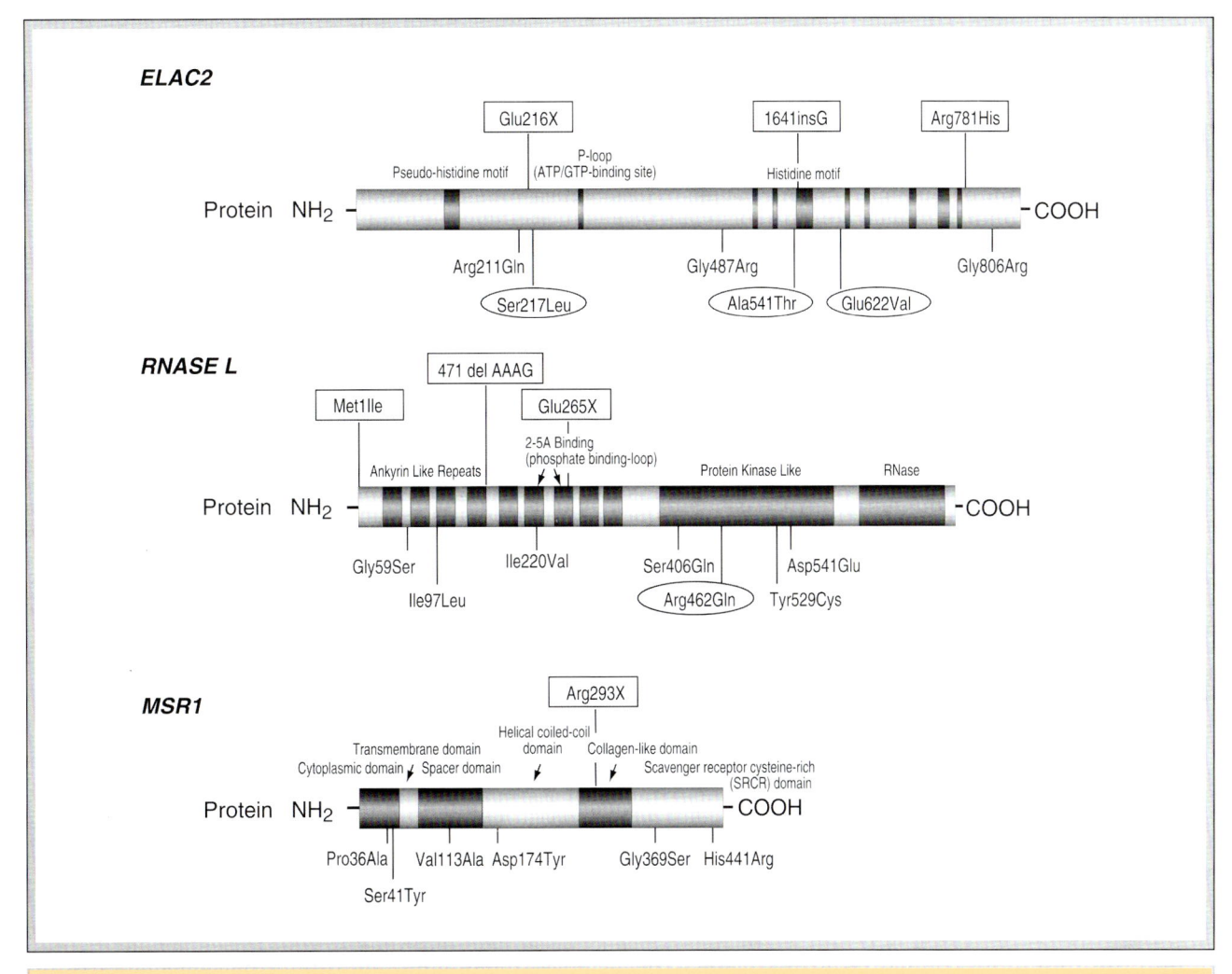

FIGURE 4: Location of sequence variants in *ELAC2*, *RNASEL* and *MSR1* genes. Dark gray boxes indicate homologies to known protein domains. High penetrance mutations of *ELAC2* are identified by a box whereas common low penetrance mutations are indicated by a circle. The significance of the other missense mutations detected in *ELAC2* is still unknown. Mutations of *RNASEL* and *MSR1*, which are identified by a box, have been suggested to be associated with increased risk of prostate cancer. The functional significance of the other missense mutations shown under the *RNASEL* and *MSR1* protein's diagrams are unknown.

carriers, PCR from microdissected tumor material indicated that LOH was present, and it was the wild-type allele that was lost. On the other hand, genotyping indicated that the Glu265X mutation has an appreciable frequency in the US Caucasian population, about 0.5%, and there was no obvious carrier frequency difference between cases and controls.

RNASEL was subsequently mutation screened in a series of Finnish familial prostate cancer cases and certain sequence variants from the gene typed in a Finnish case control series[63]. The Glu265X nonsense mutation was found in 5 of 116 patients with familial prostate cancer and seemed to be most common in families with 4 or more cases. Genotyping in the case-control series revealed that the nonsense mutation was most common in familial cases (q = 0.022), at intermediate frequency in sporadic cases (q = 0.010), and least common in controls (q = 0.009). The difference between cases and controls was significant (OR = 4.56, P = 0.04). In addition, one of four common missense variants, Arg462Gln, also trended towards being more common in cases than controls (OR = 1.96, P = 0.07).

Mutation screening of *RNASEL* in a series of Ashkenazi prostate cancer patients revealed a founder mutation, 471delAAAG, at appreciable allele frequency in that ethnic group[64]. In a small case control series, the frequency of this variant was highest in cases (q = 0.035), intermediate in population controls (q = 0.020), and lowest in elderly cancer-free men (q = 0.012). Although the carrier frequency difference between cases and controls was not significant (OR = 3.0, P = 0.17), cases who carried the variant were younger at diagnosis than cases who did not (65 vs 74.4 yrs., P < 0.001).

In addition to the Finnish group, two other groups have published association studies of the Arg462Gln missense variant. Importantly, Casey et al. compared the *in vitro* enzymatic activity of protein encoded by the two alleles on a synthetic substrate, finding that the Gln462 variant had only about 30% of the activity of the more common Arg462 allele[65]. In their association study, which was carried out on a series of discordant sibling pairs including 423 cases and 454 controls, they found a trend of increasing risk from Arg462 homozygotes to Gln462 homozygotes (odds ratios of 1.46 and 2.12, respectively, trend test P = 0.011) [65]. In contrast, in their analysis of a case control series derived from the Mayo pedigree resource, Wang et al. found exactly the opposite trend: odds ratios were 0.83 and 0.54 (P = 0.02) for heterozygotes and Gln462 homozygotes, respectively. In addition, the protective effect of the Gln462 variant was most apparent in early onset cases, with odds ratios of 0.63 and 0.29 (P = 0.0008) for heterozygotes and Gln462 homozygotes diagnosed at = 64 years, respectively[66].

In summary, published analyses of the three inactivating mutations so far described in *RNASEL*, Met1Ile, 471delAAAG, and Glu265X, trend towards evidence that these variants confer risk of prostate cancer, with best evidence in earlier onset cases as predicted from the nature of the linkage evidence at *HPC1*. Data with respect to the missense change Arg462Gln are clearly conflicting. As 471delAAAG appears to be an Ashkenazi founder mutation with an appreciable allele frequency in that population, Glu265X appears to have an appreciable frequency in European populations, and Arg462Gln is a common missense change, it should not take very long time for independent follow-on studies to tightly determine the risk conferred by these sequence variants and thereby clarify the role of this gene in hereditary prostate cancer.

3.3 MSR1 (chromosome 8p region)

One of the "Group 2" linkages described in the section 2.2.2 is at chromosome 8p. As part of the justification for scrutinizing 8p was longstanding evidence for a prostate cancer tumor suppressor in the region, there is some expectation that any susceptibility gene underlying the linkage should be a tumor suppressor and therefore subject to inactivating mutations. In addition, as this is a region of linkage, one would expect to see such germline mutations at higher frequency in familial as opposed to sporadic cases. Similarly, as the majority of the linkage evidence for the region seems to come from pedigrees with older average age at diagnosis, one would expect to see a germline mutation bias towards older (or at least not markedly towards younger) age at diagnosis cases.

Very recently, mutation screening of candidate genes from the 8p region in index cases from the Johns-Hopkins family resource revealed a number of rare mutations in the gene Macrophage Scavenger Receptor 1 *(MSR1)*[50]. From the first 159 prostate cancer pedigrees screened, one nonsense mutation and six rare missense mutations were found. After genotyping for these variants was completed on the initial 159 pedigrees plus a second set of 31 prostate cancer pedigrees, a total of 13 of the pedigrees were found to harbor one or another (and in some cases two) of these rare variants. There were individual pedigrees where the sequence variant segregated quite closely with prostate cancer, and others where the pattern of segregation was equivocal. Overall, a family based linkage/ segregation test provided evidence that there was disproportionate segregation of these variants with disease (P = 0.0007). From the point of view of follow-up studies, a very useful point was that 6 of the 13 pedigrees in which a mutation was found, all of European descent, harbored the nonsense mutation Arg293X. That nonsense variant was also found to be more common in "non-hereditary" prostate cancer cases than in disease-free male controls (8/317 v. 1/256, FET P-value = 0.047).

MSR1 is a transmembrane protein that functions as a homotrimeric receptor for a number of polyanionic ligands including a variety of bacteria (Figure 4). The Arg293X mutation would remove most of the extracellular ligand binding domain as well as the conserved extracellular scavenger receptor cystein-rich domain. Thus the Arg293X nonsense mutation would clearly interfere with *MSR1* function. Overall, the initial report presented modest but plausible evidence that *MSR1* is a prostate cancer susceptibility gene. If the allele frequency of the Arg293X turns out be in the range of 1.0% to 1.5% in prostate cancer cases of European ethnicity, as indicated from the initial mutation screening and association evidence, then that specific variant should provide an accessible and powerful tool to evaluate the genetic role that this gene plays in prostate cancer susceptibility.

4. RISK OF PROSTATE CANCER IN *BRCA1* AND *BRCA2* CARRIERS

Epidemiological studies of prostate and breast cancer have revealed that clustering of these cancers occurs in certain families[67,68]. Anderson and Badzioch observed a doubling of breast cancer risk in families with prostate cancer history [68]. An estimated relative risk of prostate cancer of 3.33 was calculated for obligate male carriers of a deleterious *BRCA1* mutation when compared to the general population in a cooperative study using 33 *BRCA1*-linked breast/ovarian cancer families[69]. In another more recent study from the Breast Cancer Linkage Consortium including 173 breast/ovarian families with a deleterious *BRCA2* mutation, a significantly increased risk (RR=4.65) for prostate cancer was observed. Furthermore, this risk was even higher before age 65 (RR = 7.33) and the estimated cumulative incidence before 70 was 7.5%-33%, depending on which reference population was used (Breast Cancer Linkage Consortium)[70]. Moreover, the founder Icelandic *BRCA2* mutation (999del5) was also associated with increased risk of prostate cancer[71, 72]. The relative risk of prostate cancer was calculated to be 4.6 in first-degree relatives and 2.5 in second degree relatives[72]. On the other hand, another population-based estimate shows a cumulative risk for 999del5 mutation carriers of only 7.6% at age 70[73]. Several analyses of germline DNA from prostate cancer cases with or without a family history have revealed that there is no increased frequency of the founder Ashkenazi Jewish *BRCA1*, and *BRCA2* mutations over that expected in this population[74-77]. However, DNA samples from affected individuals in 38 prostate cancer familial clusters were analyzed for germline mutations in *BRCA1* and *BRCA2* genes to assess the potential contribution of each of these genes to familial prostate cancer[78]. No germline mutations were found in *BRCA1*, but two novel deletions were found in *BRCA2*. These authors proposed that germline mutations in *BRCA2* may therefore account for about 5% of prostate cancers in familial clusters. A recent study in a Swedish family in which the father and four of his sons were diagnosed with prostate cancer at the exceptionally early ages of 51, 52, 56, 58 and 63, respectively, supports an increased risk of prostate cancer in *BRCA2* carriers[79]. Finally, in another study, *BRCA1* and *BRCA2* mutation screening was performed on the prostate cancer proband and on an additional family member affected with breast or prostate cancer from each of the 22 cancer families[80]. None of the 43 samples screened contained a protein truncating mutation in either *BRCA1* or *BRCA2*. It is important to note that, in contrast to the UK study described above, these American families were selected from a large collection of high-risk prostate cancer families (at least three cases of prostate cancer) for having at least two cases of breast or ovarian cancer, in order to maximize the odds of detecting mutations in *BRCA1* or *BRCA2*[78].

5. COMMON LOW-PENETRANCE ALLELIC VARIANTS OF GENES INVOLVED IN ANDROGEN BIOSYNTHESIS AND ACTION

In the general population, we observe an inter-individual variability in the susceptibility to cancer, however little is known about the underlying genes contributing to this variability. Although a number of rare highly penetrant loci contribute to the Mendelian inheritance of prostate cancer as described above, some of the familial risks may be due to shared environment and more specifically to common low-penetrance genetic variants, which alter predisposition to prostate cancer. Prostate cancer has proven to be the most hormone-sensitive cancer to hormonal manipulation[2]. It is not surprising that analyses of genes encoding key proteins involved in androgen biosynthesis and action, led to the observation of a significant association between common genetic variants and a susceptibility to prostate cancer[6, 7, 81, 82]. Such analyses provided some understanding of how common low-penetrance polymorphisms present in a number of these candidate genes were involved in prostate cancer onset, progression and response to treatment for the disease.

5.1 Androgen Receptor

Because androgen action in prostate cells is mediated through an interaction with AR, it was first suggested that abnormalities in the AR gene, which is located on Xq11-12 (~50cM centromeric to *HPCX*), could play a key role in prostate cell proliferation and differentiation as well as in carcinogenesis (Figure 5). In this regard, the precise molecular events leading from androgen-sensitive prostate cancer to androgen-refractory prostate cancer are of special interest (see [83-86] for reviews). Indeed, some of the pathways identified appear to directly involve the modulation of AR's ability to respond to specific ligands. Briefly, mutations in the AR hormone

1. Prostate Cancer Susceptibility Genes

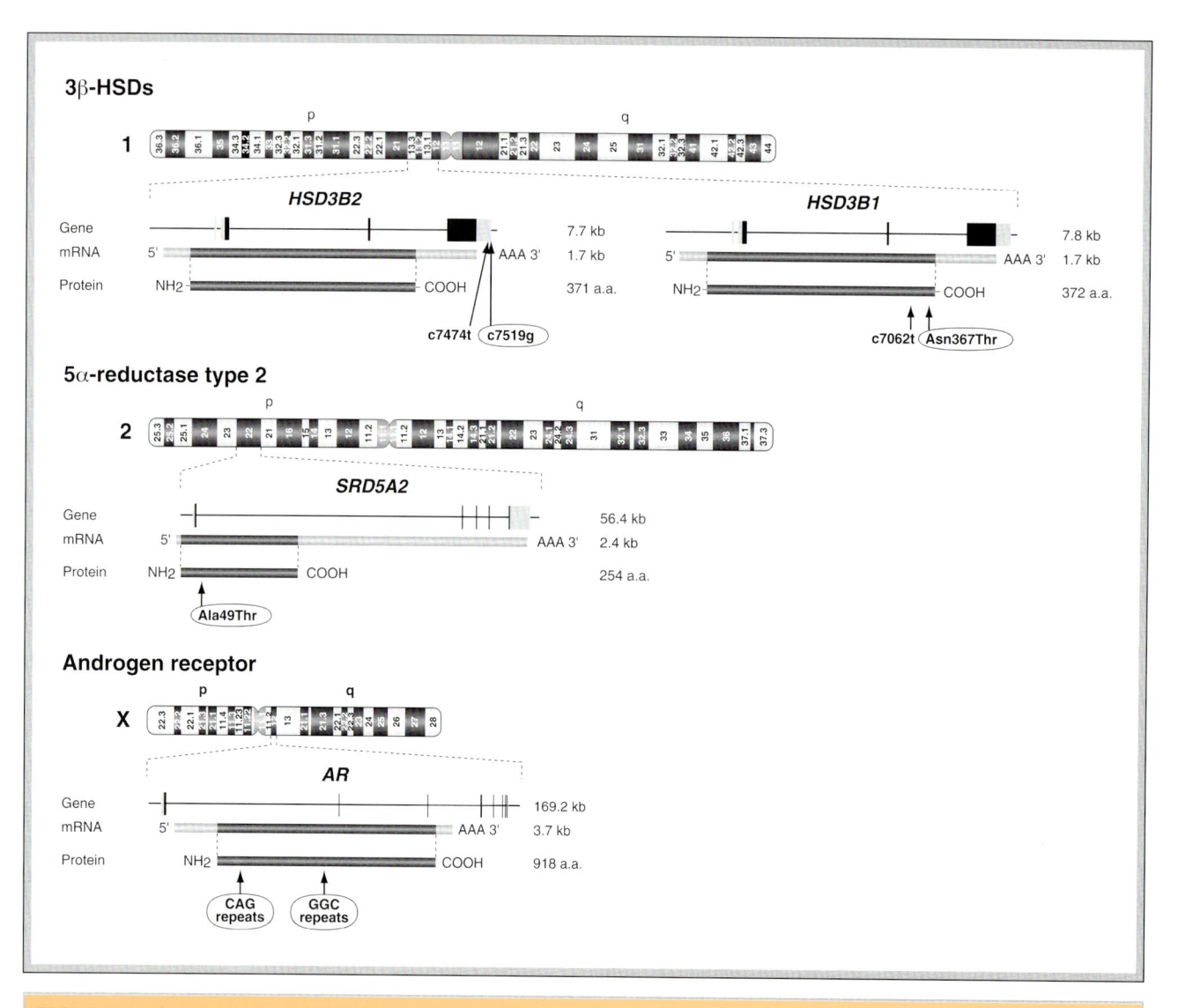

FIGURE 5. Chromosomal localization and schematic representation of *HSD3B1*, *HSD3B2*, *SDR5A2* and *AR* genes, mRNA species and corresponding proteins. Exons are represented by black boxes indicating the coding regions, whereas open boxes represent the non-coding regions. Introns are represented by black bold lines. Positions of sequence variants are shown by an arrow in reference to nucleic or amino acid sequences on the genes or proteins. Polymorphisms which have been suggested to be associated with increased risk of prostate cancer are encircled.

binding domain, or amplification of the AR gene could result in an increased sensitivity to androgens made locally in the prostate from the inactive steroid precursors, dehydroepiandrosterone (DHEA) and its sulfate (DHEA-S). These androgens of adrenal origin do not bind to the AR, but exert androgenic action after their conversion into active androgens in target tissues. Thus, recurrent hormone-refractory tumors may not always be androgen-independent, as often thought, but rather, clonal expansion of hypersensitive cells that are able to grow due to intracrine formation of androgens originating from adrenal precursors and which are converted to bioactive DHT in the prostate tissue may cause failure to monotherapy.

Second, the occurrence of mutations in several portions of the AR could allow this receptor to respond to other steroids or to some antiandrogens. Alternatively, coactivators may increase the sensitivity of the AR to androgens and even to other nonandrogenic molecules[84]. Furthermore, there are accumulating evidence that additional mechanisms, that do not result from mutations in the AR, may involve stimulation of AR transactivation by various factors and cytokinesindependently of androgens, thus facilitating the growth of prostate cancer cells despite maximal androgen blockade or acquisition of metastatic phenotype[84].

Accounting for more than half of the AR, the NH2-terminal transactivation domain is encoded by the exon 1. Within this domain, there are two polymorphic microsatellite trinucleotide repeats located ~1.1 kb appart, namely a CAG repeat and a downstream GGN polymorphism encoding variable length polyglutamine and polyglycine regions, respectively. The CAG repeat varies in length between 11 and 31 repeats in the germline DNA of normal men (see [83] for a review) and shows an inverse relationship between the length of repeats and the transcriptional activity of the AR[87-89]. A recent study using the rat probasin promoter, an androgen- and prostate-specific reporter, further supported the inverse relationship between AR transcriptional activity and the number of CAG repeats (15 vs 31 CAG) and provided evidence that this finding was cell specific, thus suggesting the involvement of accessory factors differentially expressed between different cell lines[89]. It is also of interest to mention that extended polyglutamine tract interacts with caspase-8 and 10 in nuclear aggregates[90] and increasing its length negatively affects p160-mediated coactivation of the AR[91]. Coetzee and Ross have suggested that enhanced activity of the AR, attributable to polymophisms in the AR gene, might alter the risk of prostate cancer[92]. Accordingly, the association of CAG repeat length and prostate cancer risk has been examined in several case-control studies but the results are inconclusive (Table 1). As several of these studies show an association between shorter AR CAG repeat lengths (a short CAG has been defined as ranging from < 17 to < 23 repeats, depending on the study) and increased prostate cancer risk, it is not entirely clear whether the association is with diagnosis of prostate cancer, response to endocrine therapy or severity of disease (Table 1). On the other hand, several other studies suggested that CAG repeat length is not associated to prostate cancer risk (Table 1), age of onset, histological grade and stage of disease at diagnosis or several clinical parameters, including response to hormonal therapy, time to progression after hor-

TABLE 1. Comparison of case-control studies of AR-CAG and AR-GGC/N polymorphism and prostate cancer risk*

Case-control studies	No. Cases/Controls	CAG comparison	OR/RR[a]	95% CI	References
Irvine, 1995	19 / 25	≥22	1.0	Referent	[783]
	38 / 24	< 22	1.25	0.88-1.73	
Giovannucci, 1997	60 / 72	≥ 26	1.0	Referent	[784]
	98 / 115	24-25	1.02	0.66-1.58	
	116 / 119	22-23	1.17	0.76-1.80	
	113 / 101	21	1.325	0.87-2.09	
	69 / 65	20	1.28	0.79-2.08	
	62 / 61	19	1.22	0.75-2.00	
	69 / 55	≤ 18	1.52	0.92-2.49	
Hakimi, 1997	53 / 359	> 17	1.0	Referent	[785]
	6 / 11	≤ 17	3.7	1.3-10.5	
Ingles, 1997	19 / 68	≥ 22	1.0	Referent	[786]
	14 / 56	20-21	0.89	0.41-1.94	
	24 / 45	< 20	1.91	0.94-3.88	
Stanford, 1997	136 / 140	≥ 22	1.0	Referent	[96]
	145 / 126	< 22	1.23	0.88-1.73	
Platz, 1998	201 / 298	> 23	1.0	Referent	[787]
	338 / 425	23	1.2	0.9-1.5	
	43 / 71	< 23	0.9	0.6-1.4	
Bratt, 1999	92 / 93	1 CAG decrement	0.97	0.91-1.04	[788]
Correa-Cerro, 1999	39 / 28	≥ 24	1.0	Referent	[789]
	30 / 22	22-23	1.02	0.49-2.13	
	34 / 35	20-21	1.43	0.73-2.82	
	29 / 20	≤ 19	0.96	0.45-2.03	
Edwards, 1999	74 / 178	> 21	1.0	Referent	[790]
	88 / 212	≤ 21	1.0	0.96-1.03	
Ekman, 1999	CAG repeats were shorter among Swedish prostate cancer patients than among Swedish controls; the Japanese prostate cancer patients had longer repeats than Japanese controls				[791]
Hsing, 2000	74 / 154	≥ 23	1.0	Referent	[1]
	116 / 146	<23	1.65	1.14-2.39	
	52 / 108	≥ 24	1.0	Referent	
	79 / 113	22-23	1.45	0.93-2.25	
	59 / 79	<22	1.55	0.96-2.49	
Lange, 2000	133 / 305	≥ 26	1.0	Referent	[792]
		≥ 18	0.73	0.31-1.69	

TABLE 1. *(Cont.)* **Comparison of case-control studies of AR-CAG and AR-GGC/N polymorphism and prostate cancer risk***

Case-control studies	No. Cases/Controls	CAG comparison	OR/RR[a]	95% CI	References
Beilin, 2001	456 / 456	Mean CAG repeats = 21.95 in both cases and controls			[793]
Latil, 2001	41 / 30	> 24	1.0	Referent	[794]
	55 / 36	23-24	1.12	0.59-2.10	
	61 / 45	21-22	0.99	0.54-1.82	
	68 / 45	≤ 20	1.11	0.60-2.02	
Miller, 2001	71 / 34	≥ 22	1.0	Referent	[95]
	66 / 35	< 22	1.13	0.54-2.37	
Chang, 2002	164 / 81	≥ 22	1.0	Referent	[795]
	162 / 99	≤ 21	0.81	0.56-1.17	
Chen, 2002	156 / 147	≥ 22	1.0	Referent	[93]
	144 / 153	< 22	0.89	0.65-1.23	
Xue, 2000	33 / 114	> 20	1.0	Referent	[796]
	24 / 42	< 20	1.97	1.05-3.72	

Case-control studies	No. Cases/Controls	GGC/N comparison	OR/RR[a]	95% CI	References
Irvine, 1995	10 / 21	16	1.0	Referent	[783]
	27 / 16	Not 16	1.18	Not given	
Hakimi, 1997	46 / 106	> 14	1.0	Referent	[785]
	8 / 4	≤ 14	4.6	1.3-16.1	
Stanford, 1997	56 / 75	> 16	1.0	Referent	[96]
	201 / 175	≤ 16	1.60	1.07-2.41	
Platz, 1998	244 / 369	Not 23	1.0	Referent	[787]
	338 / 425	23	1.2	0.97-1.49	
Edwards, 1999	64 / 116	> 16	1.0	Referent	[790]
	98 / 168	≤ 16	1.06	0.57-1.96	
Hsing, 2000	147 / 239	≥ 23	1.0	Referent	[1]
	39 / 56	< 23	1.12	0.71-1.78	
Miller, 2001	51 / 25	> 16	1.0	Referent	[95]
	82 / 44	≤ 16	0.98	0.46-2.06	
Chang, 2002	100 / 72	≥ 17	1.0	Referent	[795]
	227 / 102	≤ 16	1.58	1.08-2.32	
Chen, 2002	115 / 100	> 17	1.0	Referent	[93]
	185 / 200	≤ 17	0.8	0.57-1.12	
	144 / 127	Not 17	1.0	Referent	
	156 / 173	17	0.79	0.57-1.09	

TABLE 1. *(Cont.)* Comparison of case-control studies of AR-CAG and AR-GGC/N polymorphism and prostate cancer risk*

Case-control studies	No. Cases/Controls	CAG and GGC/N comparison	OR/RR[a]	95% CI	References
Irvine, 1995	34 / 28	≥ 22, 16	1.0	Referent	[783]
	23 / 9	< 22, not 16	2.1	Not given	
Stanford, 1997	22 / 32	≥ 22, > 16	1.0	Referent	[96]
	32 / 41	≥ 22, ≤ 16	1.15	0.56-2.35	
	97 / 93	< 22, > 16	1.54	0.83-2.86	
	98 / 77	< 22, ≤ 16	2.05	1.09-3.84	
Platz, 1998	66 / 119	> 23, not 23	1.0	Referent	[787]
	90 / 133	> 23, 23	1.17	0.77-1.77	
	75 / 116	21-23, not 23	1.39	0.93-2.06	
	152 / 185	21-23, 23	1.22	0.82-1.83	
	103 / 134	< 21, not 23	1.49	1.02-2.15	
	96 / 107	< 21, 23	1.62	1.07-2.44	
Hsing, 2000	53 / 120	≥ 23, ≥ 23	1.0	Referent	[1]
	19 / 29	≥ 23, < 23	1.48	0.76-2.88	
	94 / 115	< 23, ≥ 23	1.85	1.21-2.82	
	20 / 26	< 23, < 23	1.75	0.9-3.41	
Miller, 2001	21 / 8	≥ 22, > 16	1.0	Referent	[95]
	45 / 26	≥ 22, ≤ 16	0.63	0.18-2.2	
	29 / 17	< 22, > 16	0.69	0.17-2.74	
	35 / 17	< 22, ≤ 16	1.06	0.25-4.46	
Chang, 2002	42 / 30	≥ 22, ≥ 17	1.0	Referent	[795]
	109 / 46	≥ 22, ≤ 16	1.62	0.92-2.95	
	50 / 39	≤ 21, ≥ 17	0.92	0.49-1.72	
	99 / 54	≤ 21, ≤ 16	1.29	0.72-2.29	
Chen, 2002	49 / 29	≥ 22, > 17	1.0	Referent	[93]
	107 / 118	≥ 22, ≤ 17	0.54	0.32-0.91	
	66 / 71	< 22, > 17	0.55	0.31-0.98	
	78 / 82	< 22, ≤ 17	0.56	0.32-0.98	

[a]relative risk
*adapted from [94] and [93]

monal therapy, disease-free survival and overall survival (see [83, 93, 94] for recent reviews). Finally, a recent study compared repeat lengths of 140 men with prostate cancer to their brothers (n = 70) without disease from 51 high–risk sibships, stratified by median age at diagnosis of affected men within each sibship. Men with both a short CAG repeat length (< 22) and a short GGN repeat (≤16) array were not at higher risk (OR = 1.06; 95% CI, 0.25-4.46) compared to men with two long repeats (CAG repeat ≥22 and a GGN repeat >16), thus suggesting that the CAG and GGN repeats in the AR gene do not play a major role in familial prostate cancer[95]. More recently, a case-control study nested within the b Carotene and Retinol Efficacy Trial including 300 cases and 300 controls showed there was no appreciable difference in the mean number of GGC repeats between cases and controls and the risk in men at or below the mean number of GGC repeats (17) was 0.80 (95% CI, 0.57-1.12)[93]. Moreover, these authors found a decrease in prostate cancer risk among men with CAG <22 and GGC ≤17, or CAG <22 and GGC >17 or CAG ≥22 and GGC ≤17 when compared with men with CAG ≥22 and GGC >17 (Table 1). These results are thus in contrast with two other studies showing that the presence of a short repeat length for either or both CAG and GGC alleles was associated with an increased risk of prostate cancer[1, 96]. Finally, using the Johns Hopkins set, a significant association was observed in the frequencies of the ≤16 GGC repeat alleles in 159 HPC (71%), 245 sporadic cases (68%) compared with 211 controls (59%), thus supporting that GGC repeats were associated with prostate cancer risk (P = 0.02)[97]. Furthermore, male-limited X-linked transmission/disequilibrium (XLRC-TDT) was also used by these authors to demonstrate the preferential transmission of short ≤16 GGC repeat alleles from heterozygous mothers to their affected sons (z'= 2.65, P = 0.008). The stronger evidence for linkage in the families with male-to-male transmission may be explained by the hypothesis that AR is a strong modifier gene that works in conjunction with autosomal susceptibility gene(s). In support of this interpretation, Cui et al.[17] observed that the two locus model, combining autosomal dominant with either an autosomal recessive or X-linked model, fit their data better than did a single-locus models in segregation analyses. Further association studies using larger cohorts of preferably >1000 blood samples from prostate cancer cases vs ethnically matched controls, and well characterized clinical data, will thus be important to clarify the role of these low-penetrance trinucleotide polymorphic repeats in prostate cancer development and progression, taking into account their potential gene-gene and gene-environment interactions, which likely cumulate to contribute to an overall prostate cancer risk and to disease characteristics.

5.2 5a-reductase type 2

One of the best candidate genes is the 5a-reductase type 2 gene *(SRD5A2)*, which catalyzes the conversion of testosterone into the more active androgen DHT and maps to 2p22-23[98] (Figure 5). Intraprostatic

1. Prostate Cancer Susceptibility Genes

DHT is the most meaningful parameter of androgen action in prostatic tissue (Figure 6). Indeed, the importance of intracrine formation of active androgens is in concordance with the observation that after elimination of

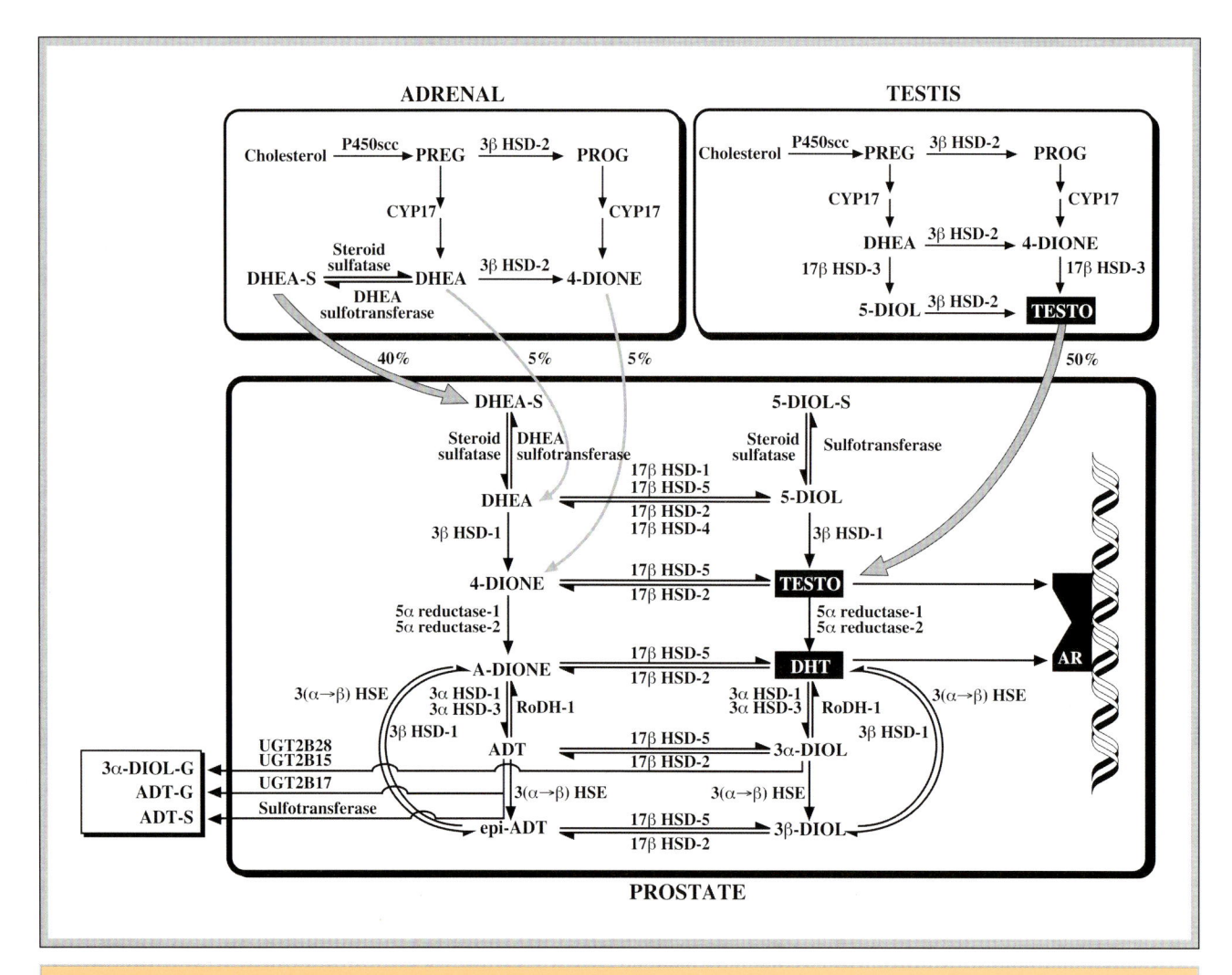

FIGURE 6. Major enzymatic pathways involved in the formation and inactivation of androgens in human and the relative importance (%) of adrenal steroid precursors in the intraprostatic concentration of DHT in adult men.
A-DIONE, androstanedione; ADT, androsterone; ADT-G, androsterone glucuronide; ADT-S, androsterone sulfate; AR, androgen receptor; CYP17, cytochrome P450c17, 17-hydroxylase/17,20 lyase; DHEA, dehydroepiandrosterone; DHEA-S, dehydroepiandrosterone sulfate; DHT, dihydrotestosterone; epi-ADT, epi-androsterone; P450scc, cholesterol side-chain cleavage enzyme; PREG, pregnenolone; PROG, progesterone; RoDH-1, retinol dehydrogenase type 1; TESTO, testosterone; UGT, UDP-glucuronosyltransferase; 3a-DIOL, 5a-androstane-3a, 17b-diol; 3a-DIOL-G, 5a-androstane-3a, 17b-diol-glucuronide; 3a HSD-1,-3, 3a-hydroxysteroid dehydrogenase type 1, type 3; 3(a→b) HSE, 3(a→b) hydroxysteroid epimerase; 3b-DIOL, 5a-androstane-3b, 17b-diol; 3b HSD-1, -2, 3b hydroxysteroid dehydrogenase/Δ^5-Δ^4-isomerase type 1, type 2; 4-DIONE, androstenedione; 5-DIOL, androst-5-ene-3b,17b-diol; 5-DIOL-S, androst-5-ene-3b,17b-diol sulfate; 17b HSD-1, -2, -3, -4, -5, 17b hydroxysteroid dehydrogenase type 1, type 2, type 3, type 4, type 5.

testicular androgens by medical or surgical castration, the intraprostatic concentration of DHT remains approximately 40% of that measured in the prostate of intact 65-year-old men, thus leaving important amounts of free androgen to continue stimulating the growth of the prostate cancer[99]. However, male pseudohermaphrodites with 5a-reductase deficiency caused by mutations in the *SRD5A2* gene exhibit external genital ambiguity and hypoplastic prostate, thus supporting the crucial role of this enzyme in normal prostate development. Modulation of 5a-reductase activity may account for part of the substantial racial/ethnic disparity in prostate cancer risk[100-102]. Furthermore, one variant, Ala49Thr has been reported to increase the catalytic activity of this enzyme[103] and is associated with an increased risk of advanced prostate cancer[104-106]. This low-penetrance allele appears to increase the risk of prostate cancer in African-Americans, Latinos and Italians by 7.2- (p<0.001), 3.6- (p<0.04) and 7.7- (p<0.11) folds, respectively[104-106] (Table 2). In contrast, the prevalence of the A49T variant in 449 Finnish prostate cancer patients was 6.0%, not significantly differing from 6.3% observed in 223 patients with BPH or 5.8% in 588 population-based controls (Table 2). Furthermore, there was no association between A49T and the family history of the patients nor with tumour stage or grade[107]. Finally, the T allele was not observed in a population-based case control study in China after the genotyping of 191 cases and 304 controls[108]. It is also of interest to know that substantial pharmacogenetic variation among the *SRD5A2* sequence variants was observed when three competitive inhibitors (Finasteride, GG745 and PNU157706) were tested, thus providing relevant information to take into account when prescribing such inhibitors for the chemoprevention or treatment of prostate diseases[103, 104].

5.3 CYP17

Another key enzyme involved in the testicular synthesis of androgens is encoded by the *CYP17* gene, namely the cytochrome P450c17, which catalyzes 17a-hydroxylase and 17,20-lyase activities (Figure 5). The *CYP17* gene is mapped to 10q24.3 and consists of 8 exons. A single-base change (a T (A1 allele) to C (A2 allele) transition) creates an additional putative Sp1-type (CCACC box) transcriptional factor binding site that was postulated to increase its gene expression. Nedelcheva Kristensen et al. showed that neither the A1 nor A2 allele could form a complex with the Sp1 protein in electrophoretic mobility shift assays[109]. Moreover, a recent study using a promoter/reporter gene construct containing sequences from -227 to +61 with either a T or C at position +27 demonstrated that this polymorphism is not associated with an altered transcriptional activ-

TABLE 2. Association of the A49T missense substitution in *SRDA2* gene with risk of prostate cancer.

African-American men

	AA	AT/TT	Relative Risk	(95% CI)	P value
Controls	257	3/1	–		–
Cases					
All	203	9/4	32.8	(1.09-11.87)	0.03
Localised	134	2/2	1.47	(0.33-6.63)	0.60
Advanced	69	7/2	7.22	(2.17-27.91)	0.001

AA= normal (wild-type) homozygotes, AT= heterozygotes, TT= mutant (A49T) homozygotes
Adapted from [104]

Hispanic men

	AA	AT/TT	Relative Risk	(95% CI)	P value
Controls	193	5/2	–		–
Cases					
All	160	10/2	2.50	(0.90-7.40)	0.08
Localised	96	4/1	1.71	(0.46-6.12)	0.41
Advanced	64	6/1	3.60	(1.09-12.27)	0.04

AA= normal (wild-type) homozygotes, AT= heterozygotes, TT= mutant (A49T) homozygotes
Adapted from [104]

Italian men

	AA	AT/TT	Odds ratio	(95% CI)	P value
Controls	112	0/0	–		–
Cases					
Sporadic prostate cancer	103	3/0	7.7	(0.39-150.54)	0.11

Adapted from [106]

Finnish men

	Prevalence of AT/TT	Odds ratio* (95% CI)	P value *
Controls	34/588 (5.8%)	–	–
Cases			
Sporadic prostate cancer	27/449 (6.0%)	1.04 (0.62-1.76)	0.89
Familial prostate cancer	5/94 (5.3%)	0.92 (0.35-2.40)	1.00
Benign prostatic hyperplasia	14/223 (6.3%)	1.09 (0.57-2.08)	0.87

*as compared to controls (blood donors and autopsy samples)
Adapted from [107]

ity[110]. Nevertheless, three independent association studies reported a small but positive association between the A2 allele and an increased risk for prostate cancer[111-113]. On the other hand, two other studies showed that the A1 allele is the risk allele for prostate cancer[114, 115]. Considering its essential role in androgen biosynthesis, a recent study was designed to further evaluate the impact of this polymorphism and to investigate what is the potential role of this gene in hereditary prostate cancer[116]. These authors performed a genetic linkage study and family-based association analysis in 159 families (Johns-Hopkins set), each of which contained at least 3 first-degree relatives with prostate cancer. It is of interest to note that a linkage analysis is insensitive to allelic heterogeneity, thus if a mutation has a high penetrance and there are multiple such mutations within a gene, a linkage study is likely to detect such a gene, whereas family-based or population based association approaches are likely to fail[116]. Thus, information concerning specific sequence variants within a gene is not necessary for a linkage study, but is essential for association studies. Their analyses suggest evidence for linkage at marker D10S222 with a LOD score of 1.03 ($p<0.01$). However, they did not observe a statistically increased risk to sporadic prostate cancer or hereditary prostate cancer in subjects with the A2 variant following genotyping of the polymorphism in 159 HPC probands, 249 sporadic cases and 211 unaffected control subjects. They concluded that *CYP17* gene or other genes in this region may increase the susceptibility to prostate cancer, whereas the polymorphism in the 5' promoter region has a minor if any effect in increasing prostate cancer susceptibility in their study sample.

5.4 3b-HSDs

The 3b-hydroxysteroid dehydrogenase/Δ^5-Δ^4 isomerase (3b-HSD) isoenzymes are responsible for the oxidation and isomerisation of Δ^5-3b-hydroxysteroid precursors into Δ^4-ketosteroids, thus catalyzing an essential step in the formation of all classes of active steroid hormones. In humans, expression of the type I isoenzyme accounts for the 3b-HSD activity found in placenta and peripheral tissues, whereas the type II 3b-HSD isoenzyme is predominantly expressed in the adrenal gland, ovary and testis and its deficiency is responsible for a rare form of congenital adrenal hyperplasia[117]. To evaluate the possible role of these enzymes encoded by *HSD3B* genes (Figure 5) in prostate cancer susceptibility, a recent study screened a panel of DNA samples collected from 96 men with or without prostate cancer for sequence variants in the putative promoter region, exons, exon-intron junctions, and 3'-untranslated region of *HSD3B1* and *HSD3B2* genes by direct sequencing[97]. Four of the eleven single nucleotide polymorphisms (SNPs) were informative. These four

SNPs were further genotyped in a total of 159 hereditary prostate cancer probands (Johns-Hopkins set), 245 sporadic prostate cancer cases, and 222 unaffected controls. Although a weak association between prostate cancer risk and a missense polymorphism *(HSD3B1-N367T)* was found, stronger evidence for association was found when the joint effect of the two genes was considered. Indeed, men with the variant genotypes at either *HSD3B1*-N367T or *HSD3B2*-c7519g had a relative risk of 1.76 (95% CI = 1.21-2.57, p = 0.003) to develop prostate cancer compared with men who were homozygous wild type at both genes, whereas the risk for the hereditary type of prostate cancer was stronger, with a relative risk of 2.17 (95% CI = 1.29-3.65, p = 0.003) (Table 3). Most importantly, the subset of hereditary prostate cancer probands, whose families provided evidence for linkage at 1p13, predominantly contributed to the observed association[97]. Additional studies are warranted to confirm these findings.

6. CONCLUSION

The clearest conclusion emerging from the linkage studies described above is perhaps that no single susceptibility locus mapped to date is by itself responsible for a large portion of familial prostate cancers, at least not with the combination of penetrance and clinical features that allowed linkage to and positional cloning of the so-far known colon and breast cancer predisposition genes. Thus, locus heterogeneity is a major parameter in the identification or confirmation of linkage for many data sets. Indeed, the possible existence of multiple prostate cancer genes may well explain why there has been limited confirmatory evidence of linkage for currently known highly-penetrant susceptibility loci/genes. As methods for statistical modeling improve, geneticists will have better tools to deal with the apparent extreme heterogeneity within data sets[7,13,21].

To clarify the role of low-penetrance polymorphisms in prostate cancer development and progression, association studies using larger cohorts of preferably >1000 blood samples from prostate cancer cases vs ethnically matched controls, and well characterized clinical data, will thus be important[6]. It will also be necessary to investigate, using various complementary genetic epidemiological approaches, the potential role of the other key steroidogenic enzymes involved in the formation and/or inactivation of androgens, such as the numerous 17b-HSDs, 3a-HSDs, UDP-glucuronosyltransferases etc. (Figure 5). We should also take into account the potential gene-gene and gene-environment interactions of low- or

TABLE 3. Frequencies and relative risk for combined *HSD3B1*-N367T and *HSD3B2*-c7519g genotypes (Caucasians only)

	No of subjects			Relative Risk* (95 % CI)		
	HPC	Sporadic	Control	HPC vs controls	Sporadic vs controls	All cases vs controls
All ages						
HSD3B1-N367T = A/A and *HSD3B2*-c7519g = C/C	30 (26%)	72 (32%)	77 (43%)	1	1	1
HSD3B1-N367T = A/C or C/C or *HSD3B2*-c7519g = C/G or G/G	84 (74%)	152 (68%)	101 (57%)	2.17 (1.29-3.65)	1.61 (1.07-2.42)	1.76 (1.21-2.57)
Older age group (.60 years)						
HSD3B1-N367T = A/A and *HSD3B2*-c7519g = C/C	17 (24%)	26 (26%)	33 (49%)	1	1	1
HSD3B1-N367T = A/C or C/C or *HSD3B2*-c7519g = C/G or G/G	55 (76%)	73 (74%)	34 (51%)	3.14 (1.52-6.49)	2.62 (1.34-5.14)	2.88 (1.59-5.23)

All odds ratios were age adjusted
Adapted from [97]

moderate-penetrance genes, which likely cumulate to contribute to an overall prostate cancer risk and to disease characteristics. In this regard, when several SNPs occur in the same gene/locus or a chromosomal region, it will be crucial to establish in each individual tested using haplotyping, if possible, an exhaustive genomic profiling for all selected sequence variants. This will allow a better estimate of their global contribution in various mechanisms involved in prostate cancer, such as in pathways involved in the fine control of intracellular androgen bioavailability and in the signal transduction of their cell-specific action.

In parallel, characterization of gene expression profiles that molecularly distinguish prostatic neoplasms may identify new target candidate genes involved in prostate cancer risk in addition to elucidate useful new clinical biomarkers leading to an improved classification of prostate cancer. This will be of special interest if such signature may help to distinguish hereditary versus sporadic prostate carcinomas, as it has recently been achieved for breast cancer[118]. Moreover, the integration of gene expression data with the knowledge of the human genome sequence as well as those of experimental models will be useful to accelerate positional cloning approaches that are often hampered by incomplete phenotypic penetrance, small pedigree size and limited access to DNA samples from affected individuals. The elucidation of transcriptomes of normal and tumoral prostate tissues can effectively focus efforts on a manageable subset of genes, thus facilitating the candidate gene approaches, especially when genetic maps cover a broad chromosomal region as frequently observed for prostate cancer susceptibility loci. Integrating both expression and functional information may further speed gene discovery via the candidate gene approach as recently suggested for retinal disease genes[119].

We are at the very early phases of functional genomics and rapid advances are also anticipated in more quantitative proteomics and bioinformatics, which should dramatically increase the likelihood of finding clinically relevant candidate genes, gene clusters and signaling pathways that will translate into better diagnostic or more targeted therapeutic strategies for men with prostate cancer.

ACKNOWLEDGMENTS

J. Simard is chairholder of the Canada Research Chair in Oncogenetics funded by the Canada Research Chair Program.

Introduction and History of PSA Screening

By Craig Berman and E. David Crawford

Prostate cancer has become a major health concern with an estimated 31,900 men who would die of prostate cancer in the United States alone in the year 2000[120]. Prior to PSA screening, many patients presented with advanced disease with an estimated 30-35% presenting with bony metastases, 45-50% with nodal involvement, and only one third having surgically organ-confined disease[121]. In 1981, Nadji and colleagues demonstrated that PSA was a potentially useful marker for prostate cancer[122].

Since the approval of the use of a commercial immunoassay for prostate specific antigen (PSA) in 1986 by the Food and Drug Administration, PSA has become a widely used screening tool for early detection of prostate cancer[123]. In 1989, a large health survey sponsored by the Prostate Cancer Education Council, found that only 50% of men over age 40 were having physical exams with only half of this group receiving a digital rectal examination[124]. Prostate Cancer Awareness Week alone has screened more than 3 million men since 1989[124]. Popularized in the United States, PSA screening guidelines have been recommended by several different medical organizations in the United States.

As the use of PSA as a marker for prostate cancer enters a fifteenth year of clinical use, the accuracy and usefulness of PSA as a screening tool for prostate cancer is still controversial and not completely accepted worldwide. Several questions are important in assessing whether PSA is

2. INTRODUCTION AND HISTORY OF PSA SCREENING

useful as a screening tool. First, is there a more accurate form of PSA or adjunctive test that will improve the accuracy of PSA testing and help differentiate malignant from benign (prostatitis, normal variation, BPH) disease and better determine who should undergo further clinical evaluation for cancer including prostatic biopsies, radiographic imaging, or further laboratory testing. Who is at higher risk and should undergo earlier screening? Is all of the expense and public health effort/concern with PSA screening detecting clinically curable cancer at a stage when the cancer can be cured? Is screening detecting cancer which, based on the natural history of the disease is either non-curable or does not need to be cured because the patient will die from comorbid disease before prostate cancer causes the patient any morbidity or mortality[125]?

This chapter will review the accuracy of PSA in detecting prostate cancer, discuss risk factors for developing prostate cancer, discuss newer advances in PSA testing, and then review the evidence both against and in support of prostate screening. In order to be effective, PSA screening must detect individuals with curable disease or incurable disease which early intervention will prolong life and/or increase a patient's quality of life.

WHAT ARE THE CURRENT SCREENING RECOMMENDATIONS

The American Urological Association recommendations for 2001 PSA screening is all men 50 years of age or older with an expected lifespan of at least 10 years and men aged 40-50 years of age who either have a first-degree relative who had prostate cancer or are of African-American ethnic background[126]. The American Cancer Society recommendations are similar, "Both the prostate specific antigen (PSA) test and digital rectal examination (DRE) is offered annually beginning at age 50 years, to men who have at least a ten year life expectancy and to younger men who are at high risk."[127]. The American Cancer Society emphasizes that patients would be informed regarding the potential risks and benefits of intervention[127]. The American Academy of Family Physicians recommends that for men, ages 50-65 years, that they be counseled about the known risks and uncertain benefits of screening for prostate cancer[128]. The American College of Physicians-American Society of Internal Medicine recommends that screening should involve physicians informing the patient of the potential benefits and known harms of screening, diagnosis, and treatment, emphasizing an individualization of the decision to screen. The recommendations emphasize that the most benefit for screening is in men age 50-69[129]. PSA screening is not universally recommended because of debate whether screening detects clinically relevant cancers and whether screening is able to influence the natural history of the disease.

NATURAL HISTORY OF PROSTATE CANCER

What is the natural history of prostate cancer, specifically what patient population may benefit from early intervention and does the intervention change the natural history of the disease? Prostate cancer is a disease with variable progression depending largely on how early the disease is detected (organ-confined or non-organ confined stage and how well differentiated the cancer is on biopsy or pathological staging. In a recent study, disease specific survival for well and moderately differentiated tumors is 87% compared to 34% for poorly differentiated tumors[130,131] looked specifically at the 5, 10, and 15 year risk of dying from prostate-specific causes in a group of 767 men treated expectantly and stratified them by age and differentiation of the tumor (Gleason sum)[130, 131]. In men aged 70-74, with a Gleason sum 7 tumor, the 5, 10, and 15yr survivals were 60%, 24%, and 9% respectively. The disease-specific survivals for this age group were 84%, 48%, and 60%. In a younger age group (aged 55-59) the disease specific survivals at 5, 10, and 15 years were excellent for low grade (Gleason 2-4 disease) with disease specific survivals 98%, 96%, and 95%, respectively. For Gleason sum 7 tumors the corresponding disease-specific survivals were 75%, 48%, and 30%, respectively. For poorly differentiated tumors, the 5, 10, and 15-year disease specific survivals were 58%, 23%, and 14% respectively.

Chodak et al (1994) performed a pooled analysis of 828 case records of patients treated for clinically localized prostate cancer with observation and delayed hormonal therapy but no surgery or irradiation[130]. They divided the tumor grade into grade 1 (Gleason 2-4), grade 2 (Gleason 5-7), and grade 3 (Gleason 8-10), an found that ten year disease specific survival was 87% for grade 1, 58% for grade 2, and 26% for grade 3. The factors that had a significant negative impact on survival were grade 3 tumors, residence in Israel or New York, and age under 61 years.

THE NEXT INVESTIGATIVE QUESTION IS HOW WELL DOES THE TREATMENT WORK FOR SCREENING POPULATIONS

Briefly, this section will review the current evidence that definitive treatments, surgery, radiation, or interstitial radiotherapy is a treatment which can cure prostate cancer which is detected by screening. How well does surgery, radiation, or interstitial radiotherapy treat moderately and well differentiated cancers.

D'Amico et al (1998) reported on a prospective analysis of 888 patients treated with a radical prostatectomy or interstitial radiation implant (with and without neoadjuvant androgen deprivation therapy) or external beam radiotherapy and looked at PSA failures[132]. The relative risk of PSA failure in low-risk patients (T1C, T2A and PSA level <=10ng/ml) compared to radical prostatectomy was 1.1 for radiotherapy, 0.5 for implant plus androgen deprivation therapy, and 1.1 for brachytherapy alone. For the, high-risk patient group (T2C, PSA>20, Gleason >=8), the relative risk compared to radical prostatectomy was 3.1 for radiotherapy, 3.1 for implant plus androgen deprivation, and 3.0 for implant alone. The author's conclusion was that comparable outcomes at 5 years is similar between all groups but that radiotherapy and surgery demonstrated lower PSA recurrence rates than implant for intermediate or high-risk disease. Gerber et al (1996) Reported on a pooled analysis of results of radical prostatectomy as a treatment for clinically localized prostate cancer in a group of 2758 men with stage T1 and T2 prostate cancer. Disease-specific survival 10 years following surgery were 94%, 80%, and 77% for grade 1, grade 2, and grade 3 tumors, respectively. Metastasis-free survival at 10 years was 87%, 68%, and 52% for grade 1, 2, and 3 tumors, respectively[133]. Pound et al (1999) also reviewed a large surgical series of 1997 men treated with radical prostatectomy alone for 3.7 years median follow-up. Actuarial metastasis-free survival for all men was 82% at 15 years. The median actuarial time to metastases was 8 years. After development of metastatic disease the median actuarial time to death was 5 years[134]. Catalona and Smith (1998) estimated that the 7-year prostate cancer specific survival rate was 97% and the all cause survival rate was 90% for patients undergoing radical prostatectomy[135]. Polascik et al (1999) compared radical prostatectomy to Iodine –125 interstitial radiotherapy for treatment of localized prostate cancer and reported that the progression-free survival following anatomic radical prostatectomy was 97.8% compared to 79% for men treated with I-125[136].

As regards brachytherapy, for clinically localized prostate cancer, Ragde et al (2000) reported the 10 year disease free survival of 229 patient with T1-T3 cancer treated with interstitial I-125 alone was 70% and for combined interstitial therapy with external beam therapy was 79%[137]. Blasko et al (2000) reported that the biochemical control rate at 9 years was 83.5%[138]. Crook et al (2001) did a literature review on brachytherapy studies and reported that brachytherapy alone series have reported a "no evidence of disease" rate varying from 63% at 4 years to 93% at five years[139]. Beyer and Priestley (1997) reported that 5-year biochemical freedom of disease was 90-94% for T1 tumors, 70-75% for T2a tumors, and 34% for T2b and T2c tumors[140].

Radiation therapy has also demonstrated clinical efficacy in treating localized prostate cancer. Shipley et al (1999) conducted a multi-institutional pooled analysis of 1765 men with stage T1b, T1c, and T2 tumors treated with external beam radiation. The PSA failure free rates at 5 and 7 years for patients, who presented with a pretreatment PSA of less than 10ng/ml were 77.8% and 72.9%, respectively[141]. High dose radiation has also demonstrated activity in treating prostate cancer. Valicenti et al (2000) reported on a ten-year disease specific survival rates of 85% for Gleason 2-5, 79% for Gleason 6, 62% for Gleason 7, and 43% for Gleason 8-10[142].

In summary, radical prostatectomy, external beam radiation therapy, and radioactive interstitial seed placement (brachytherapy) are able to cure localized prostate cancer and warrant screening intervention aimed at detecting clinically localized prostate cancer. These treatments demonstrate better cure rates for earlier detected cancers.

There are definitive treatments for early cancer and, depending on the differentiation of the disease (Gleason score) as presented above, the cancer can be cured. The other population that screening may aid is in detecting advanced disease which may benefit from earlier detection. The question is does earlier intervention with hormonal ablation, XRT, or chemotherapy prolong survival or decrease morbidity in these groups.

The natural history of patients who have PSA recurrence after definitive treatment with radical prostatectomy who received no adjunctive treatment or hormonal ablation until development of distant metastatic disease demonstrated that the actuarial metastasis-free survival for all men was 82% at fifteen years after surgery[134]. The median actuarial time to metastasis was 8 years from the time of PSA elevation. From the time that the patients developed metastatic disease, the median actuarial time to death was 5 years[134]. This analysis did include 27% of men who received adjuvant radiation therapy and had a continued elevation of PSA. Within this group of men, Gleason score 8-10, PSA recurrence within 2 years, and a PSA doubling time of less than 10 months were independent predictors of a decreased survival[134].

Whether early hormonal ablation versus late hormonal ablation would change the natural history of the progression of prostate cancer is an important question in terms of what age to stop screening of PSA. Initial studies, specifically, the VACURG study, demonstrated that there was no advantage to early treatment of men with metastatic prostate cancer. This would lead to recommendations to stop PSA screening at the age which the patient no longer had a risk of dying from localized prostate cancer. After that age, which based on Swedish studies is age 70-72, patients would be treated with the intention to prolong life and decrease morbidity of advanced disease. Within this parameter, then PSA would only be useful to determine the risk of having locally advanced or metastatic disease if there was an intervention which prior to development of symptoms of metastatic disease would decrease disease specific morbidity or disease specific mortality. In other words, if the intention to treat a patient with a less than fifteen year life expectancy with hormonal ablation or chemotherapy only at the time point in the disease which the individual develops symptomatic metastatic disease then screening PSA has no clinical value in this population.

Walsh et al (2001) provide a nice review of the studies which support and argue against early hormonal ablation[143]. In the VACURG I study, patients with locally advanced or metastatic disease were treated with placebo or orchiectomy. In the study, there was no difference in cancer specific survival[144]. Other studies including the Medical Research Council (MRC) demonstrated evidence of an advantage for early versus late hormonal ablation in treating non-metastatic locally advanced disease (32% death rate in the immediate treatment group compared to 49% for the delayed group)[145]. In the Eastern Cooperative Oncology Group (ECOG) which randomized men with node positive disease to either immediate or delayed androgen ablation demonstrated a survival advantage at 7.1 years of follow-up favoring immediate androgen ablation[146].

While inconclusive as to whether early hormonal ablation imparts a survival advantage or delays onset of symptoms of metastatic disease, these studies demonstrate evidence of decreasing mortality for patients treated with early hormonal ablation. At what age should we consider stopping screening? A reasonable age is 72-75 years in patients with a less than 10 year life expectancy and in patients who have been followed with serial, yearly PSAs and have no prior results of an elevated PSA.

ACCURACY OF PSA

Arguments in other sections have been made that PSA is useful as a screening tool both to detect and treat early stage cancer and also to direct early hormone ablation in more advanced stage cancer. The next aspect of PSA screening to be discussed is current PSA testing, focusing on the accuracy of PSA, variability of assays, PSA density, PSA velocity, age-specific PSA, an free PSA testing. One of the concerns with using PSA as a screening test is that the test has a significant false positive rate, largely due to the fact that PSA can be elevated from benign processes (prostatitis, benign prostatic hypertrophy, and normal variation). Another problem is that our current detection of prostate cancer is largely based on transrectal ultrasound guided biopsies which have positive predictive values that range from 44% for patients who had an abnormal transrectal ultrasound, abnormal DRE, and an abnormal PSA to only 24% for patients with an abnormal PSA[147]. A biopsy study by Catalona demonstrated a biopsy positive rate, even for a selected population sent to a tertiary referral center of 25%. In an analysis of date from the Prostate Cancer Awareness Week, Crawford and colleagues analyzed 22,014 men who had an abnormal DRE or abnormal PSA and 17,561 men who had both abnormal. The positive predictive values of abnormal PSA alone, abnormal DRE alone, and combined abnormal PSA an DRE tests were 27.7%, 17.7%, and 56.0% respectively. Sensitivities were 34.9%, 27.1%, and 38.0%, respectively. Specificities were 63.1%, 49.0% and 87.9% respectively. Sensitivity and specificity, using current screening recommendations of DRE and PSA was only 38.0% and 87.9%.

VARIABILITY OF SERUM ASSAYS

Several different factors can lead to variability among different commercially available assays including antibodies with various affinity and specificity for different PSA epitopes, variable calibration of the assay method, assay procedure specifics (incubation time, equilibrium or kinetics), lot-to lot variations in assays, and interference from autoanti-PSA-antibodies[148]. The authors recommend that clinicians request information from the laboratory including assay method used and notification of any change in assay, validity of reference range, molar response ratio (the ratio by which complexed and free-PSA is detected by the assay) and analytical sensitivity[148]. We completed a comparison of the Hybritech Tandem-R PSA test and the Abbott AxSym PSA test and found that both assays are highly correlated in all PSA level ranges[149].

PSA DENSITY, PSA VELOCITY, AGE SPECIFIC PSA, FREE PSA

In order to increase the sensitivity and specificity of PSA several different techniques have been used including PSA density, PSA Velocity,

2. Introduction and History of PSA Screening

and free PSA. PSA density, described in 1990 was based on the theory that a prostate gland with cancer would have a higher concentration of PSA production versus size. In addition to calculating PSA density for the entire gland, investigators have defined PSA density for the transition zone in order to normalize PSA density to the portion of the prostate gland in which BPH develops.

PSA velocity was derived from work by Carter et al (1992) in the Baltimore Longitudinal Aging Study. Using PSA velocity is based on the observations in the study that men with prostate cancer developed a more rapid rate of PSA change within five years prior to diagnosis of prostate cancer[150]. Using a cutoff of PSA velocity change of greater than 0.75 ng/ml per year they demonstrated a sensitivity of 75% and a specificity of 90%. Other investigators have not been able to reproduce these results and conflicting studies have both supported and refuted that PSA density increases the accuracy of abnormal PSA value alone[151-154]. (40-43) Age specific PSA levels was first proposed by Oesterling and Dalkin in 1993[154, 155]. Oesterling proposed normal levels of 2.5ng/ml in men aged 40-49, 3.5 ng/ml in men aged 50-59, 4.5 ng/ml in men aged 60-69, and 6.5 ng/ml in men aged 70-79[154]. Several studies have supported the use of age specific reference ranges of PSA. Oesterling demonstrated that using age specific PSA cutoffs, the sensitivity of PSA for detecting prostate cancer decreased by 9%, the specificity increased by 11% and the positive predictive value increased by 5%. Several different researchers have proposed different age specific PSA reference ranges.

Catalona et al (1997) found that the use of age specific reference ranges resulted in a 45% increase in biopsies in men aged 50-59 years and decreased the biopsy rate in men older than 70 years by 44%[156]. Bangma et al (1995), using age specific PSA cutoff values reported that 39% of cancers would be missed and Crawford et al (1999) reported that there was no significant increase in PPVS for PSA, DRE, and combined DRE with PSA using age specific reference ranges as compared to using a PSA cutoff of 4.0ng/ml, alone[157, 158]. Partin et al (1997) found that using ASRRs in younger men led to a higher detection rate of favorable cancer in younger men (age <60 years) and that 95% of the missed cancers in older men had favorable histology, leading to a recommendation of the use of ASRRs only in men aged 60 or less[159]. Other investigators have found unacceptably high levels of unfavorable cancer missed in older patients using ASRRs[160].

PSA density was first described by Bensen et al (1992) as a tool to help differentiate PSA elevations due to BPH from PSA elevations caused by prostate cancer[161]. PSA density is defined as the PSA value divided by the volume of the prostate as determined by transrectal ultrasound, with an abnormal value of greater than 0.15). The use of PSA density to increase the accuracy of PSA in detecting prostate cancer and differentiating cancer from BPH currently does not have much support due to conflicting results in the literature. Investigating the use of PSA density to help direct repeat biopsies, Catalona et al (1997) using PSA density cutoffs of 0.100 and 0.080 would have detected 90% and 95% of diagnosed cancers, respectively and avoid 31% and 12% of repeat biopsies[156]. Noguchi et al (1999) demonstrated that in comparison of men undergoing a repeat biopsy who had cancer diagnosed on the second biopsy to men who had no cancer diagnosed on repeat biopsy, that DRE, PSA, prostate volume, PSA density, and PSA velocity had no clinical usefulness in detecting cancer on repeat biopsy[162].

The overall question is whether PSA density and PSA have increased the accuracy of PSA alone. Fowler et al (2000) investigated whether total PSA, PSA density, change in PSA, percentage free PSA, and PSA velocity was useful in subsequently detecting cancer in patients who had an initial negative biopsy. In the subset of patients for whom free/total PSA results were available, only patient age and free/total PSA was predictive of subsequent positive biopsy [163]. Mettlin et al (1994) reported on the sensitivity and specificity of PSA as compared to age-referenced PSA and PSA density[164]. Investigating specificity in 2011 men without prostate cancer and sensitivity in 171 men with prostate cancer, the study determined the sensitivity and specificity to be as follows: PSA alone had a specificity of 90.0% and a sensitivity of 71.9%. PSA density (with an abnormal value greater than 0.1) had a specificity of 85.3% and a sensitivity of 74.7%. Age-referenced PSA had a specificity of 90.9% and a sensitivity of 67.3%, and PSA change (abnormal value defined as greater than 0.75 ng/ml per year had a specificity of 95.5-96.4% and a sensitivity of 45.7 to 54.8%. Overall conclusion of the study was that "none of the alternative indexes commonly used in general early detection practice demonstrated particular advantage when compared with normal PSA concentration, defined as no more than 4.0 ng/ml[164].

Investigators have also looked at further limiting PSA density to PSA density for the transition zone only. Some studies have supported and others have refuted whether transition zone density has added to the accuracy of PSA alone. Djavan et al (2000) looked at a group of men from a screening population with PSA levels between 4 and 10ng/ml and found that PSA density for the transition zone using a cut-off of 0.26 detected 78% of cancers and would have spared 52% of subsequent biopsies but did not demonstrate any advantage over free-total PSA values[165]. As Knowles et al describes in a recent review article on PSA density, measuring the transition zone volume is more difficult than measuring overall prostatic volume[166].

2. Introduction and History of PSA Screening

Recent work with PSA has demonstrated that 70-90% of PSA in serum is complexed to alpha 1-antichymotrypsin(ACT) and other proteins that are thought to be clinically non-significant and 10-30% of the PSA in serum in uncomplexed and is referred to as free PSA[167, 168]. The percentage of free PSA has been reported to increase the sensitivity and positive predictive value of PSA. Several studies have supported the use of free PSA along with PSA to for prostate cancer. For total PSA values in the 4.0 to 10.0ng.ml range, Catalona et al (1998) reported on a multi-institutional study of 773 men and determined that using a free PSA cut-off of <=22% achieved a sensitivity and specificity of 90 and 29%, respectively. Using a cutoff of <= 25%, the sensitivity was increased to 95% but the specificity decreased to 20%. Using a cutoff of 22% free PSA percentage, the study found that almost a third of unnecessary biopsies could be avoided[135]. Other studies have found that, within the range of 4-10ng/ml that free PSA adds little to improve the accuracy and clinical usefulness of a straight abnormal PSA cutoff.

A more widely utilized use for free PSA is helping decide on further management and evaluation of a patient who has a PSA greater or equal to 4ng/ml and a resultant negative prostatic biopsy. Catalona et al (1997) identified 163 men out of the Washington University PSA-3 prostate cancer screening study who had PSA levels from 4.1 to 10.0ng/ml. Of these men 99 underwent repeat biopsy. The study found that that the use of percent free PSA cutoffs of 28 and 30% would have detected 90 and 95% of cancers, respectively and avoided 13 and 12% of b biopsies, respectively. They also looked at PSA density cutoffs and found that cutoffs of 0.10 and 0.08 would have detected 90 and 95% of cancers, and avoided 31 and 12% of biopsies, respectively[156]. The unanswered question is whether the men would have been rebiopsied based on continued elevation of PSA and would missing 5-10% of cancers in a high at risk population be acceptable. The study had small numbers of patients but did point out that the rebiopsy positive rate was only 20% in this screening population.

COMPLEXED PSA

A recently advancement in PSA testing is PSA complexed to alpha-1-antichymotrypsin(ACT)[169]. PSA forms complexes with protease inhibitors such as alpha-1-antichymotrypsin and alpha 2-macroglobulin[170]. The assay developed by Matsumoto et al (2000) is an enzyme-linked immunoassay (ELISA) which utilizes three different monoclonal antibodies for three distinct PSA epitopes and simultaneously blocks free-antigen PSA[171].

Several researchers have investigated whether PSA-ACT, PSA-ACT (ACTD) density, and free-PSA/complex-PSA% have clinical usefulness to distinguish benign from malignant disease[172]. Kuriyama et al (2001) analyzed sera from 907 men with benign and malignant urologic disease and found that PSA-ACT was more accurate than total PSA but not significantly more than the free-to-total PSA ratio[173]. Hara et al (2001) investigated whether PSA-ACT and ACTD could predict organ confined versus extraprostatic disease. In 62 patients, PSA-ACT and ACTD provided better sensitivity for detecting organ-confined disease. There was no association between PSA-ACT and ACTD and Gleason score . Further studies will help determine the clinical usefulness of PSA-ACT (complexed PSA) in distinguishing benign from malignant disease.

WHICH GROUP OF PATIENTS IS AT INCREASED RISK?

The Population at Risk

The general recommendation for screening to target patients for curative therapy is men over the age of 70 who have at least a ten year life expectancy. Screening also targets patients of African American descent and patients with a first degree relative with the disease. Black men have been found to have a higher incidence rate of prostate cancer than white men from similar socioeconomic backgrounds and survival rates, when controlled for stage of presentation, are lower than for black men compared to white men[174, 175]. Increased risk based on relatives is related to the number of first degree relatives who are affected and the age that those relatives presented with prostate cancer[10, 176]. If a man has a first degree relative who presented with prostate cancer at age 50, 60, or 70, and the man has an additional affected first degree relative with prostate cancer, then the relative risk of developing prostate cancer is 4, 5, and 7 respectively. Conversely, a person related to a person who develops prostate cancer at age 70 or greater and has no additional first-degree relatives with prostate cancer has no increased risk of developing cancer[10]. An autosomal dominant inheritance of prostate cancer has been estimated in 5-10% of prostate cancer cases[177]. Current research is focused on investigating specific tumor suppressor genes and androgen receptor genes which may allow further directed screening at population groups who are at risk for prostate cancer[178]. Currently screening recommendations target the general population between the age of 50-75, with earlier screening targeted at African American and patients with a strong family history of prostate cancer.

WHAT IS THE OPTIMAL SCREENING INTERVAL

The Baltimore Longitudinal Study of Aging demonstrated that men with an initial PSA less than 2.0 ng/ml had a four percent chance of converting to a PSA of 4.1 to 5.0ng/ml during four years of follow-up. Men with a PSA level of 2.1 to 5.0 had a 27-36% chance of converting to a PSA of 4.0 to 5.0ng/ml within four years[179]. Data from the Prostate Cancer Awareness week, found that PSA became elevated in <5% and cancer detected in <1% of men on subsequent year who had an initial PSA<2.0ng/ml[180].

WHAT IS THE EVIDENCE THAT PSA SCREENING IS USEFUL

Is Screening Detecting Insignificant Cancers?

In defining insignificant cancers for patients, the general definition used is low grade (Gleason sum <4) and low volume <0.5cc. In studies looking at the final pathology of T1C cancers (cancers detected by PSA elevation alone with a normal DRE), <10% of tumors were found to be insignificant by these criteria. (Seminars in Urologic Oncology. Smart et al (1998) reported from the Surveillance, Epidemiology, and End Results (SEER) program analyzed 208, 234 patients diagnosed with prostate cancer between 1973 and 1993. The increase in prostate cancer seen from 1988 to 1992 was largely grade 2(significant) and not in grade I (insignificant) tumors[181]. The cancers detected by PSA screening are significant, potentially life-threatening cancers if not treated as described in the section on the natural history of cancer described above.

STAGE MIGRATION

A strong determinant of the usefulness of PSA screening is evidence that a higher percentage of patients presenting for treatment of prostate cancer present with localized disease which are curable with current treatment modalities. The percentage of patients in radical prostatectomy series having organ-confined disease is reported to be between 62 and 84%. This rate of organ confined disease compares to the pre-PSA era in which only 20-30% of patients presented with pathologically confined disease[182]. Newcomer et al (1997) reported on the Seer data reported that the incidence of distant stage disease peaked in 1986 and then declined by over 60% by 1994[183]. Mettlin et al (1998) reporting on the National Cancer Data Bank on 103,979 patients in 1992, and 72,337 patients diagnosed in 1995, reported that the proportion of patients diagnosed with localized disease from 1992 to 1995 was increased from 69.3% to 76.7%[184].

GRADE OF DISEASE MIGRATION

As Orenstein et al (2000) point out in a review of PSA and Early detection, the cancers that screening would most impact are moderate grade cancers since low-grade cancers may not need treatment and high-grade cancers tend to respond poorly to current treatment modalities[185]. Historically, moderate grade cancers accounted for 35% of cases compared to 58% in the SEER database. Presentation of high-grade cancers decreased from 33% to 17%[186].

DECREASED MORTALITY AND REVIEW OF RANDOMIZED SCREENING TRIALS

Initial reports on screening determined that the mortality of prostate cancer increased to a peak in 1994. Newcomer et al (1997) reported reported that mortality in the Seattle area increased from 49/100,000 in 1974 to 67/100,000 men in 1994[183]. Roberts et al, reported on the effect of PSA screening on mortality rates for Olmstead County, Minnesota. They reported an increase in age-adjusted mortality rates from 25.8/100,000 men in 1980-1984 to 34/100,00 men for the period of 1989-1992. The mortality rates fell 22% to 19.4/100,000 men in 1993-1997[187]. The National Cancer Database program of the American College of Surgeons and the American Cancer Society has reported that there has been an approximate 1% decrease in prostate cancer mortality since 1990[184].

Labrie et al (1999) reported on the results of the Quebec Prospective Randomized Controlled Trial which was a prospective randomized controlled trial of 46,193 men randomized to screening or no screening. They found 137 deaths due to prostate cancer out of the 38,056 unscreened men compared to only 5 deaths among the 8137 screened men. The prostate cancer death rates were 48.7 and 15 per 100,000 man-years in the unscreened and screened groups[188]. As discussed by Ornstein et al (2001), one of the concerns of the Laval University Study is that there was a high dropout rate among men in the screening arm[185].

Other studies that are currently ongoing to answer whether PSA screening is both cost effective and lowers the prostate cancer mortality rate is the European Randomized Study of Screening for Prostate Cancer and the National Cancer Institute's Prostate, Lung, Colorectal, Ovarian (PLCO) screening program. The results of these programs will be forthcoming.

OUR RECOMMENDATIONS FOR SCREENING (WHO SHOULD GET A PSA AND WHO SHOULD NOT)

In summary, PSA screening has shown evidence of being useful in that patients are now presenting with earlier stage disease, a higher percentage of moderate or low-grade disease, and there is some evidence of decreased mortality. At what age to stop PSA screening is largely dependent on whether the practitioner believes that early versus late hormonal ablation has a benefit in terms of decreased morbidity and delayed mortality. The use of free PSA, PSA density, PSA velocity, and age-specific PSA values are of questionable value in differentiating between benign and malignant disease on subsequent biopsies for the population that has an initial negative biopsy. Evidence supports that PSA screening can be conducted biannually for men with a PSA < 2.0 and annually for men with a PSA >2.0. The high-risk screening groups include African American men and patients with a first degree relative diagnosed with prostate cancer before age 70. The patients who should not be screened are anyone who has comorbid disease and a life expectancy less than 10 years. Even with widespread metastatic disease, the average life expectancy with hormonal ablation is 6-7 years.

In patients who are older than 75 with an elevated PSA, detection of prostate cancer is important in that early hormonal ablation has shown evidence to decrease both morbidity and mortality in this patient population. In a 73-76 year old man, we advocate a biopsy with the intention to treat high-grade cancer and follow low-grade cancer with a watchful waiting intention.

The answers to whether PSA screening will lower the incidence of cancer mortality should be answered in the next 5-10 years.

Prostate Specific Antigen and Other Kallikreins in Prostate Cancer

By Carsten Stephan, George M. Yousef, Klaus Jung and Eleftherios P. Diamandis

ABSTRACT

Prostate cancer is the most common malignancy in males in North America and is responsible for more than 30,000 deaths annually in the U.S. alone. Prostate specific antigen (PSA) is the first FDA-approved tumor marker for early detection of prostate cancer through population screening. The discovery of different PSA molecular forms in serum (free PSA, PSA complexed with various protease inhibitors like alpha1-antichymotrypsin) in the early 1990s renewed clinical research to enhance the specificity of PSA. Also, the use of another homologous prostate localized antigen, human glandular kallikrein 2 (hK2) may further reduce the number of unnecessary prostate biopsies. Recent promising data is emerging regarding molecular forms of free PSA (proPSA, BPSA, "intact" PSA) and other members of the expanded human kallikrein family which may add substantial clinical information for early detection and differential diagnosis of prostate cancer.

Prostate specific antigen (PSA) is a serine protease produced by the prostate gland at very high concentrations. This protein was first identified in 1970[189], purified, characterized and named as PSA in 1979[190], and detected in serum in 1980[191]. PSA is secreted into the seminal plasma in high concentrations (0.5-5 g/L), where it plays a role in semen liquefaction. The retrograde release of PSA into the bloodstream is a rare event in young, healthy men occurring with a frequency of less than one PSA molecule per million secreted PSA molecules leading to a concentration of <4 ng/mL PSA in serum. Perturbation of the prostate gland architecture often results in excessive escape of PSA into the circulation. Prostate cancer, benign prostate diseases, as well as physical trauma of the prostate, can result in significant increases of serum PSA. Thus, an elevated serum PSA is a sensitive marker of prostate gland pathologies including prostate cancer and many other conditions affecting the integrity of the prostate gland. These non-cancerous alterations have severely challenged the usefulness of PSA as a tumor marker for the early detection of prostate cancer. This disease is the most common malignancy in men with an estimated 198,100 new cases and 31,500 deaths in 2001[192]. Several calculated parameters, such as PSA density, PSA transition zone density, PSA velocity or age- and race-specific PSA ranges were only partially successful in enhancing the specificity of PSA, thus reducing somewhat the number of unnecessary prostate biopsies[193,194]. The discovery of different PSA forms, like free PSA and PSA bound to alpha1-antichymotrypsin (PSA-ACT) in the early 1990s renewed the clinical research on this biomarker[167,168].

This review will summarize the current clinical use of free PSA and focuses on new developments regarding the molecular forms of PSA and the promising role of additional kallikreins (especially hK2) for prostate cancer detection.

THE NEW KALLIKREIN GENE FAMILY

Until recently, only 3 human kallikrein genes were identified: the pancreatic/renal kallikrein (KLK1, encoding for hK1), the human glandular kallikrein 2 (KLK2, encoding for hK2) and PSA (KLK3, encoding for hK3 which is widely known as PSA)[195, 196]. Recently, 12 new members of the human kallikrein family have been characterized[197]. This family of proteases now consists of 15 members (Figure 7) which are classified with a new nomenclature[198]. The kallikrein genes (named KLK1 to KLK15; encoding for hK1 to hK15) share significant homologies, genomic motifs, and other similarities and all cluster within a 300-kb region on human chromosome 19q13.4. All genes have 5 coding exons and significant sequence homologies at the DNA and amino acid levels (40-80%) and at least 12 of the kallikreins are regulated by steroid hormones[197]. Besides PSA, hK2 has already shown in preliminary clinical studies to add significant information for detecting prostate cancer especially at low PSA

3. PROSTATE SPECIFIC ANTIGEN AND OTHER KALLIKREINS IN PROSTATE CANCER

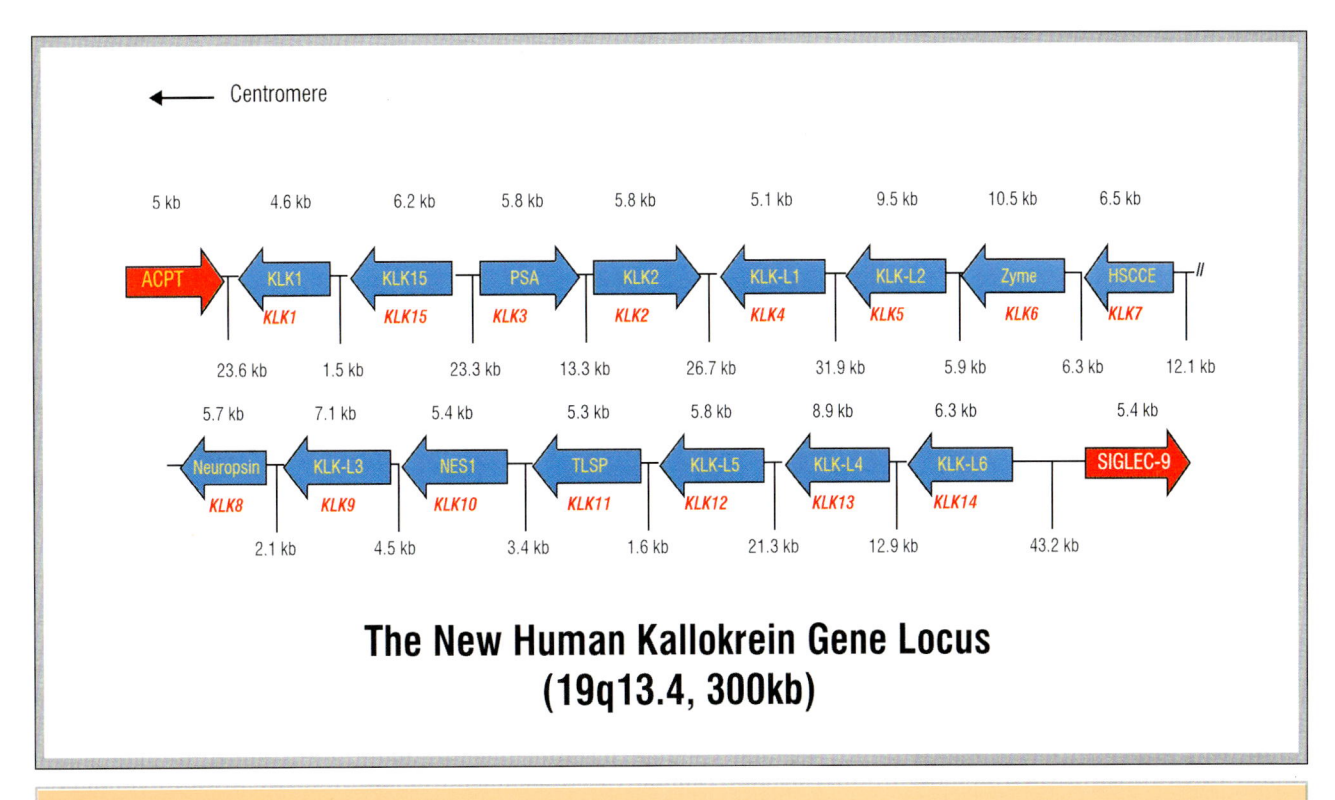

**The New Human Kallokrein Gene Locus
(19q13.4, 300kb)**

FIGURE 7. The new gene locus of the kallikrein family around chromosome 19q13.4 at an approximate 300-kb region. The direction of transcription is illustrated by blockarrows. Boxes represent the former gene names and below the boxes the new nomenclature (KLK = kallikrein) is indicated. The genomic length of each gene, in base pairs, is designated above the related boxes. Distances between genes, in base pairs, are shown between boxes. The Siglec and ACPT (testicular acid phosphatase) genes frame the kallikrein gene family but do not belong to this family. This figure is not drawn to scale. For full gene names and details see Ref. 11.

values[199-201]. Additionally, it has been shown that hK2 can activate the conversion of pro-PSA to active PSA and that these 2 kallikreins may act in concert in extraprostatic locations[198,202-204]. Very recent immunoassay studies for the kallikreins hK6 and hK10 have indicated possible roles as serum biomarkers for non prostate diseases, especially ovarian cancer[205-208]. It is quite possible that several kallikreins, in addition to PSA may add clinical information for various cancers including prostate cancer.

MOLECULAR FORMS OF PSA (HK3)

PSA circulates in serum in free (unbound) and complexed (bound to protease inhibitors) forms[167, 209, 210]. Approximately 65-95% of the PSA is bound to ACT (PSA-ACT) whereas free PSA represents, on average, only 5-35% of the total PSA (tPSA) concentration. The relative amount of free PSA tends to be increased in benign disease compared to prostate cancer. The ratio of free to total PSA is now being used routinely to increase specificity for prostate cancer and to reduce unnecessary biopsies. Other PSA complexes with alpha2-macroglobulin (PSA-A2M) and with alpha1-protease inhibitor (PSA-API) are now measurable in serum as well[211-213]. Complexed PSA is being evaluated in numerous studies to determine its clinical utility. The Bayer complexed PSA assay measures both PSA-ACT and PSA-API and has been proposed as a single assay, alternative to the free and total PSA assays[214-216]. Other existing PSA complexes are so far not measurable in serum (reviewed in Ref.[217]). Free PSA has recently been shown to exist in three molecular forms; proPSA[218], BPSA[219], a special clipped form of free PSA and inactive "intact" PSA (fPSA-I)[220]. Figure 8 gives an overview of the molecular forms of PSA.

The reason for the differences between BPH and prostate cancer regarding the molecular forms of PSA, and especially the higher PSA-ACT amounts in cancer patients in serum are so far not completely understood. It is assumed that due to the loss of tissue architecture in prostate cancer the intracellular active PSA gains quicker access to the circulation

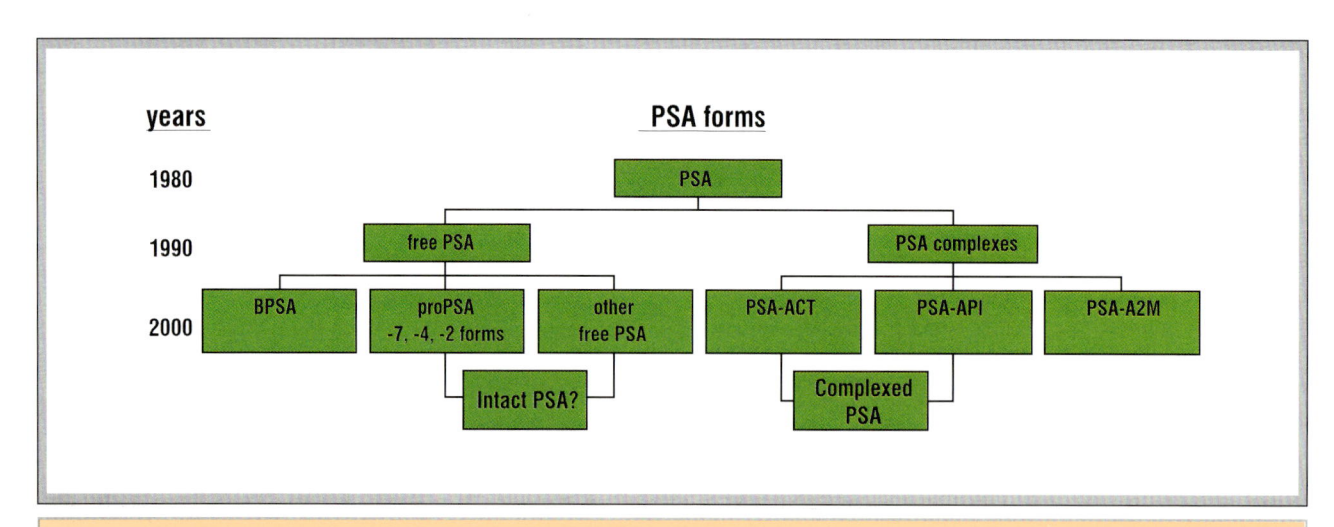

FIGURE 8. Survey of the research development of the molecular forms of PSA. The approximate years of discovery are indicated on the left side. Each box represents a different molecular form of PSA. The Bayer Complexed PSA measures the PSA-ACT and the PSA-API. Key: BPSA = BPH-associated free PSA; proPSA = precursor form of free PSA; "intact" PSA (fPSA-I) = other inactive and intact PSA, which also detects proPSA; PSA-ACT = PSA bound to alpha1-antichymotrypsin; PSA-API = PSA bound to alpha1-protease inhibitor; PSA-A2M = PSA bound alpha2-macroglobulin.

and the protease inhibitors like ACT and A2M can complex to PSA more easily[221]. If PSA reaches the circulation from normal or BPH cells, it first has to leak backwards into the extracellular space, where it is susceptible to proteolytic degradation[221]. After degradation, the inactive PSA can still form complexes with A2M but only to a very small degree with ACT[222]. This may explain the decreased capability of PSA to form complexes with ACT in BPH patients but also the higher amounts of PSA-A2M in BPH patients[221].

The earlier hypothesis[223] that higher intracellular ACT production in the prostatic epithelium leads to higher serum PSA-ACT concentrations in prostate cancer patients compared to BPH patients could not be confirmed, as prostatic tissue PSA is present almost exclusively as uncomplexed PSA[218,224,225]. On the other hand, the recent studies demonstrating distinct molecular forms of free PSA in the transition zone and prostate tumor tissue may provide a rationale for the source of free PSA in blood[218,226].

CLINICAL USE OF PERCENT FREE PSA

The use of percent free PSA (%fPSA), which is the ratio of free to total PSA, has already been established as a clinical routine parameter since the mid 1990s[227-230]. Various retrospective studies (reviewed in Refs. 6, 31) and prospective studies have demonstrated a significant improvement in specificity for the 4-10 ng/mL PSA range and for lower PSA values <4 ng/mL[231-233]. Generally, with %fPSA cutoffs ranging from 17-30%, to obtain 90-95% sensitivities, the number of unnecessary biopsies could be reduced by approximately 20% with a minimum loss in sensitivity in detecting prostate cancer. However, for a more efficient interpretation of %fPSA values, possible influencing factors like prostate volume, total PSA, stage and grade of the cancer, PIN and race as well as sample stability, prostate manipulations or drug treatment history should be considered and have been comprehensively discussed (6, 31). We will briefly summarize some of these factors.

In two recent studies on 1709 patients[234] and on 1622 patients[235] the authors confirmed the earlier findings of positive correlation of %fPSA to prostate volume[227, 230, 236, 237]. In the relevant tPSA range 4-10 ng/mL, this relationship seems to be stronger for higher PSA levels[235].

The %fPSA tends to be inversely correlated to tPSA. A significant downward trend of %fPSA for the tPSA ranges <4 ng/mL, 4-10 ng/mL and >10 ng/mL could be shown[233, 234]. One study on patients with nonmalignant prostate diseases within the tPSA range 2.6-9.9 ng/mL revealed no influence of total PSA on %fPSA[238].

For predicting the pathological stage of prostate cancer, the use of %fPSA is controversial. Some authors described an inverse relationship of %fPSA to the pathological stage[239-241]. Other studies noted no significant improvement in staging using %fPSA[242-245].

Regarding the histological grade and Gleason grade, it appears that low %fPSA values are more associated with higher grades[241, 246, 247]. A prospective multicenter clinical trial demonstrated that %fPSA, followed by the Gleason sum, was the strongest predictor for the pathological outcome[248]. Moreover, aggressive cancer may be detected much earlier using %fPSA instead of tPSA[249].

Several new investigations have focussed on the impact of isolated prostatic intraepithelial neoplasia (PIN) as precursor of prostate cancer on %fPSA[250-255]. The release of PSA into the blood may be different due to the integrity of the basal cell layer in PIN tissue contrary to cancer tissue. Significant higher mean %fPSA levels in patients with exclusively PIN lesions compared to prostate cancer patients were found[250, 253, 254]. Therefore a decrease of %fPSA values in PIN patients should be considered as a possible concomitant evidence of prostate cancer.

It has been proposed to use %fPSA as a priority decision tool for first time biopsy in men with unsuspicious digital rectal examination within the tPSA range 4-10 ng/mL as well as for lower PSA values[256, 257]. This will further enhance the number of detected cancers per biopsy. Additionally, artificial neural networks (ANN) which include clinical relevant data can add substantial information for staging and outcome of prostate cancer and its differentiation to BPH[233, 258-263]. There is a need to evaluate these ANN for clinical routine use. However, there are only limited data on %fPSA cutoff recommendations for tPSA <4 ng/mL[232, 233, 256]. With cutoffs of specificity values of 90 to 95% the number of unnecessary biopsies can be reduced using %fPSA at low tPSA concentrations but many cancers will be undetected[256]. The most recent data from Catalona et al.[264] on 841 biopsied men with PSA concentrations ranging from 2.6-4.0 ng/mL and a high cancer detection rate of 29% argue for high % fPSA sensitivity or even a general biopsy within this total PSA range. More studies have to be done to find an appropriate conclusion for this low PSA range. But it is at least clearly visible that expanding the range of additional free PSA measurements from 4-10 ng/mL to 2 or 2.5-10 ng/mL could be beneficial for detecting significant cancer at low PSA values.

TABLE 4. American Urological Association Screening Recommendations.
*All Men >= age 50 with expected lifespan >= 10 years
*Men age 40-50 with first-degree relative with prostate cancer or of African-American ethnic background
*Patients offered screening with a Prostate Specific Antigen and Digital Rectal Examination
Adapted from Thompson et al (2001).[8]

Use OF Other molecular forms of PSA

PSA-ACT and complexed PSA

For the measurement of different PSA isoforms, only assays for PSA-ACT (Roche Diagnostics, Mannheim, Germany) and complexed PSA (Bayer Diagnostics, Tarrytown, USA) have been commercially available. It is known that the complex of PSA-ACT is the predominant form of PSA in prostate cancer patients[167, 168]. Early analytical problems regarding an overestimation due to the nonspecific binding of ACT-cathepsin G-complex, loss of immunoreactivity or complex dissociation have now been solved[265]. To date, no study has shown a clear advantage of measuring the PSA-ACT alone or calculating the PSA-ACT to tPSA ratio compared to %fPSA to enhance specificity of prostate cancer detection[266-270].

The complexed PSA (cPSA) assay (Bayer Immuno 1) utilizes a blocking antibody to free PSA and detects the PSA-ACT and PSA-API but not the PSA-A2M complex[271]. Proposals to use the cPSA test alone have been debated but in general the use of the cPSA/total PSA ratio has resulted in similar sensitivity and specificity data compared with %fPSA. In studies with an overrepresentation of BPH patients at lower PSA levels and of prostate cancer patients at higher PSA levels, cPSA enhanced the specificity of tPSA to levels equal or even better than %fPSA[214-216]. However, other studies using more equal tPSA distributions in BPH and prostate cancer patients could only show a slightly better diagnostic performance of cPSA alone compared to tPSA[268, 272, 273]. Only the ratio of cPSA to tPSA could reach specificity levels comparable to %fPSA[217,274,275]. Preliminary data of a cPSA multicenter study has revealed better performance of the cPSA/tPSA ratio in the 4-10 ng/mL tPSA range compared to cPSA alone but in the lower range of 2-6 ng/mL cPSA outperformed the cPSA/tPSA ratio[276]. Studies on the use of the PSA complexes (PSA-ACT and cPSA) for low PSA values below 4 ng/mL are rare but these results indicate a possible use and warrant further prospective evaluations[277, 278].

TABLE 5. The distribution of the efficiency of abnormal PSA alone, abnormal DRE alone and combined abnormal PSA and DRE using a 4.0 ng/ml cutoff PSA in age cohort groups. Prostate Cancer Awareness Week 1992-1995.

	Abnormal PSA Normal DRE	Normal PSA abnormal DRE	Abnormal PSA abnormal DRE
Age 40-49			
Biopsies rate(%)	16.7	5.0	18.6
PPV(%)	21.4	25.0	33.3
SE(%)	25.0	66.7	8.4
SP(%)	87.4	14.9	97.7
FPR(%)	12.6	85.1	2.3
Age 50-59			
Biopsies rate(%)	21.3	15.2	33.0
PPV(%)	26.3	14.9	65.8
SE(%)	33.9	37.0	29.0
SP(%)	70.4	34.3	95.2
FPR(5)	29.6	65.7	4.8
Age 60-69			
Biopsies rate(%)	19.9	16.6	36.8
PPV(%)	28.4	18.3	54.8
SE(%)	35.5	27.4	37.1
SP(%)	63.1	49.5	87.4
FRP(%)	36.9	50.5	12.6
Age 70-79			
Biopsies rate(%)	18.4	15.1	30.5
PPV(%)	27.6	20.3	55.5
SE(%)	34.9	22.4	42.7
SP(%)	57.3	58.7	84.0
FPR(%)	42.7	41.3	16.0

Reproduced with permission from Crawford et al[48]

PSA-A2M and PSA-API

The measurement of the PSA-A2M complex in serum has been demonstrated using PSA immunoadsorption followed by pH manipulations to release the encapsulated PSA from the 25-fold larger molecule A2M[211]. PSA-A2M represents a considerable proportion of tPSA in serum and the ratio of PSA-A2M to PSA is higher in BPH patients (12%) compared to prostate cancer patients (8%) However, the previous report of a high proportion of about 60% of PSA-A2M could not be confirmed. It was also shown that the sum of %fPSA and PSA-A2M could further enhance the specificity of tPSA and %fPSA[279].

A method to analyse PSA-API has also recently been reported by the same investigators[212]. In a study of cancer and non-cancer patients, the amount of PSA-API was 1.6% of tPSA in BPH patients and 0.9% of tPSA in prostate cancer patients[280].

Both complexes, PSA-A2M and PSA-API show, like %fPSA, higher amounts in BPH patients but were not correlated to free PSA in contrast to the PSA-ACT complex which is higher in cancer patients.

BPSA

The BPSA is a specifically clipped subform of free PSA, which is highly associated with the transition zone containing BPH nodules in prostate tissue[219]. A dual monoclonal assay with a detection limit of 0.06 ng/mL was tested in serum of BPH patients with symptomatic BPH and urologically referred patients without clinical BPH as well as healthy control subjects[281]. In the control group BPSA was almost undetectable. The median BPSA values for the clinical BPH group was significantly elevated and BPSA discriminated clinical BPH patients better from non-BPH patients than %fPSA.

TABLE 6. Age - Specific PSA Levels by Ethnic Group.

Age Range (yrs)	Reference Range (ng/ml)		
	Asians	African-American	Caucasians
40-49	0-2.0	0-2.0	0-2.5
50-59	0-3.0	0-4.0	0-3.5
60-69	0-4.0	0-4.5	0-4.5
70-79	0-5.0	0-5.5	0-6.5

Copied with Permission from Thompson et al[8].

ProPSA

Recently, proPSA forms were isolated in serum and tissue from prostate cancer patients[218, 226]. The complete natural proPSA protein contains 244 amino acids (-7) compared to free PSA (237 amino acids). The proPSA in serum and prostate tissue exists as a mixture of different designated forms including the (-7), (-5), (-4) forms and partially the (-2) and (-1) forms[282]. Interestingly, Mikolajczyk and co-workers (personal communication) found the (-4) and (-2) form to be the predominant form in serum samples from prostate cancer patients with total PSA values less than 20 ng/mL. Combined measurements of these different cancer associated proPSA forms and the BPH associated BPSA could further enhance both sensitivity and specificity of PSA.

Very recently, there has been reported a newly developed assay with a detection limit of 0.035 ng/mL for non-clipped free PSA called "intact" PSA[220]. The "intact" free PSA (fPSA-I) assay detects both proPSA and other inactive non-clipped free PSA. Whereas the absolute concentrations of fPSA-I did not differ in 383 patients with negative or cancer positive biopsies, the ratio of fPSA-I to free PSA was significantly higher in cancer patients[220].

Taken together, a new area may be emerging for free PSA molecular forms, which may substantially help improve the differentiation between BPH and prostate cancer.

HK2 for early detection OF prostate cancer

PSA and hK2 share the highest homology with 78% and 80% identity at the amino acid and DNA level in the human kallikrein family which is composed of 15 distinct genes[197]. Both kallikreins have been detected in relatively small quantities in non-prostatic tissues and biological fluids[197, 217]. The hK2 mRNA amounts to 10-50% of the PSA mRNA in the prostate tissue but in serum and seminal plasma, hK2 has a concentration of only 1-3% of PSA. The picogramm/mL levels in serum posed analytical challenges for hK2 immunoassays but reliable prototype assays are now available in several research laboratories[283-285].

In 1998 Kwiatkowski et al.[199] reported first that the ratio of hK2 to free PSA enhances the discrimination of prostate cancer patients and BPH patients. In a larger study with 937 serum samples Partin et al.[201] described an enhanced prostate cancer detection rate using both ratios %fPSA and hK2/fPSA within the PSA ranges 2-4 ng/mL and 4-10 ng/mL. Other studies confirmed the advantage of the additional use of hK2 and its ratios to fPSA and %fPSA especially at low PSA concentrations for detection of prostate cancer[200, 286, 287]. The higher expression of hK2 in malignant than in benign tissue revealed by immunohistochemistry[288, 289] was hypothesized to be responsible for the higher ratios of hK2/fPSA in cancer than in BPH patients[221]. Using quantitative measurements of hK2 in matched prostate cancer samples, Magklara et al.[290] found that hK2 is decreased in malignant versus benign tissue but the degree of down-regulation is somewhat lower than for PSA. In preliminary studies hK2 was found to discriminate between high and low grade tumors and between stage 2 and stage 3 tumors[291-293].

In two very recent reports, hK2 was shown to be the most accurate marker to decide a repeat biopsy[294] and to describe the amount of Gleason grade 4/5-cancer in prostate cancer patients[295]. Until now, the Gleason grade 4/5-cancer volume is the only independent predictor of biochemical failure after radical prostatectomy and therefore a serum marker is critically needed[296].

Analogous to PSA, hK2 was also found in different molecular forms in serum but contrary to PSA, free hK2 is the predominant form and hK2-ACT represents only 4-19% of total hK2[277]. The proform of hK2 (prohK2) is also present in serum and increased in prostate diseases [297](113). The measurement of complexed hK2 may be used for additional improving of prostate cancer specificity[298]. A novel complex of hK2, hK2-PI6 has been shown to be highly associated with prostate tumor tissue relative to transition zone and peripheral zone normal cells[299]. Apparently, the hK2-PI6 is formed as a consequence of tumor necrosis[299].

OTHER KALLIKREINS AND KALLIKREIN-RELATED PROSTATE CANCER MARKERS

A differential regulation of kallikrein genes or other genes in cancerous and non-cancerous prostatic tissue might indicate potential new serum-markers. Among all kallikreins, at least 8 (KLK2-4, KLK 10-13 and KLK 15) are expressed in relatively high amounts in prostatic tissue[197]. Despite a high expression of KLK4 in prostate tissue[300] there are so far no reports about the usefulness of this kallikrein for prostatic diseases. The newly developed hK10 immunoassay shows elevated serum concentrations for ovarian cancer (median 1.9 g/L) but lower and similar concentrations in prostate cancer patients compared to healthy males[208]. KLK11, KLK12 and KLK13 are also highly expressed in prostate tissue but so far there are no further studies available[197, 301-304]. KLK14 is, like PSA and hK2, downregulated in prostate cancer tissue compared to non-cancerous tissue of the same gland[305]. The regulation of KLK15 was analysed in matched prostate tissue samples from 29 patients[306]. Almost half of the patients had higher KLK15 levels in the cancerous tissue and only 3 showed a downregulation. A KLK15 positive expression was found in all pT3 staged patients and all patients with grade 3 tumors whereas only 2/3 of the low grade and low stage patients showed this upregulation[306].

In addition to these kallikreins, 5 novel prostate specific genes have recently been cloned including Prostin[307], which has subsequently shown to be identical to hK15, Prostein[44], PSGR[308], a new member of the G protein-coupled olfactory receptors, Trp-p8[309] and Part-1[310]. Prostin (hK15) is more active than hK2 in the proteolytic conversion of proPSA to active PSA[307]. Prostein showed an exclusive expression in the prostate but there was no difference between normal versus cancerous tissue[44]. The PSGR-gene was analysed in matched prostate cancer tissue from 52 patients and an overexpression was observed in 62% of tumor specimens, no change in 27% and a down-regulation in 11.5% of the specimens[308]. A comparison of grade or stage of the cancers was not performed. The Trp-p8[309] and the Part-1 genes[311] were overexpressed in cancerous tissue compared to non-cancerous prostate tissue. In 3 very recent gene expression profiles studies, 3 genes were found to be overexpressed in prostate cancer tissue compared to normal tissue[312-314]. Hepsin, a transmembrane serine protease was reported in all 3 analysis to be highly overexpressed[312-314]. Also, the macrophage inhibitory cytokine MIC-1 (130) and a serine/threonine kinase pim-1 are overexpressed in cancerous prostate tissue[314]. These newly cloned and recently analysed genes which are prostate localized and/or members of the kallikrein family, will be intensively studied in the future as potential new markers for prostate cancer detection.

CONCLUSIONS

As the first fully clinically evaluated molecular form of PSA, the %fPSA has shown its effectiveness in improving specificity over tPSA alone. Artificial neural networks may further predict the need of a biopsy but the number of unnecessary biopsies is still very high. There is a need for the evaluation of the new promising molecular forms of PSA like proPSA, BPSA, "intact" PSA, PSA-A2M and PSA-API as well as for the hK2 and its molecular forms like hK2-PI6 and prohK2. The development of antibodies for various kallikreins and new prostate specific proteins will be of great interest. For the future, one of the most important goals for prostate cancer serum marker development is the search for a marker which can predict the Gleason grade 4/5 which is so far the only independent prognostic factor for a biochemical failure after radical prostatectomy. None of the hitherto existing serum markers fulfill this most important clinical need yet. The molecular forms of free PSA and hK2 show a potential to clarify this issue. Other kallikreins and new prostate specific genes and their related proteins remain potential candidates.

ACKNOWLEDGMENTS

We gratefully acknowledge Harry Rittenhouse (Hybritech Beckman Coulter, San Diego, CA) for his corrections and helpful suggestions.

PROSTATE CANCER SCREENING AND EARLY TREATMENT: THE ONLY POSSIBILITY FOR A MAJOR IMPACT ON SURVIVAL IN PROSTATE CANCER

By Fernand Labrie, Bernard Candas, Leonello Cusan, José Luis Gomez, Jacques Lévesque, Éric Chevrette and G. Brousseau

SUMMARY

Although combined androgen blockade significantly prolongs life in advanced metastatic prostate cancer, a major impact on survival requires the possibility of treatment at an early stage of the disease. Using PSA alone as first line screening test, 99% of cancers can be diagnosed at the clinically localized stage and are thus potentially curable. In a prospective screening trial started in 1988 in Quebec City, among 46,486 men aged 45 to 80 years, the follow-up at 11 years shows a 62% decrease in prostate cancer deaths among those who were screened and treated early compared to standard medical practice. These data are in agreement with the recent finding of a 37 to 81% decrease in deaths from prostate cancer when long-term and continuous androgen blockade is applied at the localized stage of the disease.

INTRODUCTION

Although prostate cancer is the most frequently diagnosed cancer and remains the second most common cause of cancer death in men[315], death from this disease has decreased in the United States and in the province of Quebec by up to 22% since 1991[187, 316-320]. Since even the best treatment for advanced metastatic disease, namely combined androgen blockade, can only prolong life by a few months[321, 322], the recent decrease in death rates from prostate cancer can only be due to the treatment of early disease which, for diagnosis, requires screening.

An important observation based on overwhelming scientific evidence is that prostate-specific antigen (PSA) can be efficiently used as a pre-screening test for prostate cancer, thus keeping the more costly and less well tolerated digital rectal examination (DRE) and transrectal ultrasonography (TRUS) as second step procedures[323-326]. Using this approach, 99% of prostate cancers can be diagnosed at a clinically localized and thus potentially curable stage, which practically eliminates the diagnosis of metastatic disease[323, 324, 326].

Definitive proof of the benefits of screening for prostate cancer can only be obtained from prospective and randomized studies comparing the incidence of death from prostate cancer in a group of men screened and treated early versus a group of men receiving standard medical care. Accordingly, the Laval University Prostate Cancer Screening Program (LUPCSP) was started in November 1988 and its first analysis was published in 1999[188]. The present report describes the results obtained after three additional years or 11 years of follow-up.

SUBJECTS AND METHODS

Forty-six thousand four hundred and eighty-six[46,486] men were randomly allocated either to the group invited for annual screening or to the control group not invited for screening at a ratio of 2:1 in favor of screening. The age and residential area were used for stratification to balance possible differences in sociodemographic factors between groups. Men in the control group not invited for screening were followed according to current medical practice. Men with a diagnosis of prostate cancer before November 15, 1988 as well as men who had previous screening were not eligible. Death from prostate cancer was the primary end-point. At first visit, all participants had measurement of serum prostatic specific antigen (PSA) and underwent digital rectal examination (DRE)[327]. These two tests were performed independently. Transrectal ultrasonography of the prostate (TRUS) was performed only in cases with positive PSA (>3.0 ng/ml) and/or abnormal DRE, except for the first 1002 men who all had the three procedures, as previously described[323, 327]. The study was approved by the Institutional Review Board of Laval University. Serum samples were taken before DRE and TRUS for measurement of PSA by immunoradiometric assay (Tandem-R PSA, Hybritech Incorporated or its equivalent).

At follow-up visits, PSA alone was used as prescreening test. Accordingly, TRUS was performed only if serum PSA had increased above 3.0 ng for the first time. In cases where PSA was already above 3.0 ng/ml at a previous visit, TRUS was performed only if PSA had increased by more than 20% compared with the value measured one year earlier (the interassay coefficient of variation c.v. being 9.6%, 10% was accepted as a possible increase attributable to the interassay c.v.) or if the serum PSA had increased by 20% or more over the predicted PSA (prPSA) calculated at a previous visit[328-330].

TRUS-guided biopsies were performed as previously described[327,328,331], at the judgment of the radiologist when an hypoechoic image was seen, if the measured PSA (mPSA) was above predicted PSA (prPSA) or if DRE was abnormal. In cases of negative biopsies at previous visits with measured (mPSA) above prPSA, the frequency of follow-up biopsies was at the judgment of the radiologist and clinician. Six sextant biopsies were performed only in 207 men with normal TRUS evaluation because of either abnormal DRE or mPSA greater than prPSA.

Evaluation of the impact of screening is based upon comparison of the incidence of death from prostate cancer between the two groups. The information on cause-specific death was obtained from the Death Registry of the Health Department of the Province of Quebec. This analysis covers the period of a little more than 11 years extending from November 15, 1988 to December 31, 1999. For the invited men who were screened, the duration of exposure to the intervention is calculated from the date of their first visit at the screening center up to the end of 1999, regardless of their compliance to follow-up screening visits and of the treatment received if cancer was diagnosed. For unscreened men not invited for screening, the period of exposure is calculated from the date of initiation of the trial, i.e. November 15, 1988. Results are expressed in events per 100,000 man-years in order to take full account of the years of exposure in each group thus avoiding the bias of different durations of exposure (Figure 9). Accordingly, the longer duration of exposure in the unscreened group is fully taken into account by dividing the number of events by the larger number of years of exposure.

Fisher's exact tests were performed to assess the significance of the differences between groups. The age at prostate cancer death was fitted using a Cox proportional hazards model including the following co-variables: screened versus not screened, age at study initiation, as well as regional location of the subject at randomization.

Laval University Prostate Cancer Screening Program
(November 15, 1988 to December 31, 1999)

46,486 men aged 45-80 years with no diagnosis of CaP

Randomization

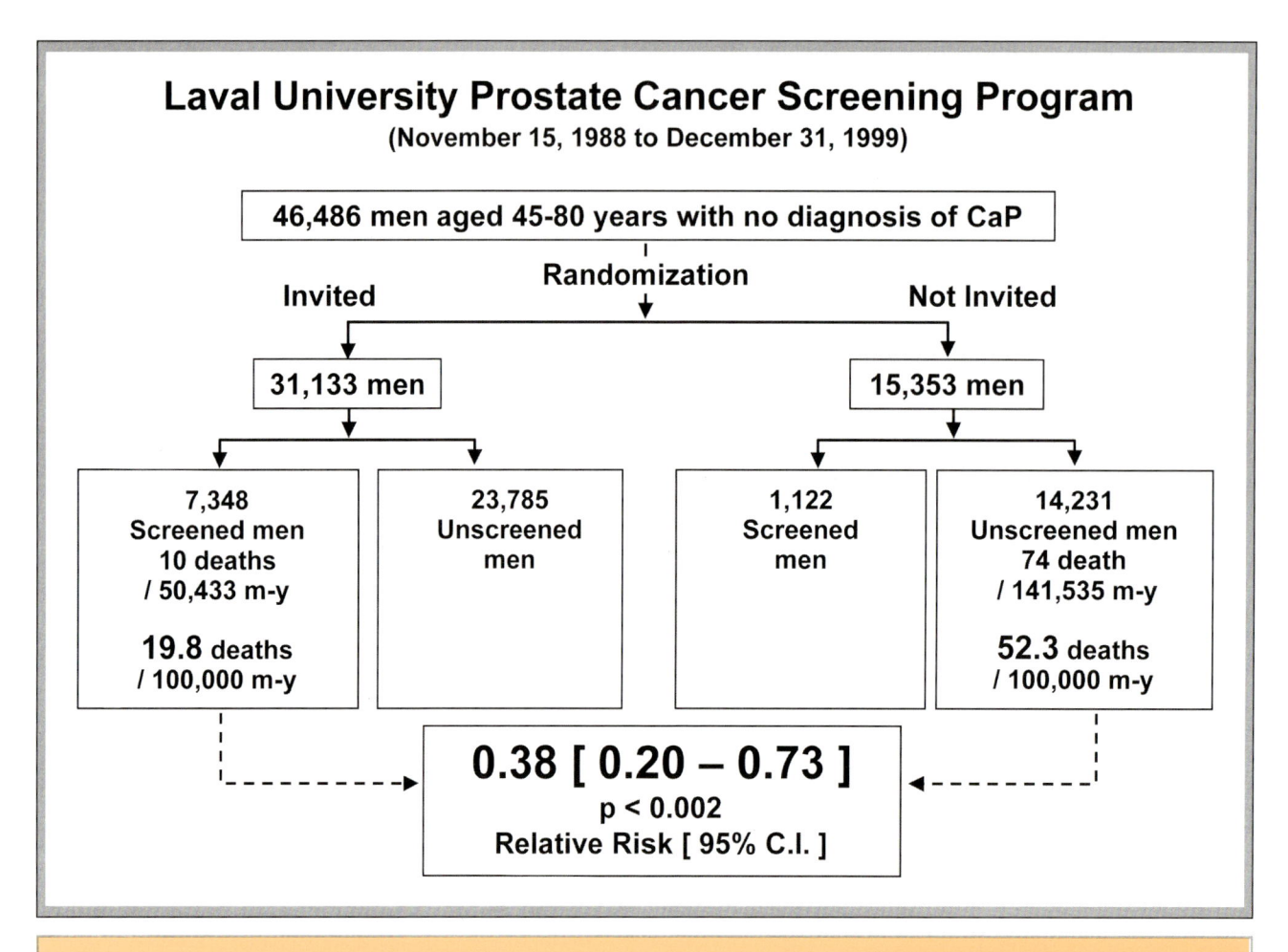

Invited → 31,133 men
- 7,348 Screened men
  10 deaths
  / 50,433 m-y

  19.8 deaths / 100,000 m-y
- 23,785 Unscreened men

Not Invited → 15,353 men
- 1,122 Screened men
- 14,231 Unscreened men
  74 death
  / 141,535 m-y

  52.3 deaths / 100,000 m-y

0.38 [0.20 – 0.73]
$p < 0.002$
Relative Risk [95% C.I.]

FIGURE 9. Trial profile of the Laval University Prostate Cancer Screening Program (November 15, 1988 to December 31, 1999), and reduction of cancer-specific death during the first eleven years in the groups of screened versus non screened men originally invited and not invited for screening, respectively.

RESULTS

Of the 46,486 eligible men aged between 45 and 80 years included in the study started on November 15th, 1988, 31,133 men were invited by letter to be screened for prostate cancer while 15,353 were allocated to the control group of men not invited for screening. These men were followed by standard medical practice. As shown in Figure 9, 7,348 men responded to the invitation and were screened at our prostate clinic from November 1988 through December 31, 1999.

4. Prostate Cancer Screening and Early Treatment

As illustrated in Figure 9, ten deaths from prostate cancer occurred among the 7,348 screened men while 74 deaths occurred among the 14,231 unscreened men. In order to eliminate potential bias due to different times of exposure in the two groups, the results are expressed in events per 100,000 man-year. The exposures in the screened and the control unscreened groups are 50,433 and 141,535 man-year, respectively. Thus, over the 11-year period, the annual cancer-specific death rate incidences are 19.8 per 100,000 man-year in the screened men compared to 52.3 per 100,000 man-year in the unscreened group (2 sided p value <0.002, Fisher's exact test) (Figure 9). The prostate cancer death rate incidence is thus 62% lower in the group of men screened for prostate cancer compared with the men of the control group who were followed according to standard medical practice (Figure 10).

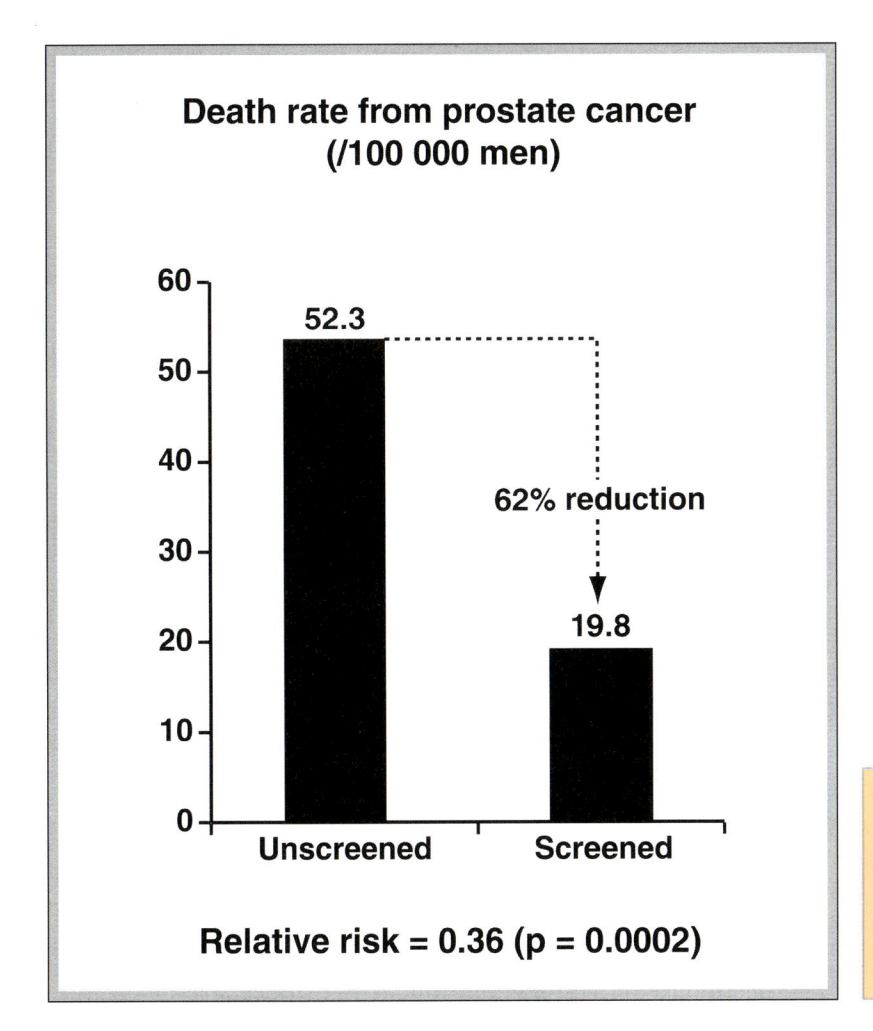

FIGURE 10. Comparison of the incidence of death from prostate cancer in the men screened compared to the men unscreened for prostate cancer during the first 11 years of the study (same data as figure 2).

4. PROSTATE CANCER SCREENING AND EARLY TREATMENT

Since a large proportion of men invited for screening were not screened, the possibility can be raised that the men who were screened were at lower risk of death from prostate cancer compared to those who did not respond to the invitation for screening. Such a possibility would necessarily translate into an increased prostate cancer death rate in the group of men who refused screening compared with the control group of 14,231 men not invited for screening and not screened. The following data, however, eliminate this possibility.

In fact, there were 143 prostate cancer deaths among the 23,785 men of the invited group who did not respond to the invitation, thus resulting in a rate of 62.0 deaths/100,000 man-year. This value is not significantly different from the 52.3 deaths/100,000 man-year found in the control unscreened group of 14,231 men described above. On the other hand, among the 15,353 men not invited for screening, 1,122 came on their own to the clinic for screening. Among these men, one died from prostate cancer, thus resulting in a death rate of 13.7 deaths/100,000 man-year, a value not significantly different from 19.3 deaths/100,000 man-year in the screened group. The present data thus show that the men not screened were not at a greater risk of prostate cancer death than those in the control non invited and unscreened group.

A comparable positive effect of screening was obtained when the data are analysed with the Cox proportional hazards model (best fitted model) presented in Table 7 which shows that screening is associated with a highly significant 61.5% ($p = 0.0025$) reduction in prostate cancer death, or a relative risk of 0.385 (95% confidence interval = 0.207-0.719). It can also be seen in this Table that the same advantage of screening was observed in the group of screened men originally invited for screening by letter compared to those who were screened despite being randomized in the group of men who were not invited, thus complementing the data indicated above showing that men who did not respond to the invitation to be screened were not at greater risk of death from prostate cancer than the control group of men not invited for screening. On the other hand, the location of men in the various areas of Quebec City had no influence on the results while age, as expected, had a small (6%) but highly significant ($p = 0.0054$) effect.

The characteristics at diagnosis and the information about the treatment received by the ten men who were screened and died from prostate cancer are shown in Table 8. It is of interest to mention that six out of the ten deaths were in men diagnosed at their first visit. Three other men who died from prostate cancer did not follow the annual visits at our clinic and were thus diagnosed and/or received unknown treatment in other institutions, including one who interrupted androgen blockade early after

TABLE 7. Analysis of the effect of screening, group at randomisation, age and area of residency on prostate cancer death using the Cox proportional hazards models.

	Intervention Model		
	Relative Risk	**95% C.I.**	**p-value**
Screened versus unscreened	0.385	[0.207-0.714]	0.0025**
Invited versus not invited	1.085	[0.822-1.433]	0.5637
Age (on Nov.15, 1988)	0.938	[0.897-0.981]	0.0054**
Regional Location			
C1	1.088	[0.833-1.421]	0.5341
C2	0.926	[0.711-1.206]	0.5697
C3	0.964	[0.741-1.254]	0.7831

C.I.: Confidence Interval

radical prostatectomy, despite having been upgraded from stage B2 to D1 and responding well to combined androgen blockade with undetectable PSA. The other man who died from prostate cancer did not accept immediate treatment and his follow-up is unknown.

Three patients had locally advanced disease and one had bone metastases at diagnosis. In fact, of the ten deaths from prostate cancer among the screened men for whom staging is known, one was diagnosed at clinical stage D2, three at stage C2, three at stage B2, and one at stage B1. Staging is unknown for one patient (Table 8). One stage C2 and one stage B2 patients at diagnosis were later upstaged to D1 at radical prostatectomy while one stage B2 patient was upstaged to C1 at surgery. A stage C2 patient failed radiation therapy, with a PSA nadir at 29 ng/ml, thus indicating advanced disease at diagnosis at first visit. It is important to mention that only four patients who died from prostate cancer were diagnosed at follow-up visits. One of these patients, as mentioned above, was upstaged from B2 to D1 at surgery. This patient stopped combined androgen blockade after only 18 months while he was responding well to therapy with undetectable PSA. Androgen blockade was stopped in order to regain sexual activity. Unfortunately, the re-initiation of androgen blockade was markedly delayed until serum PSA reached 189 ng/ml thus resulting, as expected, in a poor response and death from the disease. The

TABLE 8. Characteristics at diagnosis and treatment received by the 11 men who died from prostate cancer among the screened men.

Identification	1st visit PSA (ng/ml)	1st visit Age (years)	Diagnosis Visit	Diagnosis Age (years)	Clinical stage	Initial treatment	Death from PCa Years after diagnosis	Death from PCa Age (years)
DE-04663	25.9	75	1st visit	75	C2	EBRT[2]. Failure with nadir PSA at 29 ng/ml	2.2	77
DE-00386	87.0	65	1st visit	65	D2	CAB[1]	2.7	68
DE-03364	4.6	66	1st visit	66	C2	Radical prostatectomy, Castration Upstaged to D1 at surgery.	4.0	70
DE-04001	3.9	66	1st visit	66	B2	Radical prostatectomy with neoadjuvant CAB[1].	6.3	73
DE-01628	15.7	60	1st visit	60	C2	EBRT[2] with neoadjuvant + adjuvant CAB[1]	7.2	67
DE-02972	2.1	58	3rd visit (PSA=5,8)	61	B2	Radical prostatectomy. Upstaged to D1 at surgery. Neoadjuvant and 1 year of adjuvant CAB[1] before stopping treatment.	4.5	65
DE-01744	3.2	69	External Follow-up			Unknown		75
DE-04334	23.0	60	1st visit	60	B2	Neoadjuvant + adjuvant CAB. Radical prostatectomy. Upstaged to C1 at surgery	7.9	68
DE-04949	6.5	74	3rd visit (PSA = 10.4)	77	B1	Deferred unknown treatment	8.0	82
DE-10041	5.4	56	External follow-up			Unknown		60
DE-05757 (Not Invited)	33.8	72	1st visit	72		Unknown	1.8	74

Combined androgen blockade 2 External beam radiotherapy

second patient diagnosed at a follow-up visit and who died from prostate cancer decided to defer treatment and the follow-up is unknown. For two other patients, the diagnosis was made at another institution and the treatment is unknown.

DISCUSSION

An argument frequently cited against screening is that screening could detect insignificant cancers. It is known that one third of men older than 50 years have incidental prostate cancer found at autopsy while, on the other hand, only 10% of men develop clinical prostate cancer during their lifetime[332]. This apparent paradox has been used to suggest that screening could detect the small and still insignificant cancers which are found at autopsy or by transurethral resection of the prostate for treatment of benign prostatic hyperplasia, thus potentially leading to unnecessary treatment. The data obtained, however, do not support this hypothesis. On the contrary, it is well recognized that the available screening techniques, namely, PSA, DRE, and TRUS do not detect such small autopsy cancers[333,334]. In fact, when random or sextant biopsies are performed only in patients having a serum PSA above the predicted PSA and/or a positive DRE in the absence of hypoechoic area at TRUS[333,334], screening detects only cancers having a diameter greater than 0.75 cm. Moreover, more than 90%[182,335] of PSA-detected cancers have features typical of potentially aggressive cancers. The evidence obtained clearly shows that only approximately 7% of cancers detected by screening are microfocal and low grade[182,336,337].

PSA used as a single test for prescreening and followed by DRE and TRUS when PSA is abnormal is highly efficient in detecting prostate cancer at a localized (potentially curable) stage in close to 100% of cases, thus practically eliminating the diagnosis of metastatic and non curable prostate cancer[323,324]. The approach used is highly reliable, sensitive, efficient and acceptable by the general population[327]. With the kits available, PSA measurement is a low cost routine procedure which requires a simple blood sampling and a minimum of expenses. Only 17% of men then need to be referred to specialized prostate cancer clinics when PSA becomes abnormal (>3.0 ng/ml), thus reducing the costs and optimizing the use of specialized health care personnel and expertise. The detection of clinically non significant as well as metastatic advanced cancers has become an exception.

In the present study, only 1 out of 159 cancers (0.6%) diagnosed at follow-up visits was metastatic, thus permitting 99.4% of patients to be

4. PROSTATE CANCER SCREENING AND EARLY TREATMENT

diagnosed at a localized stage[324]. Similarly, in the screening program of the American Cancer Society National Prostate Cancer Detection Program (ACS-NPCDP), only one of a total of 51 cancers diagnosed at follow-up visits was at a clinically advanced (C2) stage[338]. Hugosson et al.[339] have found that 97% of the cancers detected by screening were clinically localized. It is thus reasonable to suggest that if one follows the recommendations of the American Cancer Society[340] and of the American Urological Association[341], namely annual screening starting at the age of 50 years for the general population at no special risk, all subsequent visits should be equivalent to the follow-up visits of the present study, thus practically eliminating the diagnosis of metastatic prostate cancer[323].

Reports from cancer registries in all the states followed by the SEER program indicate that prostate cancer incidence rates have begun to fall[316]. In Olmsted County, a 22% decline in prostate cancer death has been observed between 1980 and 1997 after PSA screening was introduced[187]. Part of the success could be attributed to the early treatment applied at the Mayo Clinic, a major treatment site in Olmsted County. This finding parallels a 6.3% decrease in prostate cancer death nationwide in the USA[319].

As mentioned above, the main argument against screening was that no proof was available about the benefits of early treatment of prostate cancer. Since 1997, however, this argumument is no longer valid. In fact, five prospective randomized trials have recently demonstrated that an important prolongation of life was observed in patients with localized prostate cancer patients treated with androgen blockade, the advantage on cancer-specific survival at 5 years of follow-up raging from 30% to 80%. In the first published study, namely the EORTC (European Organization for Research and Treatment of Cancer) trial performed in stage T3 patients, death from prostate cancer at 5 years of follow-up was decreased by 77% by androgen blockade added to radiotherapy versus radiotherapy alone[342]. On the other hand, a 37% improvement in cancer-specific survival at five years has been found in RTOG trial 08351 in the subgroup of high Gleason score patients who received androgen blockade (LHRH agonist) indefinitely or until progression with radiotherapy compared to radiotherapy alone[343]. In another study, a 54% decrease in cancer-specific death has been found in patients with an 8-10 Gleason score who had androgen blockade in addition to radiotherapy[344], while Granfors et al.[345] have found a 39% decrease in cancer-specific death when androgen blockade was added to radiotherapy compared to radiotherapy alone.

In a study of 98 men staged T2 at diagnosis but who had pelvic lymph node metastases at radical prostatectomy, 47 were randomized to receive immediate hormonal therapy while 51 had delayed treatment[146]. After a median follow-up of 7.1 years, a 81% decrease in deaths from prostate cancer has been observed in men who had immediate androgen blockade.

It is reasonable to suggest that the recently observed decrease in deaths from prostate cancer mentioned above[187, 317-319] is due to earlier diagnosis with serum PSA[323] and transrectal echography of the prostate[346] coupled with improved treatment of localized disease by surgery, radiotherapy, brachytherapy and endocrine therapy[146, 342-344, 347-352].

Coupled with treatment of localized disease, the present approach demonstrates, in the first prospective and randomized study, that early diagnosis and treatment permit a dramatic decrease in deaths from prostate cancer. If the present trend continues, the present data suggest that among the male population in the United States, the present approach could save 2.0 million lives of the 3.0 million presently living in the United States and expected to die from prostate cancer if no significant change in diagnosis and/or treatment occurs.

Two other randomized screening trials for prostate cancer are ongoing, namely the Prostate, Lung, Colon, and Ovarian trial (PLCO) and the European Randomized Study of Screening for Prostate Cancer (ERSPC). Results from those trials are not expected before year 2005. Moreover, their relatively late start carries the high risk of a significant contamination of the control group by screening.

In the United States, it has been estimated that the health care costs for the treatment of prostate cancer are $4.5 billion annually[353]. These costs are largely related to the treatment of advanced disease. The calculations performed leave little doubt that the strategy based upon efficient screening and early treatment, namely androgen blockade, surgery, radiotherapy or brachytherapy alone or in combination with androgen blockade should play a key role in the successful fight against prostate cancer while decreasing the costs for the health care system and society[334, 354-360].

As strong support for the crucial role of early diagnosis and treatment, this first prospective and randomized prostate cancer screening study, shows that early diagnosis combined with treatment of localized disease decreased death from prostate cancer by 62%. The present data are also in agreement with the 42% decrease observed in 1998 in the prostate cancer death rate in the Tyrol area where PSA screening was made available since 1993 compared to the rest of Austria where PSA screening was not offered[361]. Since about two thirds of men were screened in Tyrol during that period, the 42% decreased death rate observed in Tyrol is similar to the 64% value measured in our study among the men who were all screened (Figures 9 and 10).

Clearly, the rational use of the presently available diagnostic and therapeutic approaches could decrease prostate cancer death by at least 50%[188,323]. As an example, between 1991 and 1999, the death rate from prostate cancer has decreased by 38% in the whole population of Quıbec City and its metropolitan area[320] while the death rate has decreased by 64% in the group of men who have been screened.

MAGNETIC RESONANCE IMAGING AND SPECTROSCOPIC IMAGING OF PROSTATE CANCER: IMPROVED THERAPEUTIC SELECTION AND ASSESSMENT

By John Kurhanewicz, Mark G. Swanson and Daniel B. Vigneron

This research was funded by the following grants: NIH R33- CA32610, R01- CA79980, R01-CA 59897 and R29-CA64667, American Cancer Society Grant RPG96-146-03-CCE and the CaPCURE foundation.

ABSTRACT

An improved assessment of prostate cancer location, extent, and aggressiveness is increasing in clinical importance due to the emergence of disease-targeted focal therapies and the growing number of patients who are selecting less aggressive and alternative approaches to living with prostate cancer. Currently, a combination of serum prostate specific antigen (PSA) measurements, digital rectal examination (DRE), and transrectal ultrasound (TRUS) guided biopsies serve as the standard for prostate cancer detection and risk assessment. Recent studies in pre-prostatectomy patients have indicated that the metabolic information provided by 3D MR spectroscopic imaging (3D-MRSI) combined with the anatomical information provided by MRI can improve the assessment of cancer location and extent within the prostate, extracapsular spread, and cancer aggressiveness. Additionally, pre- and post-therapy studies have demonstrated the potential of MRI/MRSI to provide: a direct measure of the presence and spatial extent of prostate cancer after therapy; a measure of the time course of response; and information concerning the mechanism of therapeutic response. These findings, combined with the fact that MRI/MRSI is a non-invasive technique that can assay the entire prostate, suggest that this method could be a valuable addition to PSA and sextant biopsy data to more accurately characterize prostate cancer in individual patients. In this chapter, we will review the current role of combined MRI/MRSI in the diagnosis, staging, and treatment planning of prostate cancer, and its future role in the non-invasive assessment of therapeutic response to existing and emerging therapies.

INTRODUCTION

Due to increased prostate cancer screening using serum prostate-specific antigen (PSA) and transrectal ultrasound (TRUS) guided biopsy, thousands of prostate cancer patients are being identified at earlier and potentially treatable stages[362]. However, the decision on how to manage prostate cancer once detected still poses a great dilemma for both patients and their clinicians. The dilemma stems from the fact that prostate cancers demonstrate a tremendous range in biologic malignancy and are treated with a broad spectrum of approaches from "watchful waiting" and hormone ablation therapy to aggressive surgical, radiation, and cryosurgical therapies[363, 364]. Prostate cancer is one of the only cancers that can grow so slowly that it will never threaten some patients, but this cannot currently be predicted in individual patients in advance[365-368]. Moreover, if the cancer does escape the prostate and reaches the bones, there is presently no cure and the cancer becomes lethal. While a number of clinical and pathologic parameters (clinical stage, digital rectal exam, and histologic grade from biopsy) and biochemical parameters (PSA, PAP) can aid in predicting disease extent and aggressiveness, staging using these parameters alone is often inaccurate or inadequate, particularly for intermediate risk patients[369]. With early detection, there has also been increased interest in focal "disease-targeted" therapies, including interstitial brachytherapy, intensity-modulated radiotherapy, and focal cryosurgery, which can potentially reduce treatment related morbidity and allow patients to maintain their quality of life[370]. Additionally, the long developmental period (natural history) of prostate cancer and the increasingly younger age of patients at the time of detection demand the need for shorter-term endpoints than survival in order to reduce the duration of therapeutic trials and the number of patients required[371, 372]. Therefore, there has been increasing interest in new imaging technologies that could more fully characterize prostate cancer in individual patients for improved therapeutic selection, treatment planning, and assessment of therapeutic efficacy.

5. MAGNETIC RESONANCE IMAGING AND SPECTROSCOPIC IMAGING OF PROSTATE CANCER

The use of a combination of magnetic resonance imaging (MRI) and magnetic spectroscopic imaging (MRSI) for the improved staging and characterization of prostate cancer represents an exciting new approach and is currently being investigated. Conventional MR imaging of the prostate relies on abnormal signal intensities that result from morphologic changes within the prostate to define the presence and extent of cancer[373]. Unfortunately, these morphologic changes observed by MRI often do not accurately reflect the presence and spatial extent of active tumor[373]. The addition of metabolic information provided by MRSI has complemented the morphologic information provided by high-resolution MRI, and has improved the discrimination of cancer from surrounding healthy tissue and necrosis[374]. A combined MRI/MRSI exam can be performed in less than one hour using a standard clinical 1.5 Tesla MR scanner and the same coils used for MRI. A commercial package has recently been released and will be clinically tested in an upcoming multicenter trial. Since this technology will soon be more globally available to clinicians, it is timely to review what is already known about the utility of combined MRI/MRSI, and how it might be used in the future.

MORPHOLOGIC IDENTIFICATION OF PROSTATE CANCER-MAGNETIC RESONANCE IMAGING

MRI uses strong magnetic fields and radio frequency waves to non-invasively obtain anatomic pictures (images) based on physical properties (T1 and T2 relaxation times) of tissue water[373]. MR images, especially high spatial resolution endorectal coil T2-weighted images, provide an excellent depiction of prostatic zonal anatomy, prostate cancer, and surrounding soft tissues (Figure 11)[375, 376]. On T2 weighted MRI, regions of prostate cancer demonstrate decreased signal intensity relative to normal peripheral zone tissue due to increased cell density and a loss of the prostatic ducts (Figure 11)[373, 376].

Currently the prostate is best imaged using an endorectal coil combined with four external coils (pelvic phased array)[376]. The use of the body coil for excitation and an endorectal coil/pelvic phased array coil system for signal reception allows for the acquisition of high spatial resolution images of the prostate as well as coverage to the bifurcation for assessment of pelvic lymph node and bone metastases within the same exam. However, the inhomogeneous reception profiles of the surface coils employed must be taken into account in interpreting the data. If uncorrected, images exhibit very high intensity close to the coil and lower inten-

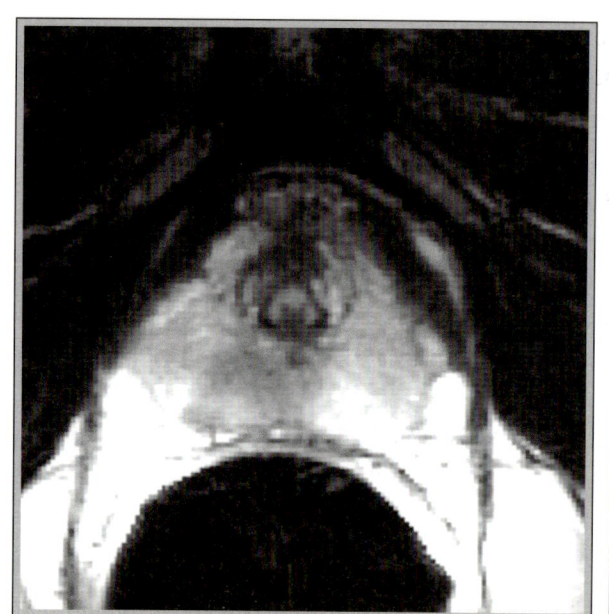

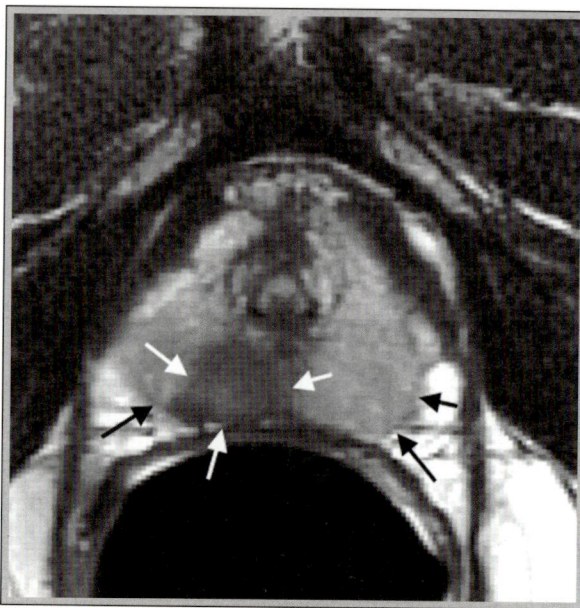

FIGURE 11. Comparison of axial endorectal coil/pelvic phased array fast spin echo prostate images A) prior to and B) after performing an analytic correction for the reception profiles of the endorectal and pelvic phased array coils. In the corrected image, the high signal intensity close to the endorectal coil has been removed allowing for improved visualization of prostate cancer (low T2 signal intensity, white arrows) as compared to adjacent healthy prostate peripheral zone (high T2 signal intensity). Additionally, important anatomical features such as the prostatic capsule (thin dark line encompassing the prostate, black arrow) can be more clearly visualized.

sity further into the prostate (Figure 11A). Even with windowing and leveling, it is difficult to interpret such images. These near–field surface coil artifacts have contributed to the inter-observer variability in staging accuracy (50-90%) reported for endorectal coil imaging. This problem has been addressed by analytically correcting the images for the reception profile of the endorectal coil, thereby eliminating near-field high signal intensity artifact and producing images in which prostatic zonal anatomy and pathology can be more easily visualized (Figure 11B)[374].

Knowledge of the spread of cancer outside the prostate is critical for determining whether focal, systemic, or a combination of both therapies is required. The use of T2 weighted fast spin echo imaging[377] and a pelvic phased-array incorporating an endorectal coil can markedly improve the evaluation of extracapsular extension (ECE: accuracy 81%; sensitivity 84% and specificity – 80%) and seminal vesicle invasion (SVI: accuracy - 96%, sensitivity - 83% and specificity – 98%) thereby improving the staging of prostatic cancer[376]. However, the detection of extracapsular extension by MRI is becoming more difficult since men are being diagnosed at earlier stages of disease, and because the microscopic spread of cancer through the capsule cannot be directly seen on MR images[373]. Additionally, there still remains great variability in the reported staging accuracy of endorectal/phased array MRI between individual readers, with one recent study reporting overall staging accuracies of 93% and 56% for two different readers within the same study[378]. The addition of objective metabolic criteria provided by 3D MRSI has demonstrated the ability to decrease this inter-reader variability[379].

In addition to staging, the assessment of prostate cancer location and extent is becoming increasingly important due to the emergence of disease-targeted therapies such as interstitial brachytherapy, intensity-modulated radiotherapy, and cryosurgery. Studies evaluating clinical data (DRE, PSA, and PSA density), systematic biopsy, TRUS, and MRI have so far shown disappointing results for tumor localization within the prostate[380-383]. High-resolution endorectal/pelvic phased array MRI has demonstrated good sensitivity (78%) but low specificity (55%) in tumor location due to a large number of false-positives[376]. These false-positives can be attributed to factors other than cancer, including post-biopsy hemorrhage, prostatitis, and therapeutic effects, which cause low signal intensity on T2 weighted images similar to prostate cancer[383, 384]. The addition of highly cancer specific metabolic information to the sensitivity of MRI has resulted in a significant improvement in the overall accuracy of cancer localization to a sextant of the prostate[385].

METABOLIC IDENTIFICATION OF PROSTATE CANCER - MAGNETIC RESONANCE SPECTROSCOPIC IMAGING

As with MRI, MRSI uses a strong magnetic field and radiowaves to non-invasively obtain metabolic pictures (spectra) based on the relative concentrations of endogenous chemicals (metabolites) that exist in the cytosol of the cell and in extracellular ducts. With MRSI, one suppresses the large tissue water and lipid signals and detects specific resonances (peaks) for the prostatic metabolites citrate, choline, creatine and polyamines from contiguous small volumes (0.3 cc) throughout the gland (Figure 12C)[386]. The peaks for these different chemicals occur at distinct frequencies or positions in the spectrum (Figure 12D and E). The areas under these peaks are related to the concentration of the respective metabolites, and changes in these concentrations can be used to identify cancer with high specificity[386]. Specifically, in spectra taken from regions of prostate cancer (Figure 12D), citrate and polyamines are reduced and

5. Magnetic Resonance Imaging and Spectroscopic Imaging of Prostate Cancer

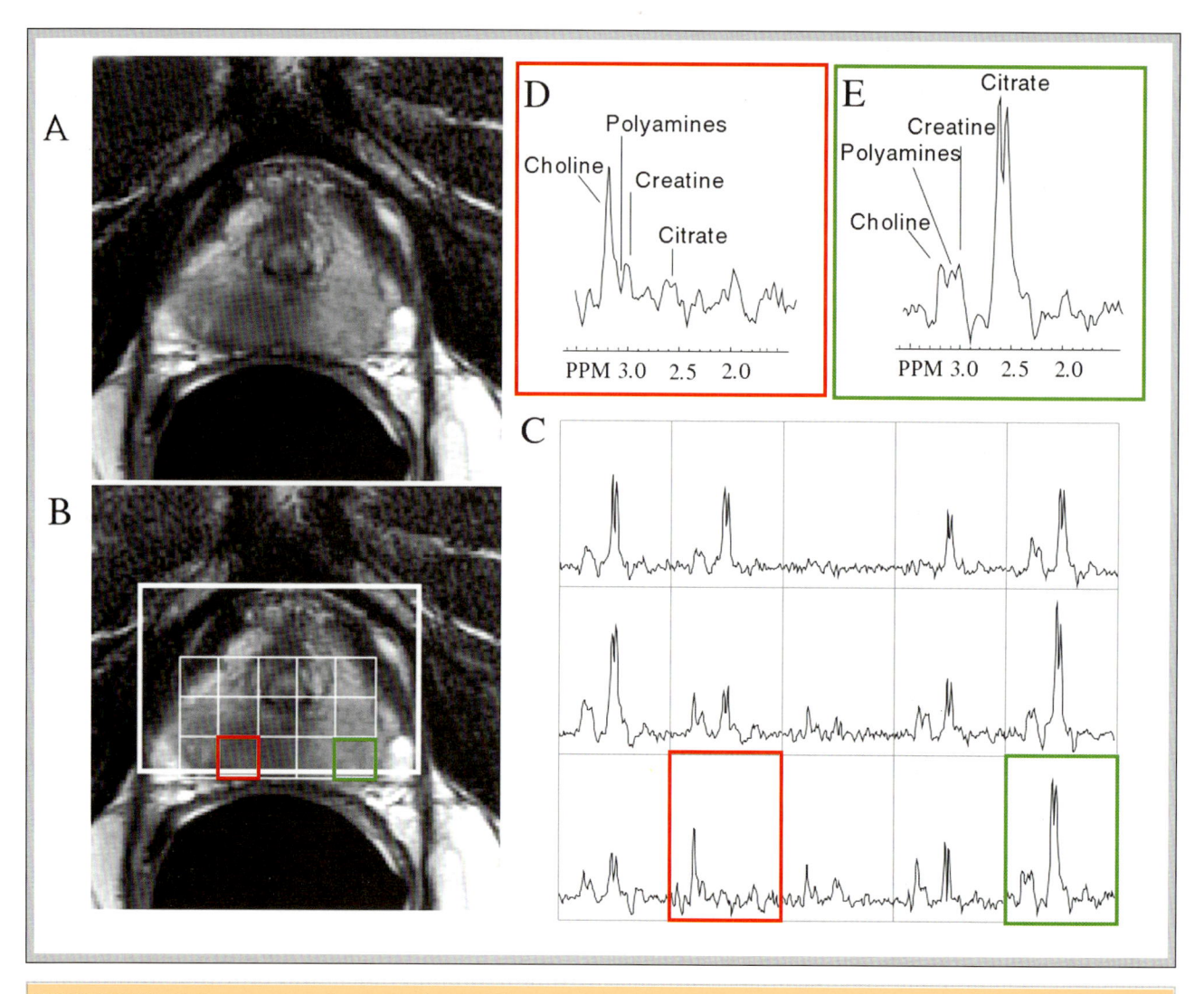

FIGURE 12: A) A representative reception-profile corrected T2 weighted FSE axial image taken from a volume data set demonstrating a large tumor in the right apex (same patient as Figure 1). The selected volume for spectroscopy (bold white box) and a portion of the 16x8x8 spectral phase encode grid from one of 8 axial spectroscopic slices is shown overlaid (fine white line) on the T2 weighted image (B) with the corresponding 0.3 cm³ proton spectral array (C). Spectra in regions of cancer (D, red box) demonstrate dramatically elevated choline reduced citrate and reduced polyamines relative to regions of healthy peripheral zone tissue (E, green box). In this fashion, metabolic abnormalities can be correlated with anatomic abnormalities from throughout the prostate and the strength of the combined MRI/MRSI exam is when there are concordant metabolic and anatomic abnormalities.

choline is elevated relative to spectra taken from surrounding healthy peripheral zone tissue (Figure 12E).

MRSI produces arrays of contiguous volumes (voxels) that can map the entire prostate, and because MRSI and MRI are acquired within the same exam, the data sets are already in alignment and can be directly

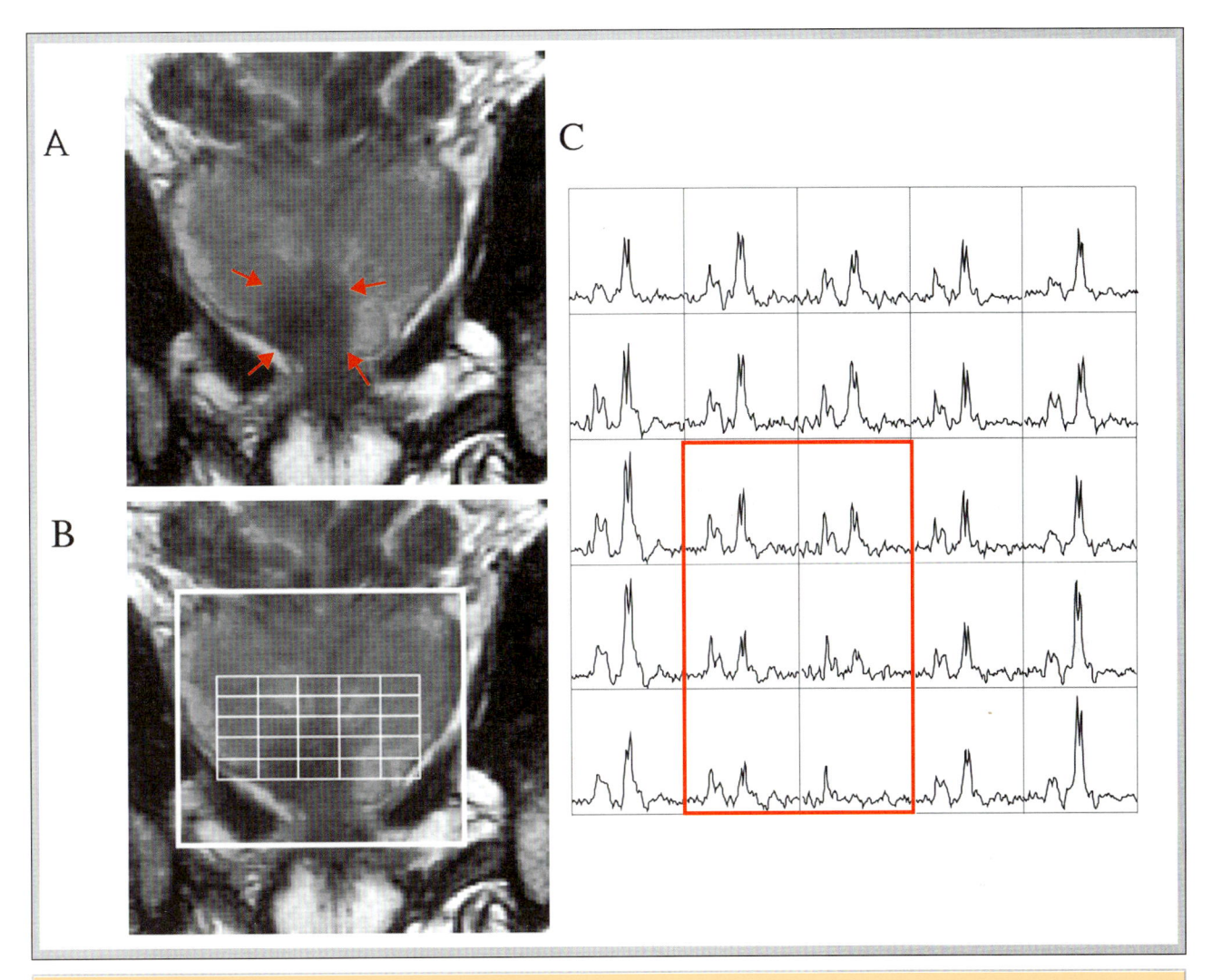

FIGURE 13: A) Coronal T2 weighted FSE image of the same prostate cancer patient shown in figure 2. **B)** Coronal image with overlying spectroscopic selected volume (bold white box) and phase encode grid (fine white line) taken from a portion of the 3-D array of spectra and **C)** corresponding 0.3 cm³ proton spectra. The coronal slice is taken at the level of the peripheral zone and MRI/MRSI (regions outline in red) are concordant for a large volume of tumor in the right midgland towards the apex and the right apex. The volume of the abnormality and irregularity in the prostatic capsule indicated early extracapsular spread which was later confirmed at radical prostatectomy.

overlaid (Figures 12-17)[386]. In this way, areas of anatomic abnormality (decreased signal intensity on T2-weighted images) can be correlated with the corresponding area of metabolic abnormality (increased choline and decreased citrate and polyamines). It is the concordance of MRI and MRSI findings that leads to the most confident identification of cancer[385,387]. Additionally, since three-dimensional or volume MRI and MRSI data are collected, the data can be viewed in any plane (axial, coro-

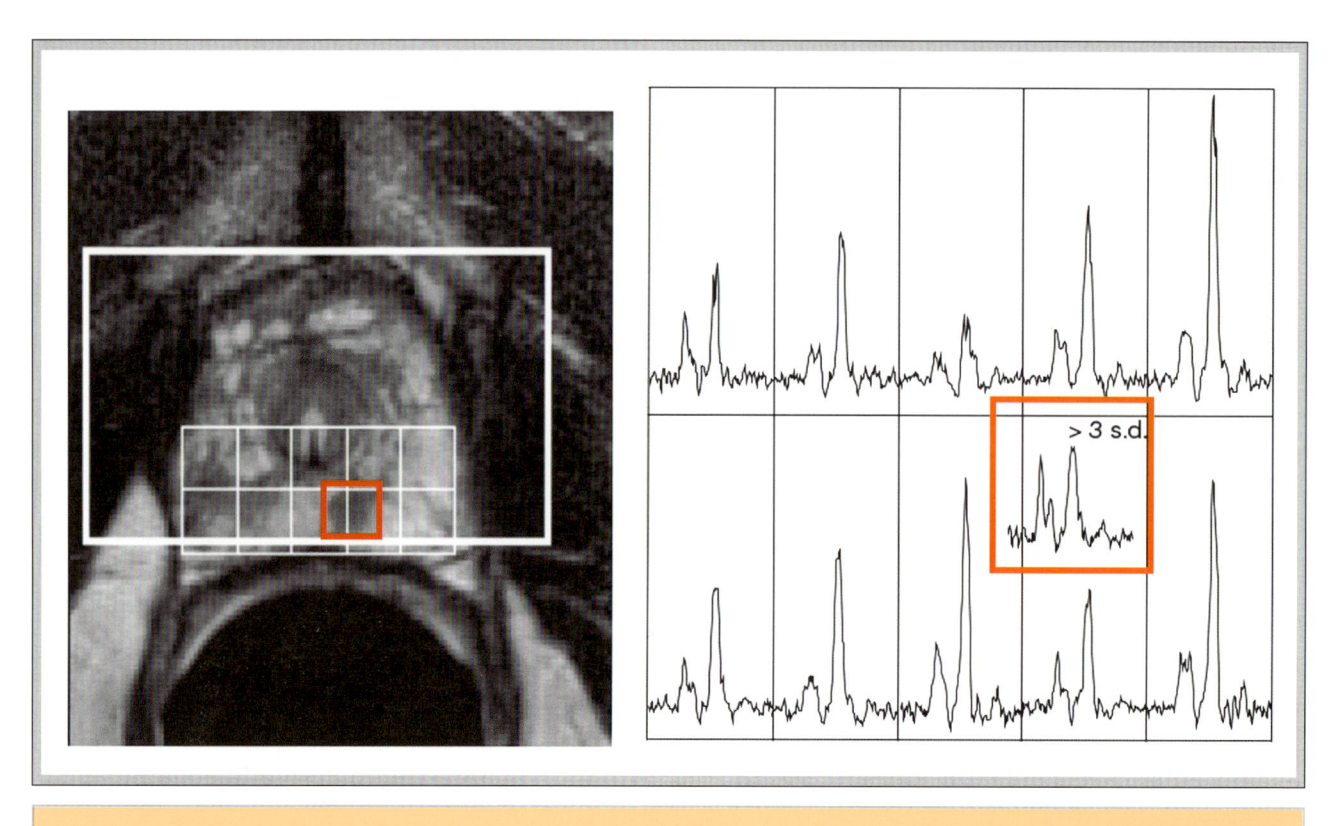

FIGURE 14: A T2 weighted axial image and corresponding spectral array from the apex of a patient who had an elevated PSA (6.8 ng/ml) but negative prior biopsy. A small foci of low T2 signal intensity in the left peripheral zone indicated cancer. On MRSI the MRI abnormality was split between two voxels yielding a borderline metabolic abnormality. During post-processing the spectral array was shifted such that the MRI abnormality was centered in a spectroscopic voxel (red box) yielding a clear-cut metabolic abnormality (choline+creatine)/citrate peak area ratio greater then 3 standard deviations of normal values). A subsequent TRUS guided biopsy confirmed the presence of cancer.

nal, sagittal) (Figure 13), and the position of spectroscopic voxels can be retrospectively changed to better examine a region of abnormality on MRI after the data is acquired (Figure 14). This sort of interactive analysis will be the way MRI/MRSI data is used in the future and should reduce interpretative errors associated with the overlapping of normal and cancerous tissues.

One of the strengths of prostate spectroscopy is that many of the biochemical mechanisms that result in the observed metabolic changes are now known and correlate with stage of carcinogenesis and response to therapy. Healthy prostate epithelial cells posses the unique ability to synthesize and secrete large concentrations of citrate[388]. The decrease in citrate with prostate cancer is due both to changes in cellular function[388] and changes in the organization of the tissue that loses its characteristic ductal morphology[389,390]. Biochemically, the loss of citrate in prostate cancer is intimately linked with changes in zinc levels that are extraordinary high in healthy prostate epithelial cells[391, 392]. In healthy prostatic epithelial cells, the presence of high levels of zinc inhibits the enzyme aconitase, thereby preventing the oxidation of citrate in the Krebs' cycle. Consequently, high levels of citrate are observed in the MRSI spectra of healthy glandular prostate tissues. Zinc levels are dramatically reduced in prostate cancer and the malignant epithelial cells demonstrate a diminished capacity for net citrate production and secretion[391, 392]. There exists strong evidence that the loss of the capability to retain high levels of zinc is an important factor in the development and progression of malignant prostate cells[391, 392]. It is also believed that the transformation of prostate epithelial cells to citrate-oxidizing cells, which increases energy production capability, is essential to the process of malignancy and metastasis[393].

As in other human cancers, the elevation of the choline peak in prostate cancer is associated with changes in cell membrane synthesis and degradation that occur with the evolution of cancer[394,395]. Phosphotidylcholine is the most abundant phospholipid in biological membranes and together with other phospholipids, such as phosphatidylethanolamine and neutral lipids, forms the characteristic bilayer structure of cells and regulates membrane integrity and function[396, 397]. High resolution 31P and 1H NMR studies of surgical prostate cancer specimens have demonstrated that many of the compounds involved in phosphotidylcholine and phosphotidylethanolamine synthesis and hydrolysis (choline, phosphocholine, glycerophosphocholine, ethanolamine, phosphoethanolamine, glycerophosphoethanolamine) contribute to the magnitude of the in vivo "choline" resonance[398-402]. There is also evidence that changes in the cytosolic levels of these phospholipid metabolites correlate with cellular proliferation[403-406] and cellular differentiation[407-409]. Additionally, changes in epithelial cell density can also contribute to the observed increase in the "in vivo" choline resonance in prostate cancer, since densely packed malignant epithelial cells replace the normal ductal morphology forming prostate cancer nodules that are often detected by digital rectal examination[390].

Another strength of prostate spectroscopy is the occurrence of multiple metabolic changes within the same voxel that indicate the presence of cancer. Historically, we have relied on two metabolic markers, choline and citrate for the metabolic detection of cancer[410]. However MRSI is still in its infancy and we are only scratching the surface of the chemical information attainable. High-resolution NMR studies of ex vivo prostatic tissues have identified several new metabolic markers of prostate cancer including polyamines, myo-inositol, scyllo-inositol, and taurine[399, 401, 402, 411-414]. Of these the most promising are polyamines which have been observed to be very high in spectra of healthy prostatic peripheral zone tissues and predominantly glandular benign prostatic hyperplasia (BPH) and dramatically reduced in prostate cancer[411, 414]. Similar to changes in choline containing compounds, changes in cellular polyamine levels have been associated with cellular differentiation and proliferation[415, 416]. Moreover, it has recently been demonstrated that the loss of polyamines in regions of cancer can be detected by 3D MRSI as an improvement in the resolution of the choline and creatine peaks (Figure 12D)[417]. Studies are underway to determine how the addition of this metabolic change further improves the detection and characterization of prostate cancer.

CURRENT CLINICAL FINDINGS AND APPLICATIONS

To date, over 3,200 prostate cancer patients have received combined MRI/MRSI exams at the University of California, San Francisco. Many of these patients subsequently underwent radical prostatectomy thereby providing a "gold standard" (i.e., step-section histopathology of the resected gland) for determination of the utility and accuracy of combined 3D MRI/MRSI in the assessment of prostate cancer. The following studies in pre-prostatectomy patients provide initial compelling evidence of the clinical potential of combined MRI/MRSI for the improved characterization of prostate cancer in individual patients.

Improved Prostate Cancer Staging using Combined MRI/MRSI

MRI alone has good accuracy in detecting seminal vesicle invasion (96%, Figure 13)[376]. However, the assessment of cancer spread through the prostatic capsule is more difficult (accuracy – 81%)[376], and is getting even harder to assess as fewer men demonstrate gross cancer spread (directly visible on MRI) due to earlier cancer detection. In a recent study of 53 patients with early stage prostate cancer, tumor volume estimates based on MRSI findings were combined with high specificity MRI criteria[418] in order to assess the ability of combined MRI/MRSI to predict extracapsular cancer spread. This study was based on prior histopathologic studies that demonstrated that tumor volume was a significant predictor of extracapsular extension (ECE) of prostate cancer[419, 420]. It was found that tumor volume per lobe estimated by MRSI was significantly ($p<0.01$) higher in patients with ECE (2.14 ± 2.3 cm^3) than in patients without ECE (0.98 ± 1.1 cm^3). Moreover the addition of a MR spectroscopic imaging estimate of tumor volume to high specificity MRI findings for ECE[418] improved the diagnostic accuracy and decreased the interobserver variability of MRI in the diagnosis of extracapsular extension of prostate cancer (Figure 13)[379].

Improved Intraglandular Cancer Localization Using Combined MRI/MRSI

It has been demonstrated that the high specificity of 3D MRSI to metabolically identify cancer can also be used to improve the ability of MRI to identify the location and extent of cancer within the prostate[385]. A study of 53 biopsy proven prostate cancer patients prior to radical prostatectomy and step-section pathologic examination demonstrated a significant improvement in cancer localization to a prostatic sextant (left, fight – base, midgland and apex) using combined MRI/3D MRSI versus MRI alone[385]. A combined positive result from both MRI and 3D MRSI indicated the presence of tumor with high specificity (91%) while high sensitivity (95%) was attained when either test alone indicated the presence of cancer (Figures 12-15). In another recent study it was found that the addition of a positive sextant biopsy finding to concordant MRI/3D MRSI findings further increased the specificity (98%) of cancer localization to a prostatic sextant, whereas high sensitivity (94%) was obtained when any of the tests alone were positive for cancer. Both of these studies used only the (choline+creatine)/citrate ratio to metabolically detect prostate cancer. The addition of other metabolic ratios (choline/creatine, citrate/normal citrate) as well as the addition of new metabolic markers such as polyamines offers the possibility of further increasing the accuracy of the metabolic assessment of cancer within the prostate.

Assessment of Prostate Cancer Aggressiveness

MRSI information may also provide new insights into tumor aggressiveness, which may lead to improved risk assessment for patients with prostate cancer[374]. In a preliminary MRI/MRSI study of 26 biopsy proven prostate cancer patients prior to radical prostatectomy, spectroscopic voxels were shifted in post-processing to be within a region of cancer as defined by step-section pathology and T2 weighted MRI. Spectra obtained from these voxels demonstrated a linear correlation between the magnitude of the decrease in citrate and the elevation of choline with pathologic Gleason score. The magnitude of the elevation in choline was the most significant predictor of Gleason score, with choline being significantly ($P<0.0001$) higher in high grade (7+8) as compared to moderate grade (5+6) cancers.

In patients prior to therapy, the improved intraglandular cancer localization, staging, and assessment of cancer aggressiveness are currently being used in two main ways. The primary reason for patient referral for MRI/MRSI at UCSF (approximately 60% of patients) has been for improved therapeutic selection. A representative example where MRI/MRSI had a impact on therapeutic selection is given by a patient interested in watchful waiting who had a PSA of 4.8 ng/ml and two of

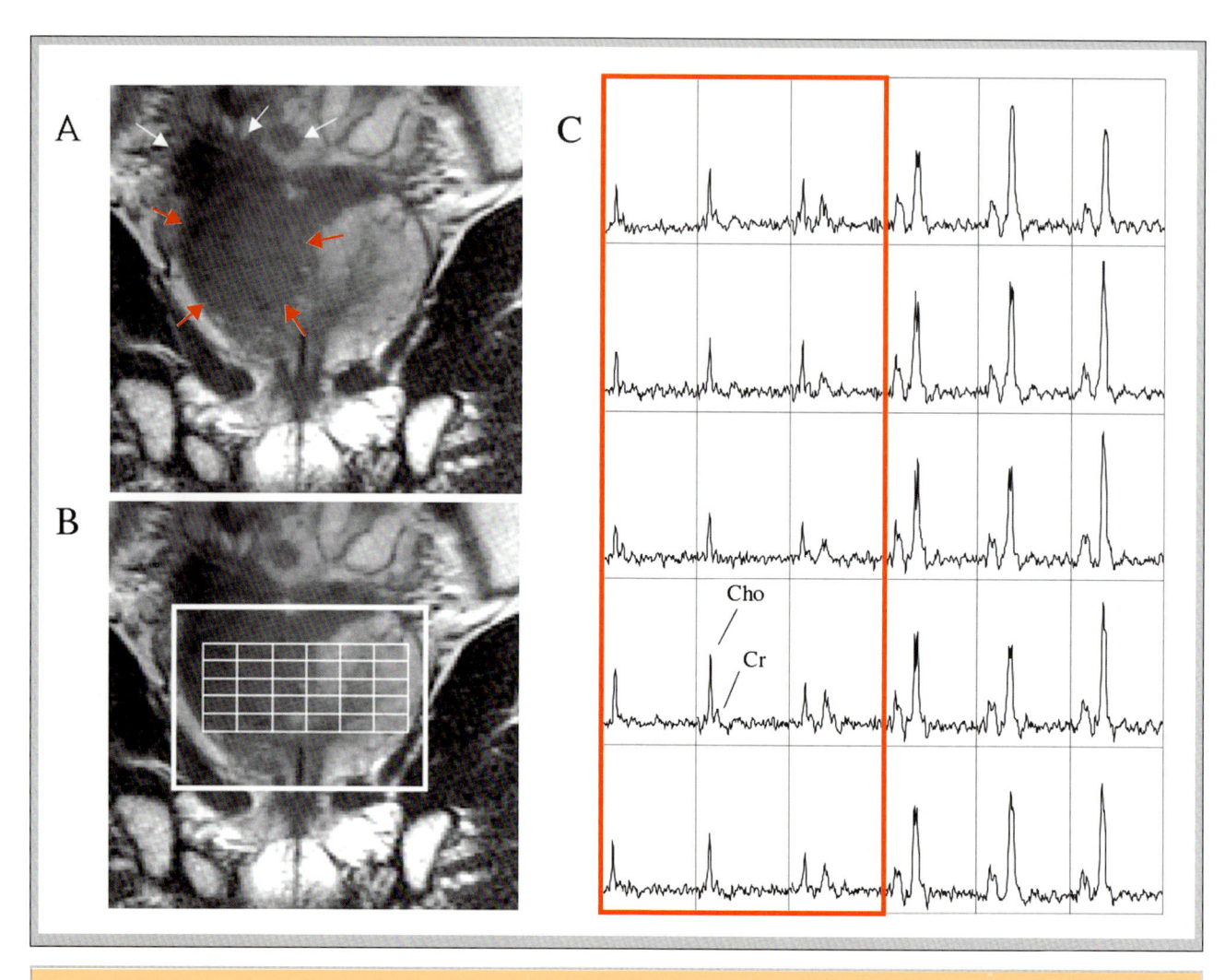

5. Magnetic Resonance Imaging and Spectroscopic Imaging of Prostate Cancer

FIGURE 15: A) Coronal T2 weighted FSE image and B) same image with overlying spectroscopic selected volume (bold white box) and phase encode grid (fine white line) taken from a portion of the 3-D array of spectra and C) corresponding 0.3 cm^3 proton spectra. The coronal slice is taken at the level of the peripheral zone and MRI/MRSI (red arrows and outlined grid) are concordant for a large volume of tumor involving all of the right peripheral zone from apex to base and extending into the right seminal vesicles (black arrows). The metabolic pattern in the region of cancer is characteristic of a high Gleason score.

twelve biopsy cores positive for Gleason 3+3 and 3+4 prostate cancer. Based upon just these clinical and pathologic findings, watchful waiting appeared to be a plausible option. However, MRI/MRSI findings were concordant for a large volume of cancer involving almost all of the right peripheral zone from apex to base (Figure 15). Based on the large volume of aggressive appearing cancer on MRSI and capsular irregularity on MRI, extracapsular extension of cancer was predicted. There was also MRI evidence of seminal vesicle invasion (Figure 15). Based on these findings it was decided that the patient should receive a combination of hormone deprivation and external beam radiation therapy as soon as possible. Another important group of patients being referred (~10% of patients) for an MRI/MRSI exam prior to therapy are those who have elevated or rising PSA levels but negative TRUS guided biopsies. These patients tend to have very enlarged central glands due to BPH, which present sampling problems for TRUS guided biopsies, or they have cancers in difficult locations to biopsy such as the apex (Figure 14)[421]. We have found in initial studies that MRI/MRSI targeting of cancer in these patients can significantly increase the positive yield of subsequent TRUS guided biopsies[422], and a study is currently underway to determine the value of MRI/MRSI targeting of cancer relative to a second systematic TRUS guided biopsy.

THERAPEUTIC FOLLOW-UP OF PROSTATE CANCER USING 3D MRI/MRSI

Growing numbers of patients (~30% of patients) receiving a MRI/3D-MRSI exam at UCSF are referred for suspected local cancer recurrence after various therapies (hormonal ablation therapy, radiation therapy, cryosurgery and radical prostatectomy). Recurrent cancer is typically suspected in these patients due to a detectable or rising PSA. However, the use of PSA testing to monitor therapeutic efficacy is not ideal since PSA is not specific for prostate cancer. Additionally, it can take one to two years or more for PSA levels to reach nadir values following radiation therapy (both external beam and brachytherapy)[423, 424]. Further, the interpretation of PSA data is more complicated for patients undergoing therapies such as hormone deprivation therapy that have a direct effect on the production of PSA. Conventional imaging methods, including TRUS, CT, and MRI, often cannot distinguish healthy from malignant tissue following therapy due to therapy-induced changes in tissue structure[425, 426]. The only definitive way to determine if residual or recurrent tissue is malignant is the histologic analysis of random biopsies, which are subject to sampling errors and are more difficult to pathologically interpret after therapy.

Studies have indicated that MRI/3D-MRSI can discriminate residual or recurrent prostate cancer from normal and necrotic tissue after cryosurgery[386, 427, 428]. In a study of 25 patients prior to and after cryosurgery, histologically confirmed necrotic tissue (N=432 voxels) demonstrated a loss of all observable prostatic metabolites. While the (choline+creatine)/citrate ratio in regions of histologically confirmed benign prostatic hyperplasia (BPH, 0.61 ± 0.21, N = 52 voxels) and cancer (2.4 ± 1.0, N = 65 voxels) after cryosurgery were not significantly different from those observed prior to therapy, but were significantly different from each other. These initial studies suggested that MRSI could discriminate successful therapy (complete loss of prostatic metabolites) from residual disease. Subsequent studies have indicated that MRSI can also detect residual disease after unsuccessful radiation[429] and hormone deprivation therapy (Figure 16)[430, 431].

In addition to the potential of MRI/3D MRSI to provide a direct measure of the presence and spatial extent of prostate cancer after therapy, there is evidence that MRI/3D-MRSI can provide a measure of the time course of response and information concerning the mechanism of therapeutic response[431]. For example, prostatic citrate production and secretion have been shown to be regulated by testosterone and prolactin[432], and an early dramatic reduction of citrate after initiation of complete hormonal blockade has been observed by MRSI[431]. Additionally, there is a time dependent loss of all prostatic metabolites in both regions of cancer and healthy tissue following the initiation of hormone ablation therapy (Figure 17A)[431]. This finding is consistent with the increased frequency of tissue atrophy that occurs with increasing duration of hormone ablation therapy and is considered to be a indicator of effective therapy[433]. There is also evidence that the same is true for radiation therapy[429]. Additionally, recent studies of patients on intermittent hormone deprivation therapy have demonstrated that the time course of metabolic recovery after cessation of therapy can be monitored by MRI/MRSI (Figure 17B). Studies are currently underway to investigate: the accuracy of MRI/MRSI in assessing the presence and spatial extent of prostate cancer after these therapies[430]; the prognostic value of the time course to metabolic atrophy; the duration of zero metabolism; and the rate of metabolic recovery, particularly of cancer. The detection of residual cancer at an early stage following treatment and the ability to monitor the time course of therapeutic response would allow earlier intervention with additional therapy, and provide a more quantitative assessment of therapeutic efficacy.

FUTURE DIRECTIONS

The studies discussed in this review provide compelling evidence that the addition of MRI/3D MRSI data to PSA and biopsy data can improve the characterization of prostate cancer prior to therapy and provide information about its response to therapy. As promising as this may seem, there

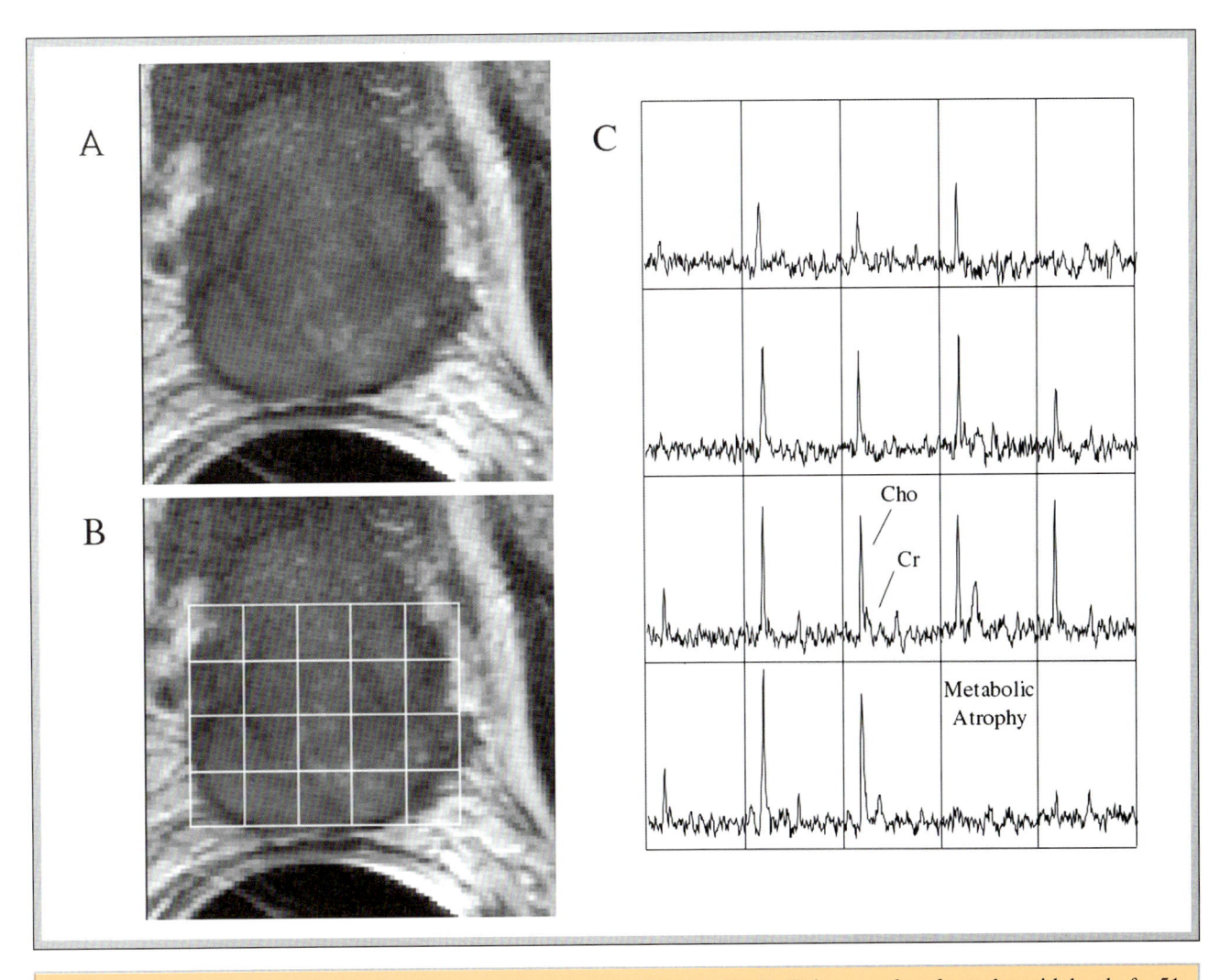

FIGURE 16: **(A)** A representative reception profile corrected T2-weighted MR image taken from the midgland of a 51-year-old prostate cancer patient who had been on long-term (21 months) hormone deprivation therapy (Flutamide and Proscar) and had a PSA of 0.7 ng/ml at the time of scan. A portion of the 16x8x8 spectral phase encode grid from one of 8 axial slices is shown overlaid on the T2 weighted image **(B)** with the corresponding 0.3 cm^3 proton spectral array **(C)**. The entire peripheral zone demonstrates diffuse low signal intensity making identification of zonal anatomy and pathology very difficult on MRI alone. Consistent with hormone deprivation therapy, most spectroscopic voxels demonstrate a complete loss of citrate. However, there are spectroscopic voxels demonstrating very elevated choline levels (choline/creatine ratio of 2 to 5) consistent with residual cancer throughout the prostate. The presence of a large volume of cancer (6/6 biopsy cores positive) was subsequently confirmed by ultrasound guided biopsies.

are currently only a few academic medical centers worldwide that have experience with this new technology. In the next stage, MRI/MRSI must be implemented and validated at multiple institutions, and large scale patient studies need to be performed to determine the true clinical value of MRI/MRSI for the improved management of prostate cancer patients.

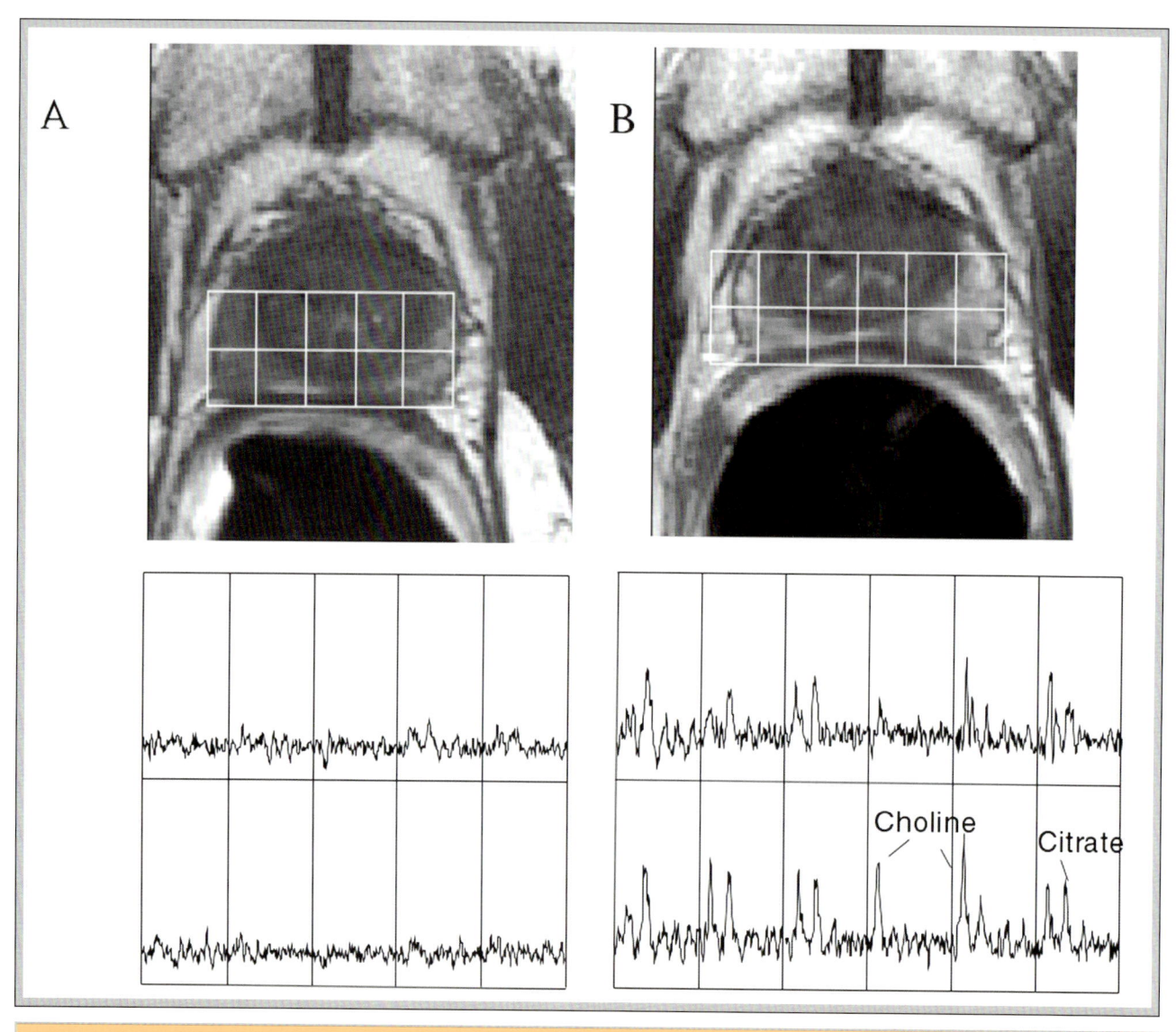

FIGURE 17: (A) T2 weighted image and corresponding 0.3cc spectral array from a 77 year old patient with bilateral Gleason 3+4 cancer after 1 year of combined (Lupron and Casodex) hormone deprivation therapy. PSA was 0.4 ng/ml at the time of the MRI/MRSI scan. (B) A corresponding T2 weighted image and spectral array from the same patient 1year after cessation of hormone deprivation therapy. Metabolism and PSA (4.5 ng/ml) have significantly recovered, and bilateral recurrent cancer is identified by MRSI.

There are also several new applications of MRI/MRSI that are currently under investigation. One area of great potential is the use of MRI/MRSI for improved radiation treatment planning. Two recent studies indicate the potential of MRI/MRSI data in combination with computed tomography (CT) to optimize radiation dose selectively to regions of prostate cancer using either Intensity Modulated Radiotherapy (IMRT)[434] or

Brachytherapy[435]. Another area of recent research is the use of MRI/MRSI to improve tissue selection for ex-vivo spectroscopic analysis and protein and genetic biomarker studies. In on-going studies at UCSF a full chemical assay of MRI/MRSI targeted tissue samples are being performed using an ex vivo high resolution NMR technique (1H HR-MAS) prior to pathologic and molecular analysis (p53, bcl-2, MIB-1, PSMA, PSA) of the same tissue. These studies have already identified potential new metabolic markers for in vivo studies and provided an improved understanding of metabolic phenotypes associated with specific tissue types and stages of cancer. Continuing improvements in MR technology such as higher magnetic field clinical scanners (3 Tesla versus 1.5 Tesla) will allow us to exploit these new metabolic markers in patients and will allow the acquisition of MRI/MRSI with higher spatial resolution and the visualization of even finer anatomic and metabolic details. This will greatly improve the ability of MRI/MRSI to characterize prostate cancer, particularly for patients with thin compressed peripheral zones or small lesions in difficult locations.

Molecular Staging in Clinically Localized and Advanced Prostate Cancer

*By Peter Lembessis, Antigone Sourla,
Constantine Mitsiades and Michael Koutsilieris*

ABSTRACT

Positive detection of the presence of PSA and PSMA mRNAs using combined nested reverse-transcriptase polymerase chain reaction performed with peripheral blood and bone marrow have a strong correlation with time-to-PSA failure after radical prostatectomy in patients with newly diagnosed and clinically localized prostate cancer. In addition, conversion of molecular staging status from positive to negative during androgen ablation therapy is associated with long progression-free survival of patients in either early stage or advanced stage (stage D2) prostate cancer. These data support the use of combined molecular staging (PSA and PSMA in the bone marrow and peripheral blood) in the evaluation of patients with early stage as well as advanced stage prostate cancer.

Dr. Michael Koutsilieris is supported by the Special Research Account, University of Athens, General Secretariat of Research and Technology of Greece (GGET; PENED II: 70/3/4874), Ministry of Development, and the Central Council for Medical Research (KESY), Ministry of Health, Greece.

6. MOLECULAR STAGING IN CLINICALLY LOCALIZED AND ADVANCED PROSTATE CANCER

1. INTRODUCTION

Prostate cancer is the most frequent malignancy in males and the second leading cause of cancer-related death in North America. Since the implementation of prostate-specific antigen (PSA)-based screening programs has contributed to earlier diagnosis of the disease, it would be intuitively expected that radical prostatectomy should (ideally) be curative for patients with no clinical evidence of extraprostatic involvement[1]. However, a substantial proportion of patients diagnosed at a clinically early stage do, unfortunately, have non organ confined disease caused either by invasion of local extraprostatic tissues (locally advanced disease) or by micrometastases, and thereby eventually develop disease recurrence. In these early-diagnosed patients with micrometastases, as well as in those newly diagnosed patients with clinically evident metastatic disease, there is overwhelming predilection for lymphatic and skeletal involvement[436-438].

The available methods for determining the clinical stage of prostate cancer, include serum prostate specific antigen (PSA) Gleason's score on specimens obtained by transrectal ultrasonography-guided biopsies (TRUS-B), computed tomography (CT) scans, magnetic resonance imaging (MRI) of the pelvis, x-rays (chest and metastatic bone survey), abdominal ultrasonography and bone scan[436, 437, 439]. Unfortunately, the overall accuracy of these staging methods with regards to the pathologic stage of disease is less than 70%[437-439]. This may be the reason why 50% to 60% of patients with clinically localized disease after radical prostatectomy (RP) have extraprostatic disease (locally advanced disease and positive lymph nodes) and eventually suffer local recurrence and/or development of distant metastases[436-439]. Similarly, >50% of patients treated by external beam irradiation monotherapy suffer a recurrence (local and/or distant metastases) within 3 to 5 years[440]. Therefore, it is of outmost importance to describe and analyze the clinical reliability of molecular tools able to provide evidence for the presence of extraprostatic prostate cancer cells at an early clinical stage of the disease.

2. NESTED RT-PCR USING SPECIFIC PSA OR PSMA PRIMERS FOR THE DETECTION OF THE EXTRAPROSTATIC TUMOR GROWTH

In relatively recent years, the expression of PSA and prostate specific membrane antigen (PSMA) genes have been used as a method for the detection of growing prostate cells outside the prostate[441-444]. Nested reverse-transcriptase polymerase chain reaction (nested rt-PCR) using specific PSA or PSMA primers (molecular staging) was proven capable of detecting in the peripheral blood (PB), bone marrow biopsies (BM), and bone marrow aspirates (BMA), the presence of extraprostatic prostate cells, a condition that was reported to correlate positively with pathologic stage[445, 446] and disease-free survival of patients with clinically localized prostate cancer treated by RP[447-449]. However, other investigators have documented an absence of any correlation of positive or negative molecular staging with organ confined disease, locally advanced disease, biochemical failure and disease outcome[450, 451]. Also, not all Pr.Ca patients who had the molecular detection of circulating prostate cells in their peripheral blood have developed clinically evident metastases during follow up, and not all the prostate cancer patients with advanced stage disease were found positive by molecular staging[452-455]. These data question the clinical significance of molecular staging in prostate cancer patients and as it is the case for all laboratory tests, the definition of the sensitivity versus specificity is of pivotal importance regarding its clinical use[454, 455].

3. SENSITIVITY VERSUS SPECIFICITY ISSUES OF MOLECULAR STAGING IN A CLINICAL SETTING

The enhanced sensitivity of nested rt-PCR detection using specific PSA and/or PSMA primers has been able to detect the presence of 1 prostate cell in 106 non-cancer peripheral blood nucleated cells. Initially, the enhanced sensitivity was thought to be an excellent approach for evaluating clinical samples due to the PSA and PSMA specificity to prostate cells[441-451]. However, PSA mRNA expression was documented in non-prostate origin cell lines and enhanced sensitivity PCR assays revealed the presence of illegitimate PSMA transcripts in peripheral blood leukocytes and other non-prostate cancer cell lines[454, 455]. Consequently, it became obvious that any further attempt to obtain enhanced analytical sensitivity PCR assays was bound to suffer a decrease in the specificity of the assays in either PB or BM, thereby compromising the clinical usefulness of molecular staging in patients with prostate cancer[453].

Recently, the clinical reliability of molecular staging was re-examined by changing the definition of positive and negative rt-PCR detection. Accordingly, a positive molecular staging was defined only by the detection of both PSA and PSMA mRNAs in each sample of peripheral blood (PB) and bone marrow (BM)[453]. Consequently, samples found to be, in a repetitive manner, of differential rt-PCR status for PSA and PSMA (PSA positive/PSMA negative or vice versa) were classified as negative. In these cases, the positive detections were attributed to illegitimate transcription[453].

Therefore, repetitive and site-specific (PB and BM) molecular staging using PCR sensitivity of 3-5 LNCaP prostate cancer cells in 10^6 peripheral blood nucleated cells was tested in patients with (a) newly diagnosed and clinically localized prostate cancer, (b) biopsy-proven benign prostate hyperplasia (BPH), and (c) advanced stage prostate cancer with frank and diffuse bone metastases. The specificity of the rt-PCR conditions was tested on total RNA extracts of young men and women under the age of 30 who were expected to test negative for PSA and PSMA. We emphasize that we used bone marrow biopsies (BM) and not bone marrow aspirates (BMA) in order to eliminate or to minimize the risk of peripheral blood contamination. Molecular staging of BMA may be misleading because, at least in our hands, always resulted in a repetition of molecular staging of the peripheral blood[453].

With the use of well defined rt-PCR assays, we analyze patients with clinically localized disease in PB and BM with reference to the time elapsed since TRUS-B (2 and 8 weeks after TRUS-B) and time elapsed from RP (2 and 12 months after RP). Under our conditions, molecular staging was negative in 30 PB samples obtained by the blood donor clinic, suggesting that the sensitivity limits of our rt-PCR could avoid illegitimate transcription (Figure 18). In addition, molecular staging was negative in BM in all biopsy-proven BPH patients (negative controls for molecular staging and additional test of the PCR conditions vis-ΰ-vis illegitimate transcription). Our conditions gave positive rt-PCR detections for PSA and PSMA in BM in all stage D2 patients (positive controls) with frank and diffuse metastatic disease into bones[453, 456].

Furthermore, in patients with clinically localized disease, repetitive molecular staging detected a notable drop of the positive rt-PCR detection 8 weeks after TRUS-B as compared with 2 weeks after TRUS-B. This is indicative of a direct association in the rate of positive rt-PCR detections and the time elapsed after TRUS-B, thus suggesting that TRUS-B can spread prostate cells into PB. In agreement with the above, we unexpectedly detected positive molecular staging in PB for both PSA and PSMA in approximately 10% of the BPH patients who had undergone diagnostic TRUS-B. Repetition of molecular staging 8 weeks after TRUS-B showed the conversion of positive to negative rt-PCR status in all the biopsy-proven BPH patients. The positive analyses of BM 2 weeks after TRUS-B remained positive 8 weeks after TRUS-B in the prostate cancer patients but not in the BPH patients, thus suggesting that molecular staging in BM is not affected by TRUS-B. Furthermore, the prostate cancer patients with

FIGURE 18: An example of nested rt-PCR analysis in known rt-PCR positive and rt-PCR negative samples at peripheral blood (PB) using specific primers for the PSA, PSMA and GAPDH. Lane 1 shows the DNA markers used in our experiments (100 bp ladders). Lane 2 shows the detection of a 521 bp rt-PCR PSA fragment corresponding in rt-PCR positive blood sample. Lane 3 shows the detection of a rt-PCR negative for PSA sample (blood donor). Similarly, lane 4 shows the detection of a 515 bp rt-PCR PSMA fragment corresponding in a rt-PCR positive blood sample. Lane 5 shows a rt-PCR negative sample for PSMA (blood donor). Lanes 6 and 7 show the detection of the 599 bp rt-PCR fragment corresponding in house keeping GAPDH of the rt-PCR negative samples of lanes 3 and 5, respectively. The latter was to confirm integrity of RNA in our rt-PCR negative samples for PSA and PSMA.

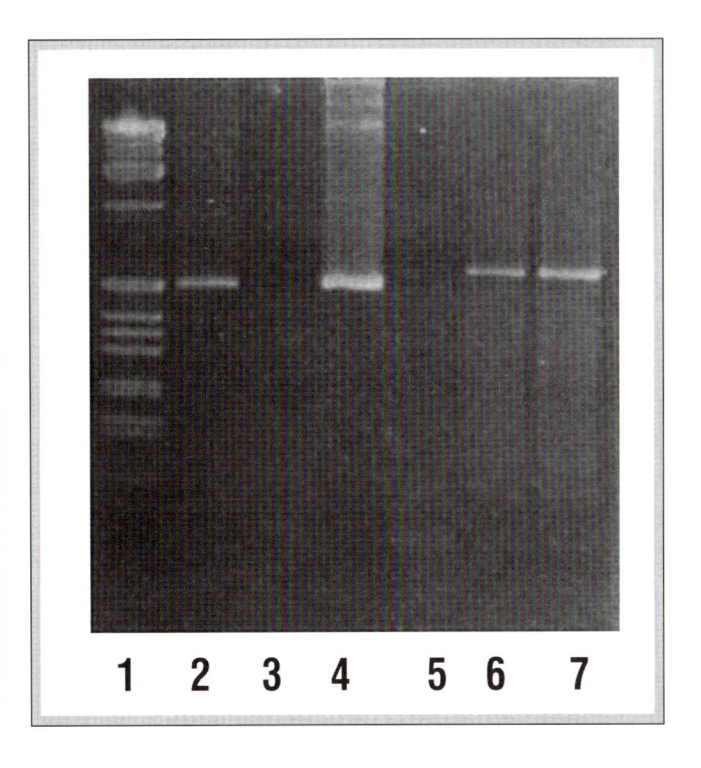

positive molecular staging at BM were also positive at PB. Consequently, BM appears to be the preferable site for molecular staging in prostate cancer patients when performed within 2 weeks after TRUS-B[453].

It is also important to note that patients with clinically localized disease and negative pre-operative molecular staging became positive for both PSA and PSMA at PB (60%) and at BM (33%) when tested 2 months after RP and 25% of these patients maintained positive at molecular staging after 12 months from RP at PB [453]. These data confirmed previous reports which show substantial dissemination of prostate cells occurs during RP[454, 455]. Until now, there is no study addressing the issue of clinical significance of positive molecular staging 12 months after RP vis-ὒ-vis disease-free progression and disease outcome[453].

Analysis of the mean values of Gleason's scores and PSA levels at diagnosis in patients with positive and negative molecular staging (Group I) were found to be significantly different from Group II (patients with negative molecular staging) ($p<0.05$). Because Gleason's score and PSA plasma levels are considered prognostic indices, it was conceivable that the positive molecular staging defines the subgroup of patients with clinically localized disease (PSA>20 ng/ml and Gleason's score >7 at diagnosis), where immediate local monotherapies (radiotherapy and RP) should be avoided because of the increased risk of extraprostatic disease[453].

Moreover, these data suggest that the clinical significance of molecular staging should be evaluated vis-ϋ-vis PSA/Gleason's score at diagnosis, pathologic staging, disease-free progression and disease outcome in prospective studies of patients stratified into groups with (a) negative analysis for both PSA and PSMA in PB and BM, (b) positive analysis for both PSA and PSMA in PB and BM, and (c) positive analysis for both PSA and PSMA at PB but negative for both in BM[453].

4. MOLECULAR STAGING AND BIOCHEMICAL FAILURE IN CLINICALLY LOCALIZED PROSTATE CANCER

Recently, we have analyzed in our laboratory (unpublished data- manuscript in preparation) the results of 153 analyses performed on patients with clinically localized prostate cancer. The analyses in PB showed 75% rt-PCR negative and 25% rt-PCR positive detections. Similar analysis inBM showed 81% negative and 19% rt-PCR positive detections. Consequently, prostate cancer patients with clinically localized disease who had undergone molecular staging could be classified into 3 groups; Group I: patients who are negative in PB and BM, group II: patients who are positive in PB and negative in BM, and group III: patients who are positive both in PB and BM. Using the Bonferonni's post-hoc tests for the PSA levels and Gleason's scores at diagnosis we observed that there is a statistically significant difference across all 3 groups ($p<0.001$). The above-mentioned data confirm the previously reported association of positive molecular staging with higher PSA and Gleason's score values at diagnosis as compared with those of negative molecular staging. Kaplan-Meier analysis and log-rank tests reveal that the median time-to-PSA failure (biochemical failure) was significantly different between groups with positive and negative molecular staging either in PB or BM ($p<0.001$). The patients of group III with positive molecular staging in both the PB and BM were subjected to either immediate radical prostatectomy (group III-1) or they were prescribed CAB for 12 months and then underwent radical prostatectomy (group III-2) only after converting the molecular staging status from positive to negative. The PSA levels and Gleason'score values at diagnosis of group III-1 and group III-2 were not different, suggesting that the formation of these 2 groups was rather random. Kaplan-Meier analysis and log-rank tests revealed that the median time-to-PSA failure (biochemical failure) was statistically significantly different between group III-1 vs group III-2, both with positive molecular staging in PB and BM ($p<0.001$).

During the follow up bone scans were now found to be positive in 20% of the patients of group III-1 (confirmed by CT-scan). These data suggest that positive molecular staging in PB and BM defined a group of patients with high risk for progression as compared with those with negative molecular staging. In addition, pre-operative administration of CAB for 12 months appear to be capable of both converting the positive molecular staging to negative and equalizing the chances for disease progression (biochemical failure and appearance of bone lesions) to those found in patients with negative molecular staging.

5. CELLULAR EVENTS PARTICIPATING IN THE DEVELOPMENT OF BONE METASTASES: CORRELATION OF MOLECULAR STAGING WITH PROGRESSION-FREE SURVIVAL IN ADVANCED STAGE D2 PROSTATE CANCER

The most important clinical manifestations of cancer which define clinical course of the disease, such as treatment approach, prognosis, and overall survival, is metastasis to organs distant from the primary tumor. The process of metastasis implies a cascade of events, involving (a) angiogenesis, (b) detachment of tumor cells from the primary tumor (cell mobility), (c) migration into the adjacent tissue (invasion), (d) adhesion to the wall and entry into the local vessels, (e) dissemination through the systemic circulation (survival in peripheral blood), (f) arrest in specific organs (seed and soil theory), (g) extravasation (penetration into host tissue), and (h) local growth within a permissive microenviroment of the host organ[457-459].

There are serious concerns stemming from the fact that bones correspond to the most prevalent site of metastases, producing mainly osteoblastic lesions[457-463] while the actual number of the metastatic foci into bones is the single most powerful prognostic factor, predetermining the lethal outcome of the disease[464, 465]. In addition, osteoblastic metastases represent the exclusive site of disease progression to terminal stage D3 of the disease (hormone refractory stage) while the actual number of skeletal metastatic foci (>6 foci) determines limited response to androgen ablation therapy and poor survival in advanced prostate cancer[465, 466]. Of note, disease progression to stage D3 occurs frequently in bones while androgen ablation therapy still provides an adequate control of tumor evolution at the primary site[459, 460, 464, 465]. Consequently, bone is not an innocent bystander that suffers locally the consequence of metastatic cell growth. The bone constitutes a favorable microenvironment of extreme biologic importance for homing prostate cancer cells[464, 467, 468]. This is secondary to interactions of prostate cancer cells primarily with osteoblasts and other cell types such as the osteoclasts, macrophages etc., promoting the growth and optimizing survival of metastatic prostate cancer cells[468, 469]. Recently, bone-derived growth factors [insulin-like growth factor I (IGF I) and transforming growth factor beta 1 (TGFβ1)] protected prostate cancer cells from chemotherapy-induced apoptosis, introducing the novel concept of therapy (anti-survival factor therapy; ASF therapy) aiming at the elimination of bone-derived survival factors[467, 468, 470, 471].

Because the prognosis is extremely poor in stage D2/D3 prostate cancer patients (bone metastases), the development of molecular tools to detect prostate cancer dissemination at the earliest possible phase in this process is a priority[460-463, 472]. Theoretically, micrometastases may become detectable at the initial phase of invasion of tumor cells into the sites of metabolically active "red" bone marrow. Initially, the invading tumor cells are more or less equally distributed into the "red" bone marrow. The actual number of invading tumor cells into the bone marrow is the most important factor determining the development of clinically evident bone metastases[458, 461, 472]. The latter is directly associated by the actual amount of "red" bone marrow of each individual bone, which in its turn, explains the increased frequency of metastases into the metabolically active bone marrow-containing bones.

At the initial stage of micrometastasis, the ability of invading tumor cells to survive while under an intense immunological surveillance of the bone marrow is directly linked with their ability to penetrate inside the bone matrix, thereby escaping or hiding from the immunologic surveillance of the bone marrow microenviroment. The bone provides the tumor cells optimal conditions for survival and growth by establishing permanent cell-cell interactions with local bone cells (osteocytes-osteoblasts). This is the step that transforms the stage of diffuse invasion of bone marrow (micrometastasis) to an eventual site for the development of clinically evident metastatic foci (Figure 19).

This opportunity is presented to the prostate cancer cells by the naturally and cyclically occurring phenomenon of bone remodelling. Therefore, the activation of osteoclasts, which direct local bone resorption, provides tumor cells the opportunity to penetrate into the bone matrix, thereby developing the initial seed of bone metastasis[462, 467, 468, 472]. Apparently, at initial stage the development of bone metastasis is directly associated with the ability of tumor cells to stimulate local attraction-activation-function of osteoclasts. Conceivably, the pharmaceutical block-

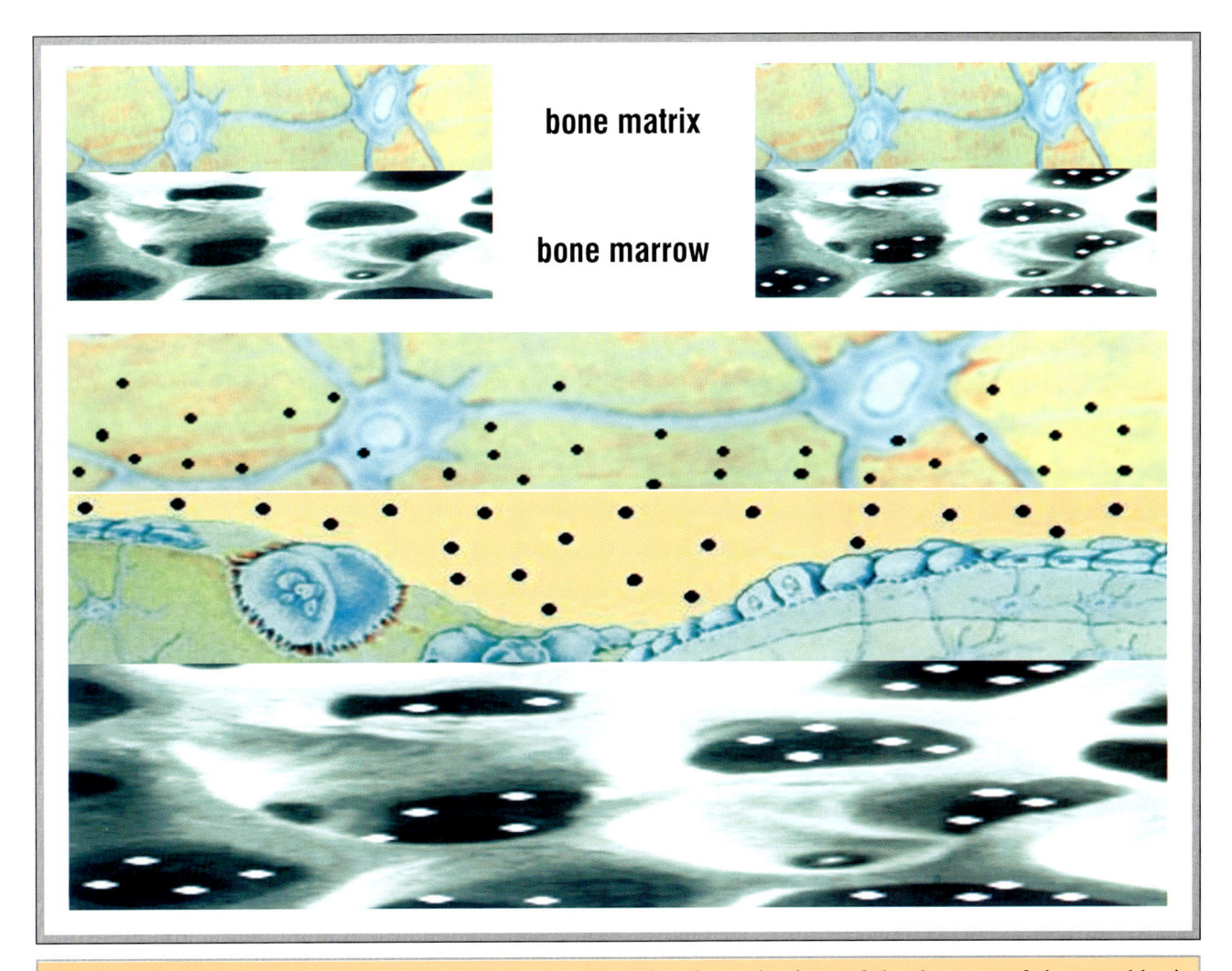

6. MOLECULAR STAGING IN CLINICALLY LOCALIZED AND ADVANCED PROSTATE CANCER

FIGURE 19: A schematic representation of the events during the early phase of development of the osteoblastic metastasis; (a) left side; upper panel: bone microenviroment-bone marrow at the quiescent phase of bone remodelling; (b) right side; upper panel: initial arrival of invading prostate cancer cells into the metabolically active "red" bone marrow, and (c) lower panel: invasion of prostate cancer cells into the bone matrix using the resorptive phase of bone remodelling which is naturally activated at bone remodelling unit; the later enables the tumor cells to escape the immunological surveillance of bone marrow and to establish fruitful local cell interactions with bone cells, mainly with osteoblasts.

ade of osteoclast-mediated bone resorption could inhibit the establishment of clinical evident metastases[473].

In addition, because the biochemical parameters of bone resorption are significantly increased in the serum and urine of patients with advanced stage disease, it is fair to conclude that active osteoclast-mediated bone resorption is taking place in bone, even at very advanced stage of disease evolution, when osteoclasts can still be a very important pharmacologic target for the treatment of patients with established osteoblastic metastases[473].

Recently, the detection of a negative molecular staging in PB and conversion of a positive detection to a negative one were associated with prolonged progression-free survival in stage D2 Pr.Ca patients on androgen blockade therapy[452, 456, 474, 475]. At diagnosis, all stage D2 patients with diffuse bony metastases were found to be rt-PCR positive for PSA and PSMA in BM[453]. It is evident then that these data have a power vis-a-vis the presence of diffuse bony metastases involving the pelvis (site of BM sampling).

Tumor cells, however, were not always present in the circulation of these stage D2 patients and 25% of them were repeatedly found rt-RCR negative for PSA and PSMA in PB. Concerning the RT-PCR status during clinical response to combined androgen blockade (CAB) in advanced stage D2 prostate cancer patients, there were patients with rt-PCR negative analysis at diagnosis who remained rt-PCR negative in PB during clinical response to CAB and there were stage D2 patients with rt-PCR positive status at diagnosis who remained positive during clinical response to CAB. Interestingly, there were also patients with positive rt-PCR analysis at diagnosis whose rt-PCR status was converted to negative during clinical response to CAB. These patients were and remained rt-PCR positive in BM during clinical response to CAB despite the fact that all experienced excellent clinical response to CAB. These data suggest that CAB-induced apoptosis of tumor cells can convert rt-PCR positive to rt-PCR negative status in PB but not in BM[456].

In addition, the majority of patients who progressed to androgen refractory stage had rt-PCR positive status for PSA and PSMA in PB, including stage D2 patients who were tested negative at diagnosis. Interestingly, 15% of stage D3 patients were found to be rt-PCR negative for both the PSA and PSMA. These data suggest that even at disease progression to an androgen refractory stage, which occurs mainly if not exclusively in bones, the presence of tumor cells in the circulation is not always evident. Interestingly, of all the stage D2 patients who had tested rt-PCR negative for PSA and PSMA during objective response to CAB, including those who converted rt-PCR status from positive to negative during CAB, showed time to disease progression >12 months. With one exception, all stage D2 patients who tested rt-PCR positive for PSA and PSMA during an objective response to CAB, showed time to disease progression <12 months. These data suggest that rt-PCR status in PB during clinical response to CAB is possibly associated with the length of clinical response to CAB[452, 456].

However, the finding that some 25% of the advanced stage patients have rt-PCR negative status for PSA and PSM at PB requires a credible explanation. This could be related to the fact that stage D2 disease, albeit hematogenously established into the skeleton, does neither require nor preclude the continuous presence of tumor cells in the circulation[452,453,456]. In addition, because PSA and PSMA gene expression is differentially regulated by androgens at the transcription level, it is expected that PSA and PSMA transcription could be also differentially affected during CAB[456]. Therefore, the conversion of rt-PCR status from positive to negative during CAB for both the PSA and PSMA at PB should not be attributed to gene transcription. Conceivably, elimination of tumor cells from the circulation produced by CAB-apoptosis during objective clinical response may be the reason[443, 446, 451].

The conversion of rt-PCR status from positive to negative was however not detectable in BM. Conceivably, prostate cancer cells having established cell to cell interactions with bone cells survive CAB-apoptosis, resulting in rt-PCR positive status in BM, even though, patients are experiencing an excellent clinical response. These data are in agreement with reports documenting the presence of bone (osteoblasts)-derived survival factors and their ability to rescue metastatic cancer cells (prostate and breast cancer cells) from chemotherapy-induced apoptosis[467]. Therefore, host tissue-mediated survival of tumor cells can explain the rt-PCR positive status for PSA/PSM in BM even during the remarkable reduction of tumor volume by CAB which is able to convert rt-PCR status in PB. In conclusion, these data suggest that rt-PCR positive analysis for PSA/PSMA at BM indicates diffuse metastases in the skeleton while the conversion of rt-PCR positive to negative status in PB during CAB is associated with a progression-free survival >12 months in stage D2 prostate cancer.

BONE MICROENVIRONMENT PARTICIPATION IN THE DEVELOPMENT OF ANDROGEN ABLATION REFRACTORINESS IN PROSTATE CANCER PATIENTS WITH BONE METASTASES: CLINICAL APPLICATION OF AN ANTI-SURVIVAL FACTOR THERAPY

*By Constantine Mitsiades, John Bogdanos,
Dimitrios Karamanolakis, Athanassios Tsintavis,
Constantine Milathianakis, Theodoros Dimopoulos,
Evaggelos Zagaras and Michael Koutsilieris*

Key words: Bone microenvironment, osteoblastic reaction, metastatic prostate cancer, IGF-1, androgen ablation therapy refractoriness, anti-survival factor therapy.

ABSTRACT

The local milieu of cancer metastases protects tumor cells from anti-cancer drug-induced apoptosis via diverse mechanisms, including soluble growth/survival factors and cytokines. The concept of anti-survival factor therapy aims at neutralizing the protective effect conferred upon cancer cells by such survival factor(s), thus increasing the sensitivity and/or reversing the resistance of tumor cells to other anti-cancer therapies. A prime example of this therapeutic paradigm has recently been applied in the setting of androgen ablation refractory prostate cancer (stage D3). At

---

Michale Koutsilieris is supported by grants from the Special Fund for Research Development, University of Athens, General Secretariat of Research and Technology, Ministry of Development, and the Central Council of Health, Ministry of Health, Greece.

this stage of the disease, which predominantly involves bone metastases, IGF-1 production (either growth hormone (GH)-dependent or GH-independent) protects tumor cells from apoptosis, despite the significant suppression of androgens. The anti-survival factor (ASF) therapeutic concept in this setting involves combination of dexamethasone (to suppresses GH-independent IGF-1) and a somatostatin analog (to suppresses "endocrine", GH-dependent IGF-1) with sustained use of LHRH analogs and a pure antiandrogen to maintain testicular and adrenal androgen suppression. In such stage D3 patients who had several adverse prognostic features and had relapsed from anti-androgen withdrawal and, sometimes, chemotherapy, the "anti-survival factor"-based strategy achieved durable objective responses and major symptomatic improvement, providing the framework for further applications of this approach. The ASF-based combination illustrates a novel paradigm in cancer treatment: anti-cancer therapies may not only target the direct induction of cancer cell apoptosis, but also the tumor microenvironment, in order to neutralize the protection of the environment on metastatic cancer cells. The favorable side-effect profile of this regimen has prompted further studies in a randomized controlled setting for metastatic prostate cancer.

1. INTRODUCTION: THE INTERACTION OF METASTATIC CELLS AND HOST-TISSUE MICROENVIROMENT AS A THERAPEUTIC TARGET

The therapeutic management of metastatic neoplasms has been traditionally based on modalities, exclusively aimed at directly inducing the death of tumor cells. Novel anti-cancer agents are generally tested in clinical trials only if *in vitro* studies have documented a sufficient degree of cancer cell killing in standard anti-cancer drug screening assays and if this effect if subsequently confirmed in pre-clinical *in vivo* models. Without ignoring the major contributions that such drug development approaches have yielded and will continue to offer in the future, it has become apparent by accumulating pieces of evidence, from both the clinical and basic research fronts, that the paradigm for the design of novel anti-tumor therapies may have to be revisited: the *in vivo* response of malignant cells to anticancer therapies is directly influenced by the host tissue microenvironment in which they metastasize[467]. In contrast, however, the almost entire spectrum of currently available *ex vivo,* as well as most *in vivo* models, for the evaluation of putative anticancer drugs, cannot serve to sim-

7. BONE MICROENVIRONMENT PARTICIPATION IN THE DEVELOPMENT OF ANDROGEN ABLATION REFRACTORINESS

ulate the potential effects of the tumor microenvironment in attenuating the response of tumor cells to the tested anti-cancer agents.

These limitations may explain why several therapeutic agents initially considered highly promising, on the basis of pre-clinical evaluation, did not fully live up to initial expectations in clinical trials of patients with advanced neoplasias: organ sites frequently afflicted by the formation of metastases, such as the bones, appear to confer to cancer cells, protection against anticancer drug-induced apoptosis. This protection is mediated by a constellation of mechanisms, including, but not limited to, soluble growth factors and cytokines released by the normal cellular constituents of the host-tissue microenvironment[468]. Such interactions between the host tissue and cancer cells may explain, at least in part, why many conventional and novel therapies yield sub-optimal responses in patients with systemic disease. Conversely, these interactions may be viewed, in and by themselves, as attractive therapeutic targets: by neutralizing the protection conferred to tumor cells by the metastatic host-tissue microenvironment, it is conceivable that responsiveness to other conventional or novel therapies can be enhanced, leading to improved outcome of patients[476].

A prime example of the importance of the host-tissue microenvironment in protecting tumor cells from anticancer therapies is the setting of androgen ablation refractory (stage D3) prostate cancer. For years, it was widely accepted that the development of resistance to androgen ablation therapy is determined exclusively at the genetic level and caused by mutations/chromosomal abnormalities that neutralize pro-apoptotic intracellular pathways and/or constitutively activate anti-apoptotic ones, in tumor cells. Yet, it is now well documented that this type of resistance can also be conferred by epigenetic, non-genetically determined, mechanisms[470]. These mechanisms involve interaction of tumor cells with the local microenvironment at the site of bone metastases, which are the almost exclusive sites for development of androgen ablation refractory disease. An important component of such microenvironment-dependent resistance to therapy is mediated by local survival factor(s) or proteins stimulating anti-apoptotic signaling cascades in tumor cells (Figure 20), thereby attenuating the clinical responses to conventional or investigational therapies and/or shortening their duration of efficacy.

Survival factors thus constitute another molecular level for therapeutic targeting and one of its first applications involves the use of such an anti-survival factor therapy in combinations with combined androgen ablation for prostate cancer patients. The novelty of such an approach is that, instead of attempting to directly induce cancer cell apoptosis, the anti-survival factor therapy aims at neutralizing the protective effect conferred upon cancer cells by bone microenvironment-derived survival factor(s).

FIGURE 20. Schematic representation of the neutralizing effects of the host tissue (bone) on the pro-apoptotic actions of anticancer treatments, such as combined androgen blockade (CAB), radiotherapy and chemotherapy in prostate cancer biology.

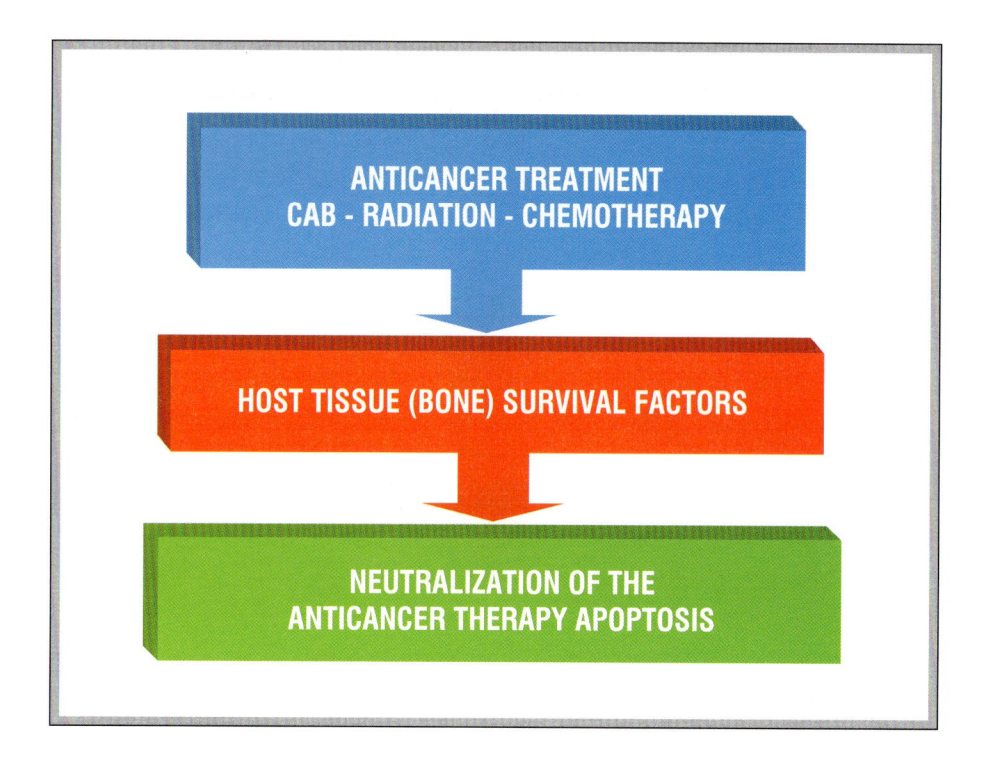

This neutralization may not necessarily induce apoptosis per se, but it can enhance the sensitivity and/or reverse the resistance of cancer cells to other anticancer therapeutic strategies[467, 468, 470].

2. THE INITIAL RESPONSE AND THE PROGRESSION/FAILURE OF COMBINED ANDROGEN BLOCKADE IN PROSTATE CANCER PATIENTS WITH SKELETAL METASTASES

Combined androgen blockade (CAB) is the first line therapy for patients with advanced stage prostate cancer (distal metastasis other than lymph nodes; stage D2). CAB therapy consists of chronic administration of a long-acting luteinizing hormone-releasing hormone analog (LHRH-A) or orchiectomy and a "pure" anti-androgen, such as flutamide, nilutamide or bicalutamide[477]. While the pulsatile endogenous hypothalamic LHRH secretion stimulates gonadotropin production from the anterior pituitary, chronic administration of the superagonistic LHRH-A rapidly down-regulates the expression of its receptor in gonadotropin-producing pituitary cells, thus suppressing pituitary production of luteinizing hormone (LH), the major stimulus for the production of testosterone (T) in the testes. Testicular testosterone, via its transformation to dihydrotestosterone (DHT) by 5α-reductase, provides about equal amounts of intraprostatic androgenic activity the other fraction being of adrenal origin (7). Thus the androgens remaining after LHRH-A treatment or orchiectomy are of adrenal origin while locally produced androgens via the transformation of adrenal steroid precursors, such as dehydroepiandrosterone (DHEA), DHEA-sulfate (DHEA-S), Δ4-androstenedione (Δ4-A)[478], can significantly enhance the growth and survival of prostate cancer cells. Therefore, to neutralize both sources of androgens, LHRH-A or orchiectomy should be combined with an anti-androgen, such as flutamide, nilutamide or bicalutamide and possibly with a 5α-reductase inhibitor[477, 478].

In newly diagnosed stage D2 prostate cancer patients, CAB achieves an overall response rate of >90%[479], with a median response duration ranging from 24 to 30 months. Unfortunately, almost all stage D2 patients eventually progress to stage D3 (androgen ablation refractory disease). Some of these progressing patients, (even up to 30% of them according to some estimates[480, 481] may transiently benefit from cessation of anti-androgen administration (anti-androgen withdrawal syndrome). Eventually, practically all CAB-treated patients become refractory to hormonal manipulations[482] and their median survival after the establishment of this resistance is approximately 9-10 months[483, 484]. Various combination chemotherapy regimens[485] or immune-based modalities[486] have been proposed as potential treatment options. However, such approaches have not been shown to significantly prolong survival[487, 488]. This has prompted major research efforts to define the molecular mechanism(s) of hormone refractoriness, in order to design modified CAB-based therapeutic strategies which may circumvent the resistance to CAB and, hopefully, further prolong the overall and progression-free survival of these patients.

Until recently, most studies on the mechanisms of resistance to anti-cancer therapies focused on chemo-resistance and used *in vitro* models of protracted exposure of cancer cell lines to cytotoxic drugs. Undoubtedly, such studies offered valuable insight into several genetically-determined mechanisms of chemo-resistance, including mutations causing reduced intracellular drug accumulation[489], overexpression or altered structure of the intracellular targets of anticancer drugs[490]. Some of these mechanisms have been targeted in clinical trials in an attempt to overcome chemo-resistance. The results obtained, though, were less encouraging than their pre-clinical background. These studies, however, gave sufficient evidence that clinical chemo-resistance is a multifactorial phenomenon and that neutralizing only one mechanism of drug resistance is unlikely to translate into substantial clinical benefits. They also reinforced the notion that the degree of cancer cell sensitivity to anticancer therapies is largely influenced by the dynamic balance between the opposing forces of proteins, which facilitate (pro-apoptotic) vs those who impede (anti-apoptotic) the process of apoptosis[491]. Importantly, in several tumor models, the relative expression and function of these pro- and anti-apoptotic mechanisms are not dictated only by intrinsic-genetically determined-mechanisms, but are also significantly influenced by extracellular stimuli from the microenvironment of the tumor: these stimuli, either in the form of soluble mediators secreted by non-tumor, host-tissue cells[470, 492] or in the form of direct contact or tumor cells with stromal cells or extracellular matrix components[493] activate signal transduction pathways that may block drug-induced apoptosis. Interrupting this tumor cell–microenvironment interaction or the signaling pathways associated with this interaction may represent a new approach to cancer therapy. These individual mechanisms can act in a concerted manner to determine overall clinical responses of cancer patients to cytotoxic chemotherapy, endocrine therapy or any other form of anticancer therapy whose effectiveness relies on the induction of cancer cell apoptosis (Figure 21).

For many years and long before the role of such microenvironmental factors became recognized, the investigation of hormone resistance in prostate cancer was evolving around the major macro-environmental stimulus for tumor cell growth, i.e. androgens: the overwhelming focus on the androgen receptor was an influence from research efforts in other endocrine-dependent neoplasias, where the status of sex steroid action was the principal determinant for growth/survival of tumor cells and a prime target for genetic changes that can affect the biological behavior of these cancer cells. Indeed, in the field of breast cancer, the lack of detectable estrogen (ER) and/or progesterone (PR) receptors has been regarded as an adverse prognostic indicator[494] and such ER-/PR- patients are poor candidates for hormonal manipulations. Extrapolation of this experience to prostate cancer leads to the initial hypothesis that refractoriness to CAB androgen ablation therapy is related to defects in the androgen receptor (AR) gene expression[495]. In particular, it was postulated that deletions or inactivating mutations of the AR gene contribute to the hormone refractory phenotype. Conceivably, such AR gene defects would be irreversible phenomena, precluding re-introduction of androgen suppression-based treatment approaches. However, down-regulation or loss of AR expression has not been documented in a significant proportion of androgen-independent prostate cancer[496, 497], thus indicating that other mechanism(s) are the main culprit(s) for the phenotypic switch to androgen ablation-refractoriness.

In fact, not only AR remains active in CAB-refractory prostate cancer

7. BONE MICROENVIRONMENT PARTICIPATION IN THE DEVELOPMENT OF ANDROGEN ABLATION REFRACTORINESS

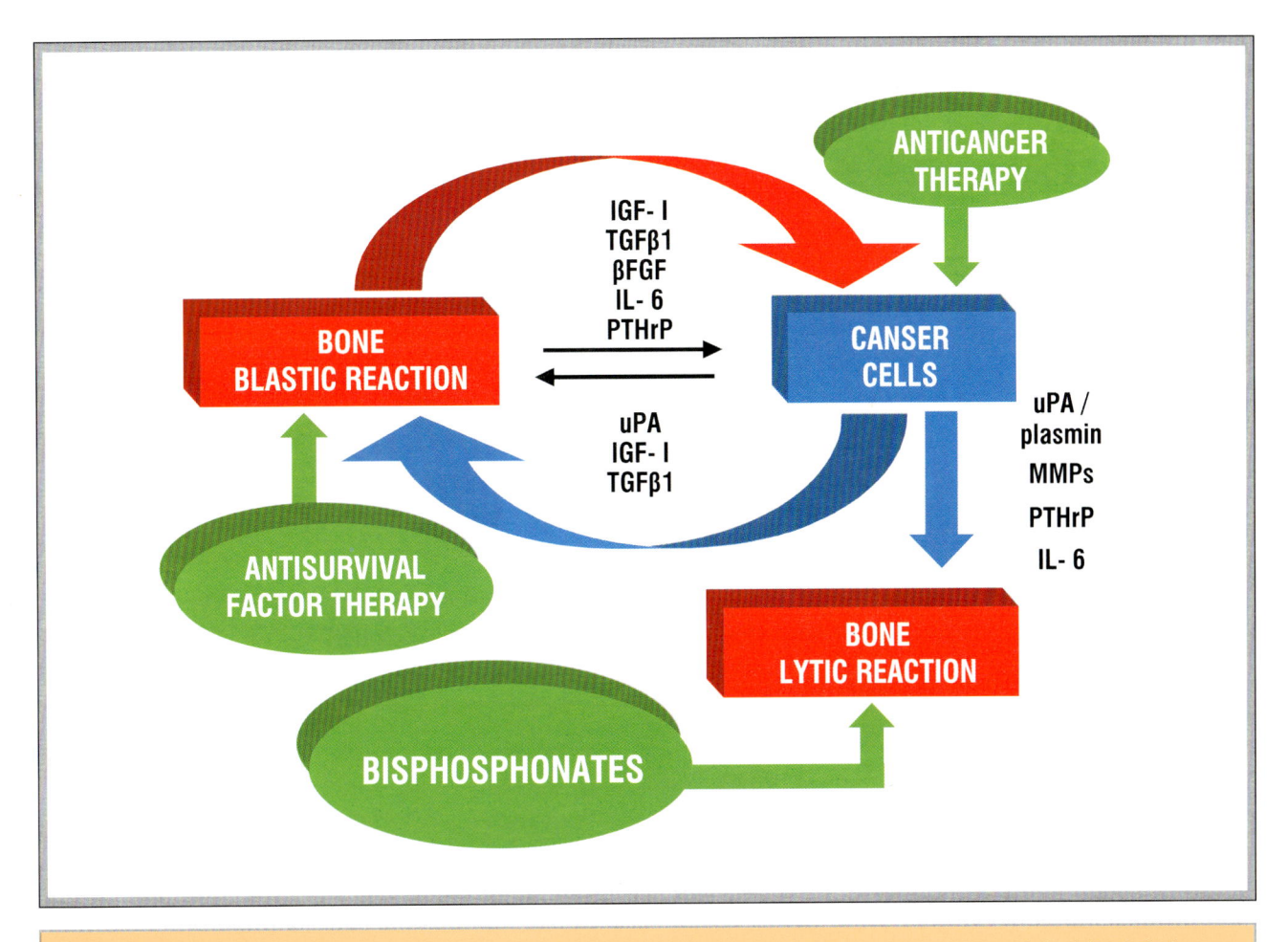

FIGURE 21. Cell-cell interactions and biochemical mediators implicated in the development of the blastic/lytic reaction in the skeleton and hormone/chemo refractoriness of prostate cancer cells growing in the bone microenviroment. The concept of a novel combination therapy, using anticancer therapy (CAB/chemotherapy), anti-survival factor therapy (dexamethasone and SM-a) and bisphosphonates.

cells, but its expression and activity are increased in several cell lines that are used as an *in vitro* models for monitoring changes during long-term androgen ablation, while relapse from CAB therapy occurs in the setting of high levels of AR expression in metastatic disease[498]. Inhibition of AR expression in LNCaP prostate tumor cells by antisense oligodeoxynucleotides (ODNs) against the AR almost completely abrogate its expression[499] and result in significant cell growth inhibition, reduction in PSA secretion, and a major increase in apoptosis. These studies not only showed that inhibition of AR expression and function is a promising potential approach for treatment of advanced human prostate cancer, but also provided strong proof-of-principle evidence that disruptions of the AR function, such as those deriving from structural defects of its gene,

115

should not be expected to confer resistance to androgen ablation, but in contrast could add to its effect.

In retrospect, the above-mentioned findings are entirely consistent with the role of AR in prostate cancer cells: the AR transmits both growth and survival signals. Therefore, disruption of its transcriptional activity would place a prostate cancer cell at a serious growth/survival disadvantage over its counterparts with normal or increased AR function. Conversely, if AR gene alterations are to play any role in resistance to CAB, they should be enhancing or even constitutively activating the AR transcriptional activity, rather than down-regulating it[472]. Therefore, research on the role of AR in CAB-resistance has shifted towards identifying mutations or other structural modifications of the AR gene that lead to more potent or constitutively active AR trancriptional activity.

Indeed, such modifications in AR gene expression or structure have been identified: point mutations at the AR ligand binding domain can alter its ligand binding specificity, creating a mutant AR whose transcriptional activity can be paradoxically activated by steroids other than its conventional ligand, or even by antiandrogens[480, 500, 501]. Such mutations could constitute a molecular explanation of some cases showing the anti-androgen withdrawal syndrome[502, 503]: mutations rendering AR transcriptionally active in the presence of anti-androgens and despite the absence of the natural AR ligand could help prostate cancer cells to proliferate in the setting of some antiandrogen therapy. Therefore, in these cases, upon anti-androgen withdrawal, these cells lose a growth/survival stimulus, which can explain the responses of some hormone-refractory patients to this manipulation, although the incidence of AR mutations in refractory prostate cancer is low.

However, prostate cells with AR gene amplification can explain the ability of some prostate cancer cells to survive in the androgen-deficient environment created by CAB therapy and the disease progression to stage D3[504-506]. These AR gene mutations and alterations are fairly frequent[507], but are present in only a subgroup of tumor samples from hormone refractory patients[500, 508-514]. This indicates that other molecular events mediate active transcription of AR-dependent pro/anti-apoptotic genes, even the presence of low concentrations of DHT[515]. One could hypothesize that other genes involved in the regulation of AR transcriptional activity (e.g. co-repressors or co-activators of AR function) may be aberrantly expressed, deleted or otherwise altered in hormone refractory prostate cancer cells, thus modulating their response to the residual androgenic activity present in patients receiving CAB. Yet, no single genetic defect or constellation of defects, have been universally identified in hormone refractory prostate cancer.

Independent confirmation of this potential mechanism comes from cDNA and tissue microarray technologies: their use in specimens from early and hormone refractory stages of prostate cancer, did show overexpression of the hsp27 gene, a gene involved in chemo-resistance against doxorubicin 2 in approximately 30% of hormone refractory prostate cancer specimens[516]. Interestingly, the IGFBP-2 gene was overexpressed in all hormone refractory prostate cancer specimens, including strong staining in the stromal tissue in close proximity with tumor cells. Because IGFBP-2 participates in the regulation of the local bioavailability of IGF and is expressed not only by the tumor cells, but mainly by host tissue cells in the microenvironment of metastases, the tissue microarray studies have indicated that every effort to explain the development of hormone refractoriness should take into account not only the genetic make-up of the tumor cells but also how their gene function is influenced by the interactions of these cells with their microenvironment. Therefore, during the last few years, new interest has been developed for a better understanding of how the metastatic prostate cancer cells interact with the bone microenvironment.

3. PATHOPHYSIOLOGY OF OSTEOBLASTIC METASTASES IN PROSTATE CANCER: THE ROLE OF THE UROKINASE (UPA)/PLASMIN/IGFS SYSTEM IN THE DEVELOPMENT OF HORMONE REFRACTORINESS

The bone microenvironment and its cellular constituents (e.g. osteoblasts/osteocytes, osteoclasts, stromal cells) are major sources of soluble mediators with significant role in the regulation of bone remodeling[461,463]. Prostate cancer cells express receptors for many of these proteins, which can therefore stimulate their proliferation[469,517-521]. Interestingly, prostate cancer cells themselves secrete many of these factors, such as interleukin-6 (IL-6), fibroblast growth factors (FGFs)[521-523], transforming growth factor beta 1 (TGF-β1)[524], bone morphogenetic proteins (BMPs), parathyroid hormone-related peptide (PTHrP)[525, 526], or endothelin-1[527, 528]. These prostate-derived mitogens can conceivably act, in either an autocrine positive feedback loop, on in a paracrine fashion on cancer cells themselves, as well as locally modulate the bone remodeling process, at sites of skeletal metastases, by stimulating the proliferation of osteoblasts and their contribution to deposition of new bone[469,517-520,528-530]. The role of these peptides in promoting the osteoblastic reaction may be synergistic or additive and it is possible that novel factors may also contribute to these intercellular interactions

7. BONE MICROENVIRONMENT PARTICIPATION IN THE DEVELOPMENT OF ANDROGEN ABLATION REFRACTORINESS

between metastatic cancer cells and the bone cells [Mundy, 1997 #506;[461, 524]].

The reaction of the bone microenvironment to metastatic prostate cancer cells predominantly involves a local proliferation of osteoblasts[458, 462]. It was therefore hypothesized that a prostate cancer cell-derived mitogen may specifically mediate this response. Indeed, such an osteoblast-specific mitogen, without substantial effect on fibroblasts, was detected in extracts from prostate cancer, benign prostatic hyperplasia and normal prostate tissues, and conditioned media (CM) of both human and rat prostate cancer cells[469, 518, 529, 531]. This mitogen is the urokinase-type plasminogen activator (uPA)[531], which is synthesized as a single chain precursor (pro-uPA) and subsequently converted to active uPA, by human kallikrein 2 (hK2) or plasmin, but not by prostate specific antigen (PSA)[532]. Active uPA consists of an α- and a β- chain (which correspond to the N- and C-terminals of pro-uPA, respectively) linked by a disulfide bridge, with the β chain possessing serine protease activity[533]. uPA interacts with its cell surface receptor (uPA.R) which lacks intracellular or transmembrane domains and is, instead, anchored to the cell membrane by a monomeric glycerolphosphoinoside (GPI) moiety. In agreement with the proposed role of uPA in promoting the osteoblastic reaction in prostate cancer metastases, purified rat and human uPAs selectively stimulate the proliferation of human MG-63 and SaOS-2 osteoblast-like cells[534].

These above-mentioned studies indicate that the osteoblastic reaction is not a non-specific local proliferation of cells from the bone microenvironment, but is instead, a specific response of the osteoblasts to the presence of metastatic prostate cancer cells, coordinated by uPA[534]. Its protease activity may, by itself, contribute to the extracellular matrix degradation processes that accompany the establishment of metastases and the blastic reaction of osteoblasts. Importantly, uPA, through its β-chain protease activity, can directly cleave fibronectin[535] and convert plasminogen to plasmin[536], which in turn orchestrates an extensive proteolytic degradation of the extracellular matrix[535]. uPAR attracts uPA at focal sites adjacent to the cell surface, but also facilitates its proteolytic activity at these sites, which are the preferred foci for uPA-mediated protein degradation[535, 536]. Indeed, competitive displacement of uPA from uPAR results in decreased matrix degradation[537]. The uPA expression and uPA-mediated extracellular matrix degradation by prostate cancer cells correlate with their metastatic behavior, *in vivo*[538]. In animal models, uPA overexpression correlates with higher, both skeletal and nonskeletal, tumor burden[539], while uPA down-regulation reduces metastatic tumor size[540, 541]. Elevated uPA levels in the peripheral blood correlates with far advanced metastatic disease and increased number of bone metastatic foci[541].

These findings further support the notion that uPA plays a key role in osteoblastic metastases and their pathophysiology. However, a key question is how a protease such as uPA can stimulate osteoblast proliferation. One hypothesis has been that uPA functions per se as a growth factor, independently of its proteolytic activity, and initiates, downstream of the uPA receptor, signaling pathway(s) stimulating cell proliferation. According to this hypothesis, prostate cancer cells produce a, yet unidentified, proteinase, which cleaves the a-chain of uPA and specifically generates the amino-terminal fragment (ATF, or ATF-uPA), which contains at its N-terminus a "growth factor domain" (GFD) sequence, which is structurally similar to the epidermal growth factor (EGF)[71, 78]. This GFD sequence was proposed to render ATF-uPA capable to act per se as a prostate-derived mitogen for osteoblasts[542, 543]. uPA-R is expressed on both prostate cancer cells and osteoblasts, and the proposed model, for such a potential direct mitogenic effect, holds that, aside intact uPA, ATF-uPA also binds to uPA-R on the osteoblast surface, thus transducing mitogenic signals[543]. Indeed, ATF-uPA does promote the proliferation of human SaOS-2 osteoblast-like cells and upregulates the expression of c-myc, c-jun and c-fos genes in a time-dependent manner[544]. Tyrosine kinase inhibitors, such as herbimycin, block these effects, suggesting that the effect of ATF-uPA on osteoblasts' proliferation involves tyrosine kinase-mediated signaling pathways[544]. However, it is not determined how the uPA receptor (a GPI-anchored receptor lacking identifiable intracellular tyrosine kinase domain), can transduce a growth signal. Apparently, in order for this hypothesis to hold true, it is implied that another, yet unidentified, novel receptor molecule, perhaps specifically binds N-terminal uPA on osteoblasts[542-544]. Ongoing investigation is addressing the involvement of such potential mechanisms.

An alternative explanation of how uPA mediates prostate cancer cell-induced stimulation of osteoblasts puts emphasis on the direct protease activity of uPA and the indirect uPA-mediated generation of plasmin, which can hydrolyze IGF-binding proteins (IGFBPs)[545]. This event releases active IGF-1, significantly increases its local bioavailability and leads to type I IGF receptor-mediated proliferative response of osteoblasts and prostate tumor cells[531, 534, 545, 546]. A significant body of experimental evidence supports this hypothesis: in agreement with the known role of tyrosine kinase signaling in the proliferative responses of osteoblasts to uPA, the type I IGF receptor is a tyrosine kinase stimulating a pleiotropic pattern of proliferative and anti-apoptotic downstream signaling pathways. The protease activity of uPA and its downstream target, plasmin, are key determinants in the osteoblastic response, because the protease inhibitors benzamidine and aprotinin, abrogate the mitogenic activity of prostate cancer cells' conditioned media (CM) on osteoblast-like cells[531, 542]. Furthermore, anti-IGF-I neutralizing antibodies block the mitogenic effect of human and rat uPA on human and rat osteoblasts, respectively[545], indicating that a significant part of the mitogenic action of uPA on osteoblasts is, in fact, IGF-mediated[544, 547]. Of note, uPA can also activate latent-TGFβ1 produced by prostate cancer cells and osteoblasts, where it exerts important regulatory functions[534, 546, 547]. Moreover, IGFBP-3, a major target of uPA-mediated proteolysis, can induce apoptosis of prostate cancer cells, via an IGF-independent mechanism[548]. Therefore, uPA-mediated hydrolysis of IGFBP-3, not only increases the bioavailability of IGF-1, but also further promotes the survival of metastatic prostate cancer cells by removing the pro-apoptotic stimulus of IGFBP-3.

The uPA/plasmin/IGF axis is therefore likely to be heavily involved in the pathophysiology of osteoblastic metastases and involves effects at multiple molecular and cellular targets to increase the proliferative stimulation of prostate cancer cells and osteoblasts, to promote the remodeling of extracellular matrix and its proteins and even protect prostate cancer cells from pro-apoptotic extracellular proteins, such as IGFBP-3. These biological mechanisms converge to provide a favorable microenvironment for metastatic prostate cancer cells and may conceivably be complemented by other cytokine-, growth factor- or cell adhesion molecule-mediated interactions that can contribute to prostate cancer cell homing in the bone[461, 463, 472, 517].

Since the uPA/plasmin/IGF axis can facilitate the establishment of osteoblastic bone metastases of prostate cancer, further research efforts focus on the potential role of this pathway in rescuing metastatic cells from hormonal therapy and development of the clinical phenotype of hormone refractoriness. At a cellular level, CAB therapy promotes *in vivo* apoptosis of prostate cancer cells by abrogating the AR transcriptional activity and its significant anti-apoptotic role for these cells. When refractoriness to CAB therapy is established, LHRH-A or orchiectomy continue to suppress testicular androgen production and the anti-androgen prevents the AR binding of residual adrenal androgens. Therefore, "failure of CAB" does not mean failure to suppress androgen production (either of testicular or adrenal origin) or to inhibit their binding to the AR. In contrast, it reflects the fact that prostate cancer cells have established alternative pathways to maintain their survival despite an almost complete depletion of androgenic stimuli. In particular, it has been proposed that bone-derived survival factors, such as IGF-1, can promote the survival of metastatic prostate cancer cells by stimulating intracellular anti-apoptotic

7. BONE MICROENVIRONMENT PARTICIPATION IN THE DEVELOPMENT OF ANDROGEN ABLATION REFRACTORINESS

signal transduction pathways, including activation of AR-dependent transcription, despite the significant suppression of androgens by CAB[471].

Bone is the predominant site where prostate cancer metastases develop and progress to hormone refractoriness[464, 472], even when CAB therapy continues to offer sustained control of the disease at its primary site or other extraskeletal sites, such as pulmonary metastases[459, 549]. This strongly implies that local environmental cues present in the bone, but probably absent or attenuated in other tissues, may be responsible for rescuing prostate cancer cells from hormonal therapy-induced apoptosis[459,470,472,550]. Indeed, in comparison to most other tissues of the body, the bone is highly active in regards to the production, by various cells of its microenvironment, of an extended spectrum of growth factors involved in regulating the cyclical bone remodeling processes[461]. Conceivably, some of these growth factors could also function as "survival" factors, mediating anti-apoptotic signals to cancer cells.

Indeed, osteoblast-derived growth factors and osteoblast conditioned media (CM) can rescue prostate cancer cells from chemotherapy-induced apoptosis, *in vitro* (). Particular focus has been placed on IGF-1 because this growth factor is a major focal point for the the uPA/plasmin pathway. IGF-1, CM from MG-63 osteoblast-like cells and TGFβ1, partially neutralized the doxorubicin-induced cytotoxic death of PC-3 cells. IGF-1 provided the most pronounced protective effect, which was enhanced, in an additive manner, by TGFβ1 and MG-63 CM[470]. Similarly, IGF-1 functioned as a survival factor for estrogen receptor negative (ER-) MDA-MB 231 human breast cancer cells against chemotherapy-induced apoptosis[551]. The studies lead to the conclusion that osteoblast-derived growth factors, particularly IGF-1, can protect prostate and breast cancer cells from chemotherapy-induced apoptosis[470, 551, 552].

Importantly, these studies were confirmed in three-dimensional type I collagen gel cell culture systems, an ex vivo co-culture model which simulates the osteoblast-prostate cancer cell interactions in a milieu simulating the local metastatic microenvironment[492, 553, 554]. In this model, inoculation of human PC-3 cells produced a local osteoblastic reaction, documented by increased number of MG-63 osteoblast-like cells and increased density of type I collagen around those MG-63 cells that were adjacent to inoculated PC-3 cells[553]. In contrast, under identical experimental conditions, cell-free medium, human breast cancer cells, endometrial adenocarcinoma cells and lung cancer cells did not produce this blastic reaction[492, 554]. This 3-D *in vitro* model confirmed that human osteoblasts and exogenous IGF-1, rescued human prostate cancer cells from induction of apoptosis, e.g. by doxorubicin[470]. These results can explain several features of known aspects of the pathophysiology of advanced prostate cancer, in particular why bone metastases are far more likely to develop resistance to androgen ablation therapy, in comparison to extraskeletal metastases[519, 555, 556].

Of note, IGF-1 is abundantly present in the circulation and in extracellular fluids throughout the body, while its local concentrations at the bone microenvironment are conceivably much higher because of the major IGF-1 production by osteoblasts. At the sites of bone metastases, the local IGF-1 bioavailability is further potentiated by the cleavage of IGFBP-3 by the uPA/plasmin cascade (Figure 21). Therefore, prostate cancer cells at the site of bone metastases are exposed to higher concentrations of IGF-1 in comparison to extraskeletal tissues, which could explain both the high predilection of prostate cancer cells for bone metastases and the selective development of hormone resistance in these metastases[460, 465, 468, 472].

4. DEVELOPMENT OF AN ANTI-SURVIVAL FACTOR THERAPY (ASF THERAPY) FOR ANDROGEN ABLATION REFRACTORY PROSTATE CANCER

Because IGF-1 is a nodal point for multiple mechanisms, which promote the establishment of bone metastases and their resistance to hormonal- or chemo- therapy, this cytokine has become an attractive therapeutic target. Conceptually, the effect of IGF-1 might be abrogated by strategies targeting its intracellular signaling pathways in tumor cells. However, no specific inhibitors of the IGF-1 signal transduction pathways are currently available for clinical use, which the design of clinically applicable methodologies aimed at down-regulating the local IGF-1 concentration at the metastatic sites would have to involve blockade of production of both growth hormone (GH)-dependent and GH-independent IGF-1 production in bones, including the uPA/plasmin cascade-mediated release of IGF-1 from IGFBPs, as well as, suppression of circulating GH-dependent and GH-independent IGF-1 of extraskeletal origin.

Major advances in structural biology, biochemistry and bioinformatics have allowed the de novo synthesis of hundreds of compounds with predicted 3-dimensional structures allowing for their appropriate binding to key active sites of various therapeutically relevant molecular targets. In theory, it would be worth pursuing the development of agents selectively inhibiting each one of the mechanisms responsible for the increased IGF-1 bioavailability at the sites of bone metastases. Such agents should, for instance, be selective inhibitor(s) of the protease activity of uPA, soluble forms of the type I IGF.R with higher IGF-1 binding affinity than the type I IGF.R on the surface of prostate cancer cells, selective inhibitors of the tyrosine kinase activity of the type I IGF.R or inhibitors of its downstream signaling pathways, e.g. inhibitors of the PI-3K/Akt pathway. Such approaches are currently underway and may, in the future, yield useful therapeutic agents, not only for prostate cancer, but also for other neoplasias responsive for the survival factor role of IGF-1 or for which uPA plays a role in the pathophysiology of their metastases. However, the role of the uPA/plasmin/IGF-1 pathway in metastatic prostate cancer had already been demonstrated a few years ago, at a time when the use of structural biology and bioinformatics for rational design of novel drugs was still at its very early stage.

I order to effectively block the survival factor role of IGF-1, we focused on the use of already available pharmacologic agents that could target the production of uPA and IGF-1. Ideally, these agents should have an acceptable toxicity, their administration should be clinically compatible with conventional treatment strategies and not interfere with the ability of acceptable disease markers such as PSA, to serve for monitoring the evolution of the disease. The development of such approaches was greatly facilitated by further ex vivo studies on the molecular constituents of the uPA/plasmin/IGF-1 pathway. Analysis of the promoter regions of the uPA and IGF-1 genes for putative transcription factor consensus binding sites reveals the presence of glucocorticoid receptor (GR) binding sites[557], thus suggesting a role of glucocorticoids in the regulation of transcription of these genes. This indicated that modulation of the GR is a potential target for anti-survival factor strategies (Figure 22).

Importantly, it was confirmed that the GR is functional in both prostate cancer cells and osteoblasts[534, 546, 558] and that dexamethasone decreases production of osteoblast-derived IGFs[546, 557, 559] and down-regulates prostate cancer cell expression of uPA[560], thus subsequently reducing the uPA/uPAR/plasmin-mediated degradation of extracellular matrix and the uPA-mediated hydrolysis of IGFBPs. Consequently, glucocorticoids significantly reduce the bioavailability of IGFs to both prostate cancer cells and osteoblasts[531, 545] and increase the pro-apoptotic effect of IGFBP-3 upon prostate cancer cells[548]. In agreement with these converging molecular events, glucocorticoids can inhibit the proliferation of androgen-insensitive rat PA-III and human PC-3 prostate cancer cells *in vitro* [546l Koutsilieris, 1992 #5143] and induce regression of PA-III prostate tumors in rat bones[560]. However, these encouraging initial responses of bone metastases to dexamethasone were short-lived. The PA-III cells used in these *in vivo* experiments expressed wild type GR[558]

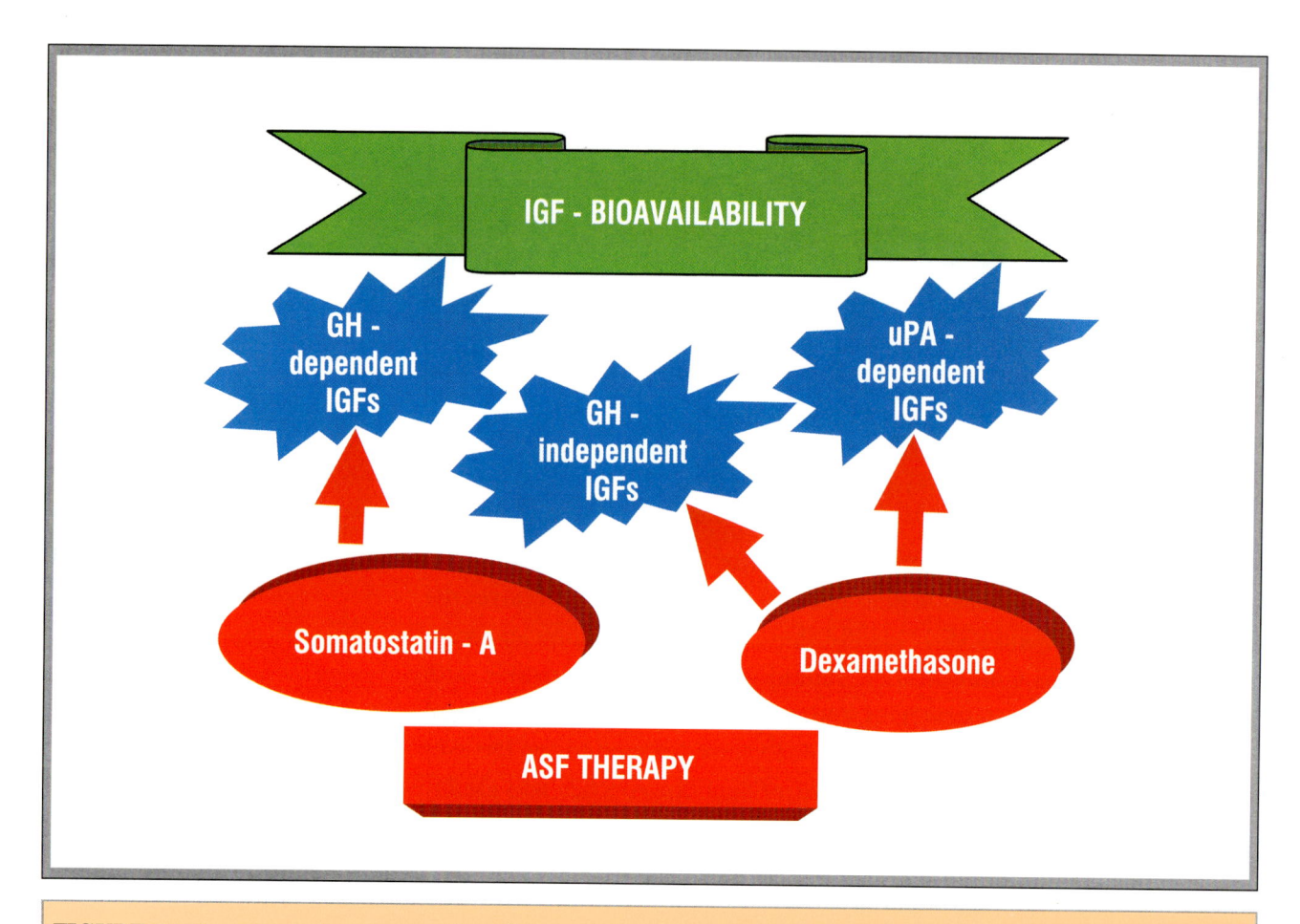

7. Bone Microenvironment Participation in the Development of Androgen Ablation Refractoriness

FIGURE 22. The schematic representation of the main target (GH-dependent and GH-independent IGF-bioavailability) of the novel anti-survival factor therapy in patients with androgen-refractory prostate cancer.

and the time-frame for the development of resistance was not suggestive of development of genetically-determined resistance. Therefore, the short lived response to dexamethasone would have to involve a mechanism implicating the tumor microenvironment and not genetic events in the tumor cells. The initial responses of osteoblastic metastases to dexamethasone-induced downregulation of local IGF-1 bioavailability were quite significant. Therefore, the recurrence of osteoblastic reactions was possibly secondary to a re-emergence of IGF-1 survival effect, even in the setting of effective suppression of osteoblast-derived IGF-1 and down-regulation of the uPA/plasmin activity by dexamethasone.

As previously mentioned, IGF-1 is abundantly present in the peripheral blood and the major source of this circulating GH-dependent IGF-1 is the liver. Glucocorticoids can locally down-regulate osteoblast-derived

IGF-1, but this effect is opposed by the incoming influx, to the bone, of circulating, growth hormone (GH)-dependent, mainly liver-derived IGF-1 and the systemic (blood) IGFBP-3/IGFs complexes[561,562]. Dexamethasone administration is thus necessary to sustain the suppression of local IGF-1 production, but it cannot neutralize the entire load of bioavailable IGFs, unless appropriate blockade of GH-dependent IGFs production is also attempted, which prompted our efforts for comprehensive suppression of IGF-1 concentrations, with additional emphasis on simultaneous suppression of GH-dependent IGF-1 production.

Somatostatin analogs are well-established and effective agents in suppressing GH-dependent IGF-1 production and have been clinically used for years in the setting of GH-secreting pituitary adenomas. In fact, octreotide or other somatostatin analogs, including, more recently, long-acting somatostatin analogs, such as lanreotide, have offered remarkable clinical improvement, associated with a decrease in circulating GH-dependent, IGF-1[563] and an increase in circulating IGFBP-1[564]. The toxicity profile of these compounds has been very favorable, including non-life-threatening and transient side effects, such as abnormal oral glucose tolerance tests, moderate elevations in blood glucose levels, cholestasis, constipation, etc., all of which were well-managed medically[563, 564]. Based on this experience, dexamethasone and somatostatin analogs were incorporated into a therapeutic protocol aiming at neutralizing the survival factor effect of IGF-1 upon prostate cancer cells (Figure 22). Such an anti-survival factor regimen would be combined with an appropriate pro-apoptotic regimen, with the objective enhancing the induction of tumor cell death, by counteracting the protective effect of the cancer cell survival factor, i.e. IGF-1 in this case.

5. INITIAL CLINICAL EXPERIENCE OF THE ANTI-SURVIVAL FACTOR (ASF) THERAPY IN ANDROGEN ABLATION REFRACTORY PROSTATE CANCER

In metastatic prostate cancer, an appropriate stage for testing the ASF manipulation is in patients that have failed both CAB and anti-androgen withdrawal. Although there is no conclusive evidence that cytotoxic chemotherapy can significantly prolong the overall survival or improve the quality of life of stage D3 patients, the first clinical applications of this anti-survival factor approach involved patients who had also failed salvage chemotherapy. In this way, all patients enrolled in that trial were refractory to every available conventional modality. In our institution, this therapeutic concept has been currently investigated, in an investigator-driven phase II study, in prostate cancer patients with: (a) disease progression to stage D3 while on combined androgen blockade (CAB; LHRH-analog plus anti-androgen, e.g. flutamide), (b) relapse under CAB therapy with a progression-free survival of less than 12 months, which is an important adverse prognostic indicator for overall survival, (c) no response to anti-androgen withdrawal manipulation or relapse after initial response to it, (d) failure to respond to salvage chemotherapy and (e) more than 6 foci of skeletal metastases, which is yet another powerful adverse prognostic indicator of survival.

The treatment schedule includes administration of oral dexamethasone (4 mg daily for the 1st month of treatment, tapered down to 2 mg daily within 2 months and a maintenance dose of 2 mg daily, thereafter) plus a long-acting somatostatin analog (lanreotide or octreotide in intramuscular injection) in combination with androgen ablation therapy (using intramuscular injections of the LHRH analog triptorelin, 3,75 mg every 4 weeks or 11,25 mg every 3 months). Currently, more than 50 patients have entered this trial with 41 patients having a follow-up of more than 6 months (Koutsilieris et al, manuscript in preparation).

In a preliminary report of the first 4 patients receiving the anti-survival factor therapy[565], we observed major improvements in objective parameters by biochemical monitoring, such as reduction in PSA and alkaline phosphatase (AP) levels, as well as significant improvements in bone pain, analgesic requirements, and patient performance status. These initial responses to ASF were confirmed in a larger cohort of patients[471], where we documented major and sustained responses of serum PSA and AP, as well as prolonged improvements in performance status and bone pain control. Further clinical trials are currently under way to define whether the combination of the anti-survival factor regimen with LHRH-A in patients who failed CAB can prolong the survival of these stage D3 patients. Definitive comparisons of the efficacy of this regimen vs conventional strategies, e.g. combination chemotherapy, will be performed only after completion of randomized controlled clinical trials, which are in progress.

It must, however, be emphasized that the first clinical applications of the anti-survival factor therapy have revealed encouraging results, which indicate that it merits further clinical evaluation. First, this is a very well tolerated regimen, which had no life-threatening side effects. The combination of dexamethasone and somatostatin analogs may contribute to insomnia, myopathy and hyperglycemia in a small number of patients (10%). However, these side effects were transient and resolved upon tapering of dexamethasone or were effectively controlled with appropri-

7. BONE MICROENVIRONMENT PARTICIPATION IN THE DEVELOPMENT OF ANDROGEN ABLATION REFRACTORINESS

ate lifestyle (e.g. diet) modifications or adjustments in insulin dosage. Second, this combination therapy led to major improvement in parameters of quality of life, such as bone pain and performance status[471], in patients who were very compromised at baseline. Third, although the majority patients with more than 12 months of follow-up have relapsed, their post-relapse performance status and bone pain were still significantly improved compared to their baseline status (i.e. at the onset of the combination therapy), even for several months after relapse. Fourth, in metastatic prostate cancer patients who developed resistance to CAB, their overall survival has historically been in the range of 10 months, even when salvage chemotherapy was administered. Patients enrolled in clinical trials of LHRH-A in combination with SM-A plus dexamethasone had already failed both anti-androgen withdrawal and salvage chemotherapy, thus suggesting that their (median) overall survival would be expected to be less than a year. However, in the initial cohort of patients receiving the combination therapy the median overall survival is clearly longer than 12 months[471], providing some evidence of a potential survival benefit offered by this combination therapy. Conversely, it may be reasonable to hypothesize that if the anti-survival factor-based combination therapy is administered at earlier stages of the disease, e.g. to patients who have just failed CAB and anti-androgen withdrawal, it may offer a more significant increase in their overall survival, as well as improved quality of life.

The responses to the anti-survival factor therapy-based combination cannot be attributed to favorable baseline clinical characteristics of our patients since all of them had diffuse bone metastases (> 6 foci) and short clinical responses to CAB (<12 months), which both correspond to strong adverse prognostic factors[464-466, 566]. Furthermore, all patients had significantly compromised performance status (median baseline ECOG score of 3). Finally, one of the most encouraging features of the anti-survival factor approach is that its combination with LHRH-As can re-introduce (in patients who had failed all available treatment options including LHRH-A based treatment) clinical responsiveness in the presence of LHRH analogs.

It is important to clarify why the responses achieved by the combination of LHRH analogs with dexamethasone and a somatostatin analog most likely constitute a "re-introduction of response to androgen ablation" rather than a response to dexamethasone only, somatostatin analog only or their combination, irrespective of the administration of an LHRH analog. First, it should be noted that neither dexamethasone nor somatostatin analog monotherapies have been shown to achieve durable responses in stage D3 patients with the aforementioned powerful adverse prognostic features (>6 bone metastases, <12 month clinical response to

CAB, median ECOG score of 3). Second, there have been no pre-clinical data to suggest that a combination of dexamethasone with a somatostatin analog would yield objective and symptomatic responses in the absence of LHRH analog-based androgen suppression. Third, the only clinical trial designs that could unequivocally prove that the ASF + LHRH-A combination is superior to both ASF alone and LHRH-A monotherapy cannot be performed. It should be remembered that dexamethasone blocks the secretion of adrenal androgens, thus reinstating a modified form of CAB.

In the past, various clinical trials have investigated the use of glucocorticoids or somatostatin analogs in prostate cancer. However, the rationale for their use was not oriented towards suppression of survival factor(s) and the schedule was often markedly different, which may also explain why the observed responses, if any, were quite short. This anti-survival factor-oriented rationale for the administration of glucocorticoids is a novel concept, totally different from the previously reported uses of glucocorticoid in the prostate cancer literature[477, 567-575]. In these studies, the administration of glucocorticoids was either empirically attempted or constituted a glucocorticoid replacement therapy in the setting of aminoglutethimide-induced "medical adrenalectomy", intending for, what was hoped to be, a more complete androgen blockade for prostate cancer. Objective responses (with a rate of 10-20%) and/or transient symptomatic improvement were recorded in some trials[477, 574, 575], although some of these studies were performed prior to the recognition of the concept of the "anti-androgen withdrawal syndrome" which could explain the results. It is, thus, unclear if the responses observed in these studies were indeed associated with glucocorticoid use or with concomitant (yet inadvertent and not documented) response due to the anti-androgen withdrawal syndrome. In fact, it is conceivable that a major part of the efficacy of adrenolytic agents (e.g. ketoconazole) in advanced prostate cancer[574], may, in fact, be due to the concomitant administration of glucocorticoids, which are necessary to prevent the side effects of adrenal failure resulting from ketonazole.

The contrast between the results of prior (non "anti-survival factor-oriented") uses of glucocorticoids and the efficacy that one might predict based on the *in vitro* effectiveness of dexamethasone to block paracrine survival factors, mainly skeletal IGF-1, is probably explained by the existence of GH-dependent sources of IGF-1, such as the liver. With regard to somatostatin analogs, they have also been previously tested in clinical trials for advanced stage prostate cancer, but the rationale for their administration was to produce either a somatostatin-receptor-mediated anti-proliferative or pro-apoptotic effect on metastatic cancer cells or to achieve a selective targeting of somatostatin receptor positive cancer cells

7. BONE MICROENVIRONMENT PARTICIPATION IN THE DEVELOPMENT OF ANDROGEN ABLATION REFRACTORINESS

using cytotoxic compounds linked to somatostatin analogs[576-582]. The unimpressive results of these efforts of somatostatin analog monotherapy, underline the importance of combined blockade of both endocrine (GH-dependent, liver-derived) and paracrine (osteoblast-derived) IGF-1. In fact, somatostatin analog monotherapy cannot offer a complete survival factor ablation in bones. Instead, a complete anti-IGF therapeutic approach should include both glucocorticoids and a long-acting somatostatin analog, in order to achieve a more comprehensive "anti-survival factor" (ASF) therapy.

An important question is whether the LHRH-A should be combined with the ASF therapy or whether the ASF strategy can account for all the activity of the ASF + LHRH-A combination. The current experience, as well as extensive pre-clinical data, suggest that LHRH-A should be a part of the combination. Although IGF-1 potently promotes prostate cancer cell survival and its suppression enhances the activity of pro-apoptotic stimuli (e.g. androgen suppression), it is unlikely that suppression of IGF-1 anti-apoptotic activity per se can suffice to induce extensive tumor responses *in vivo*. In fact, testicular androgens are more potent stimulators of growth and survival for prostate cells than IGF-1 and their levels would gradually rise if LHRH-A use were to be discontinued following progression from CAB therapy. Although such a return of testicular androgens to their baseline levels following discontinuation of LHRH-A therapy might be delayed (mainly due to prolonged prior testicular suppression in this group of, often elderly, patients), such an increase in circulating androgens would provide cancer cells with a potent growth and survival stimulus, capable of overriding the potential therapeutic benefit conferred by the suppression of IGF-1. The bone metastases of prostate cancer at stage D3 are resistant to androgen ablation, but not unresponsive to any androgenic stimulus to which they may be exposed. The available data, therefore, support the notion that the ASF therapy must be combined with LHRH-A.

Prostate cancer remains an "androgen-responsive" disease even when it acquires an "androgen ablation-refractory" phenotype. It may therefore be tempting to hypothesize that some part of the activity of the ASF regimen might be due to a decrease of residual androgen levels. The prolonged LHRH-A use in these patients leaves almost no room for significant further reduction of testicular androgens. In term of adrenal androgens, glucocorticoids can indeed suppress the production of anterior pituitary-derived adrenocorticotropic hormone (ACTH), which is the stimulus for adrenal androgen secretion. However, several pieces of information indicate that the activity of the ASF regimen is not likely to be primarily due to adrenal androgen suppression: since all patients enrolled in these studies have previously relapsed from CAB, which included an anti-androgen, e.g. flutamide. This implies that adrenal androgens were no longer having a major contribution to the mechanisms whereby cancer cells acquired hormone refractoriness. A role of the antiandrogen itself is however a possibility. Contrary to the pre-treatment low levels of circulating DHEAs, the mean serum IGF-1 levels (which were not suppressed at baseline) are significantly decreased, as a result of the ASF therapy, to levels at or well below the lower limits of normal[471]. Ongoing studies are expected to define the exact extent to which the IGF-1 suppression can account for the activity of the ASF-based combination. The currently available data, though, suggest that IGF-1 is a main target for this therapy, and that other, if any, mechanisms of action are having a supporting role to the one of IGF-1 down-regulation.

Other mechanisms which might contribute to the clinical responses to ASF-based combination include other known growth and survival factors locally produced in the bone microenvironment, namely PTHrP, interleukin-6 (IL-6) or fibroblast growth factors (FGFs). IL-6, a multifunctional cytokine produced by multiple sources in the bone microenvironment e.g. bone marrow stromal cells[583, 584], osteoclasts[585] or osteoblasts[586] can also confer resistance against cisplatin and etoposide-induced cell death in PC-3 and DU-145 prostate cancer cells[587]. Serum IL-6 levels are significantly elevated in hormone-refractory prostate cancer patients, compared to earlier stages of the disease or to benign prostatic hyperplasia patients [588]. The precise role of IL-6 in the establishment of the hormone refractory phenotype *in vivo* remains to be elucidated. The fact that glucocorticoids can also down-regulate the IL-6 production from osteoblasts[589-591] might suggest a role for IL-6 as a potential target for the ASF-based combination therapy.

It should be mentioned that for prostate carcinoma cells, at equimolar concentrations of IL-6 and IGF-1 is a more potent growth and survival factor than IL-6 *in vitro* (Koutsilieris M., unpublished observation), while, moreover, the serum IL-6 levels in advanced prostate cancer[588] are much lower than those of IGF-1. Basic FGF (bFGF), an angiogenic cytokine associated with *in vitro* epigenetic resistance to a wide range of cytotoxic drugs[592], could potentially be a target of the ASF-based combination. However, similarly to IL-6, bFGF achieves a protective effect comparable to the one of IGF-1 only at levels significantly higher than those found in the serum or bone marrow aspirates of patients with prostate cancer[593, 594] or various osteotropic neoplasias[595] serum levels of bFGF are again considerably lower than those of IGF-1, an observation which further reinforces the notion that the role, if any, of growth/survival factors other than

IGF-1, in the mechanism of action of the ASF-based combination therapy appears less significant.

Another question, which can be raised, is whether it is possible that other, non-survival factor-related, properties of the combination therapy could account for the observed objective and symptomatic responses. It must be noted that glucocorticoids have been reported, either to increase[596, 597] or not to change[598, 599] the PSA expression in human prostate cells. Such data indicate that the PSA decline observed during ASF-based combination therapy cannot merely be attributed to dexamethasone-induced suppression of PSA transcription. Furthermore, the PSA decline observed during responses to ASF therapy were accompanied by decreases in alkaline phosphatase and improved bone pain control and performance status. Conversely, at relapse, the PSA rise was associated with increasing alk. phosphatase and deteriorating performance status and bone pain. These events indicate that PSA changes during ASF therapy are closely paralleled by the changes in other parameters of objective and symptomatic responses, further indicating that PSA is a reliable marker of tumor burden in the setting of the ASF-based therapeutic approach. Importantly, the anti-inflammatory properties of dexamethasone per se, are unlikely to explain the clinical responses of our study, because bony metastases in prostate cancer are predominantly associated with deposition of woven bone tissue rather than the presence of inflammatory infiltrates[460].

Despite the encouraging and durable responses to the ASF-based regimen, almost all patients who have been followed for more than 12 months eventually relapse. However, even when there is disease progression, performance status and overall quality of life remained significantly improved, for several months post-relapse, in comparison to the patients' baseline (at onset of ASF combination therapy). It is of interest to investigate the molecular mechanisms responsible for disease progression from this combination therapy, with the goal to define clinically applicable methodologies that could extend the duration of patients' responses. It is possible that relapse from ASF therapy has multi-factorial etiology. Obviously, all patients enrolled in this clinical trial were at far advanced stages of their disease and had failed all available conventional treatment modalities. In these patients, tumor cells are likely to have acquired a more aggressive biological behavior, than at earlier disease stages, a situation which may in turn contribute to more aggressive growth and survival of the cancer cells, despite major suppression of IGF-1. Furthermore, IGF-1, at least in terms of its circulating levels, is significantly suppressed by the ASF combination, but not completely shut down. This suggests that there may be room for improving the efficacy of ASF therapy, by more comprehensive neutralization of IGF-1 survival factor activity, e.g. by combining dexamethasone and somatostatin analogs with other investigational agents capable of blocking down-stream events of IGF-1 / IGF-1R signaling in tumor cells. It may also be reasonable to explore potential strategies to block the survival factor effect of other molecules such as IL-6, bFGF, et.c. These latter molecules may be less efficient growth/survival factors for prostate cancer cells than IGF-1. However, their presence may confer a residual anti-apoptotic activity critical for sustaining the tumor cell survival when IGF-1 is significantly, suppressed.

It remains to be determined which of these or other putative mechanisms may be more responsible for the relapse from this current application of the ASF concept. Further clinical studies should also address the potential role of this combination therapy at earlier stage of prostate cancer. Importantly, it must be emphasized that, the "anti-survival factor therapy" concept is neither confined to only one survival factor (e.g. IGF-1), no matter how significant its role for tumor refractoriness may be, nor should it be focused entirely on a single strategy for neutralizing each survival factor's activity. Instead, the applications of the ASF concept should involve the targeting of multiple potential survival factors and at multiple levels of their mechanisms of anti-apoptotic action. Achieving the former goal will require the full characterization of the array of paracrine/autocrine and/or endocrine survival factors for prostate cancer or any other neoplasia where this therapeutic concept may be applicable.

Particular emphasis should be placed on defining the "hierarchy" of survival factors, i.e. to evaluate which are the major anti-apoptotic molecules on which each type of tumor primarily depends on for its protection from anti-cancer therapies, as well as to define secondary survival factors which may confer some residual degree of protection and substitute for the lack of "major" survival factors, if and when their activity is decreased. In some respect, the development of the currently tested IGF-1-oriented ASF-based therapy for prostate cancer was based on exactly this conceptual framework. Indeed, one may consider androgens to be the "primary" survival factor for prostate cancer cells. Once their concentrations are inhibited by CAB therapy, IGF-1, a less potent anti-apoptotic factor than androgens, but quite abundant in the bone microenvironment, can substitute for their absence and even activate the AR transcriptional activity, as previously reviewed[467]. To address the need for targeting the survival factors at multiple levels of their actions, future research efforts should investigate the regulation of their production, bioavailability, as well as their intracellular signaling pathways in cancer cells. These steps should facilitate the design of clinically applicable strategies to comprehensively neutralize as many of the aforementioned steps as possible.

Importantly these strategies should be designed in a manner that will selectively increase the sensitivity of cancer cells to pro-apoptotic therapies, both conventional and investigational, but spare normal tissues, or at least achieve an acceptable toxicity profile.

6. THE ROLE OF OSTEOCLASTS IN THE BONE METASTASIS OF PROSTATE CANCER: THE POTENTIAL USE OF BISPHOSPHONATES AS PART OF ASF THERAPY FOR STAGE D3 PATIENTS

Within the multi-step process of prostate cancer cells metastases to the bone, tumor cell invasion into the bone marrow is a critical event: it initially involves a diffuse pattern of tumor cell invasion into the bone marrow sinusoids (metastases), predominantly in bones with metabolically active "red" bone marrow. At this stage, the critical factor determining whether these invading prostate cancer cells shall establish metastatic sites, is directly associated with local tumor cell survival. While failure of immunologic surveillance is an important prerequisite for the development of metastases in any organ, their establishment in bones of prostate cancer patients, is directly linked with the ability of tumor cells to penetrate into the bone matrix, where conditions for growth/survival are more favourable, not only in terms of less pressure from immune surveillance, but, importantly, because of the opportunity to establish cell-cell interactions with bone cells (Figure 21).

The transition of prostate cancer cells from the bone marrow sinusoids to the bone matrix is a key step in the progression from the "seeding" of tumor cells to the actual establishment of the favourable "soil" for generation of a metastatic site. The entry of metastasing cells in the bone matrix is facilitated by osteoclast-mediated bone resorption which is an indispensable part of the naturally-occurring bone remodeling in the metabolically active bones. Alternatively, it has been hypothesized, that tumor cells can stimulate local resorption or can recruit osteoclasts, locally, and then stimulate their function. Using either mechanism, bone resorption (osteoclast-mediated or tumor cell-induced) promotes the first seed of what will eventually become the site of a bone metastasis. Therefore, inhibition of bone resorption at this particular stage of the disease could conceivably impede or decelerate the establishment of clinically detectable bone metastases.

Furthermore, biochemical markers of active bone resorption are significantly increased in the serum of prostate cancer patients with osteoblastic metastases[600-602], thus reinforcing the notion that osteoblastic metastases are associated with an extensive bone resorptive component[603, 604] that is caused primarily by osteoclasts[605]. Recent data indicate that prostate cancer cells directly stimulate osteoclastogenesis from osteoclast precursors in the absence of underlying stroma *in vitro*, by producing a soluble form of receptor activator of NF-B ligand (RANKL), a potent stimulator of osteoclastogenesis[606].

The above-mentioned data suggest that active osteoclasts may continue to play a role in sustaining the evolution of clinical evident bony disease in prostate cancer. Therefore, agents reducing bone resorption may modify the natural history of osteoblastic bone metastases. Bisphosphonates, a class of agents with known activity in reducing bone resorption in the setting of both neoplastic diseases[607, 608] and osteoporosis[609-612], including loss of bone density due to androgen ablation therapy in prostate cancer patients[613]. This experience has already prompted forthcoming studies on combinations of the ASF approach with bisphosphonates. The rationale of such a combination is that the bisphosphonates may complement the anti-survival factor approach by targeting the survival factor effect conferred upon cancer cells within the context of the resorptive process in the bone microenviroment in stage D3 disease. In addition, the 3rd generation bisphosphonate zolendronic acid exhibits direct cytotoxic activity against prostate[614] and breast cancer cells[615] *in vitro*. These multiple molecular and cellular levels of potential synergistic interactions between zolendronic acid and the ASF therapy has provided the framework for upcoming clinical trials of this combination for stage D3 prostate cancer patients.

It must be recognized that neither the prostate cancer cell genome and its alterations nor the bone microenvironment of a metastatic tumor, can completely control the behavior of the tumor. Instead, it is the dynamic interplay of these forces and of the components of the circulation that shape the tumors' biology. Therefore, future clinical applications of the ASF therapeutic strategy may have to be individualized to match the distinct pattern of genomic abnormalities in each patient's tumor cells while taking into account other cellular components of the bone microenviroment. Though challenging, this task will, in due time, become progressively more feasible, thanks to the major progress recently achieved in the fields of high-throughput global analyses of the genomic, and proteomic make-up of tumor cells.

COMBINED ANDROGEN BLOCKADE WITH NON-STEROIDALD ANTIOANDROGENS FOR ADVANCED PROSTATE CANCER: A REVIEW OF THE EVIDENCE OF EFFICACY AND TOXICITY

By Derek Nathan B.A., and Charles Bennett, M.D. Ph.D.

INTRODUCTION

Prostate cancer is the second leading cause of cancer death in men[120]. An estimated 21% of all newly diagnosed prostate cancer patients present with advanced disease, and the primary hormonal treatment for this stage of cancer has been castration[616]. It has been hypothesized that counteracting adrenal androgens can improve survival, which has been evaluated in 20 studies of combined androgen blockade therapy with non-steroidal anti-androgens[466, 617-634]. Although very close, the Southwest Oncology Group (SWOG) trial (NCI 0105) of combined androgen blockade with orchiectomy plus flutamide versus orchiectomy failed to reach a statistically significant increase in survival with combined androgen blockade[624, 635], while an earlier SWOG study (NCI 0036) of patients randomized to combined androgen blockade with flutamide plus daily leuprolide injections versus daily leuprolide injections found a 24% increase in survival[466]. Smaller trials and several overviews[322, 616, 636, 637] have found conflicting results. A 1995 meta-analysis did not find a statistically significant increase in survival with combined androgen blockade[637], while recent overviews, found a 3-5% statistically significant increase in five-year survival with combined androgen blockade when non-steroidal anti-androgens were used[322, 616, 636]. An evidence report recently prepared by the Blue Cross and Blue Shield Association Evidence-Based Practice Center questioned the clinical significance of this magnitude of difference, in light of the limited published data at 5 years and the increased adverse effects associated with combined androgen blockade[616]. A subsequent overview from the Prostate Cancer Trialists Collaborative Group stated that the "collaborative group makes no comment on whether, if real, a difference of a few percent in 5-year survival should be considered clinically significant."[322] Comment on these findings ranged from supporting a shared decision making approach[638] to suggesting that there is no role for combined androgen blockade[639]. In this review, we summarize the available information on efficacy and toxicity of combined androgen blockade.

DATA AND METHODS

This review was designed to evaluate the relative efficacy and toxicity of combined androgen blockade using any non-steroidal anti-androgen compared to castration alone for advanced prostate cancer.

For efficacy, randomized controlled trials of non-steroidal antiandrogen therapy in addition to castration compared to castration alone were reviewed. For toxicity, randomized and nonrandomized studies were included. Trials were included if they enrolled men with advanced prostate cancer who were not previously treated with hormonal therapy. The following groups were included: a) disseminated and/or symptomatic metastases; and b) asymptomatic metastatic disease or advanced, non-metastatic, disease. Sensitivity analyses were restricted to studies that provided separate data for stage D2 (M1) patients.

The efficacy data were based on reviews of CAB produced by the Blue Cross and Blue Shield Association Evidence-Based Practice Center[616], the Cochrane Controlled Trials Register, the CENTRAL register, and the VA Cochrane Prostate Disease and Urologic Malignancy register were searched for trials focused on non-steroidal anti-androgens for prostate cancer. Toxicity data were obtained from clinical trial adverse event reports and review of data obtained from MedWatch, the Food and Drug Administration's passive surveillance program.

ANALYSIS

Pooled odds ratios for survival were derived from: 1) directly abstracted information from individual studies providing the "number of surviving patients" at each time period or 2) the "percent survival" listed

8. COMBINED ANDROGEN BLOCKADE WITH NON-STEROIDAL ANTIANDROGENS FOR ADVANCED PROSTATE CANCER

in the report or calculated from the hazard rate. Second, the "number of patients at risk" and the "number reaching each endpoint" at 1, 2, or 5 years were obtained based on the provided "number at risk at baseline" and the "percent survival" at the corresponding time interval as calculated from the individual study hazard rates. The number at risk at follow-up was assumed to be equal to the number at risk at baseline, providing an underestimate of survival in trials with relatively few patients. It is unlikely to effect differences in survival between treatment arms.

Sensitivity analyses were conducted. Odds ratios for these studies did not vary by more than 10%. Additionally, the effect size and statistical significance of our results were compared to those in the evidence report from the Blue Cross and Blue Shield Association Evidence-Based Practice Center[616]. Data were analyzed with the random-effects model. If sensitivity analyses indicated that smaller or less well-designed studies changed the results, the studies were analyzed separately.

Adverse events included in clinical trial reports were categorized by system and pooled to estimate the frequency of event occurrence. Adverse events related to pneumonitis were also evaluated based on review of files from MedWatch, the FDA's passive reporting system. For this toxicity, we estimated occurrence rates based on number of MedWatch reports with this toxicity (numerator) and usage data for cases associated with bicalutamide and flutamide (denominator), as no cases were identified in clinical trials with these agents. Nilutamide-associated pneumonitis rate was based on phase III clinical trials adverse event reports.

OVERVIEW

EFFICACY

1. Clinical trial results

We identified 27 randomized controlled trials that compared survival with monotherapy to the outcomes of combined androgen blockade. Seven trials were excluded because a steroidal anti-androgen, cyproterone, was used. One trial comparing four regimens for combined androgen blockade was excluded because there was no comparison to monotherapy[640]. Twenty trials with 6,320 patients were included in this review.

Most patients (n=6,095) had distant metastases. Eight studies (n=3,271) included only patients with distant metastases[466, 617, 621, 624, 625, 630, 641]. Two studies had no information about percentage with M1 disease (n=225)[632]. In the remaining trials most patients (mean weighted percent=78%) had M1 disease (n=2,824).

8. Combined Androgen Blockade with Non-Steroidal Antioandrogens for Advanced Prostate Cancer

Twelve trials (n=4,672) used flutamide, eight (n=1,648) nilutamide, and none bicalutamide. Of the 6,320 enrolled patients, 5,523 were randomized to treatment or control and 5,432 (98.4%) were analyzable. Nineteen trials were 2-arm trials. One of these trials was a two-by-two factorial design[632]. For this review, the two monotherapy arms were pooled together as were the two combined androgen blockade arms. One 3-arm study compared monotherapy to two combined androgen blockade arms, each with a different dose of nilutamide[620]. Among the 20 eligible trials, the monotherapy was orchiectomy in nine studies (n=2,671), a LhRH agonist in ten studies (n=2,959); and orchiectomy or a LhRH agonist (n=690) in one study. All trials with flutamide used 250 milligrams three times daily. All but one of the trials with nilutamide used 300 milligrams daily. In one study and in one of the three arms in a second trial a dose of 150 milligrams daily was used[620, 623]. Data were available to calculate: overall survival at 1, 2, and 5 years in 13 studies (N= 4970 patients), 14 studies (N= 5286 patients), and 7 studies (N= 35 patients) respectively; progression-free survival at 1, 2 and 5 years in 7 studies (N= 2278 patients), 5 studies (N= 2141 patients), and 2 studies (N= 1017 patients), respectively; and cancer-specific survival at 1, 2 and 5 years in 5 studies (N= 1270 patients), 4 studies (N= 1232 patients), and 2 studies (N= 781 patients), respectively.

Eight studies specified the method of randomization[466,617-619,622,623,627,629]. Allocation was adequately concealed in six studies[466, 617-619, 622, 623]. Higher quality studies were defined as those that both blinded patients and investigators to group assignment and used intent-to-treat analysis of outcomes[466, 617, 620, 623, 626, 630, 632, 634].

2. Meta-analysis

Three studies reported a statistically significant increase in survival that favored combined androgen blockade with a 5-year survival advantage ranging from 3% to 9%[466, 622, 623]. The remaining 17 trials reported no significant difference. The proportion of patients surviving with combined androgen blockade compared to control was 84.6% vs 84.0% at 1 year, 58.6% vs 55.6% at 2 years, and 30.1% vs 24.9% at 5 years. The pooled estimate of the odds ratio for overall survival progressively increased with time (Odds Ratio=1.03 (95% CI: 0.85 to 1.25) at 1 year, odds ratio=1.16 (95% CI: 1.00 to 1.33) at 2 years, and odds ratio=1.29 (95% CI: 1.11 to 1.50) at 5 years). When only studies with more than 90% M1 disease were included, the point estimate of the odds ratio for overall survival was significant only at 5 years. The odds ratio was 1.08 (95% CI: 0.86 to 1.38) at 1 year, 1.12 (95% CI: 0.94 to 1.32) at 2 years, and 1.25 (95% CI: 1.05 to 1.48) at 5 years. When analysis was limited to studies identified as being of high quality, the pooled odds ratio for overall survival progressively increased but was not significant at any follow-up interval. The odds ratio was 1.02 (95% CI: 0.67 to 1.55) at 1 year, 1.21 (95% CI: 0.93 to 1.32) at 2 years, and 1.34 (95% CI: 0.96 to 1.87) at 5 years.

Studies used varying definitions for progression-free survival, generally based on either PSA failure, bone scan changes, or clinical evaluation. The pooled odds ratio for progression-free survival was determined for specific follow-up time intervals and progressively decreased at 2 years and 5 years. There were no differences detected in progression-free survival at later follow-up. The pooled odds ratio at 1 year was 1.38 (95% CI: 1.15 to 1.67), 1.19 (95% CI: 0.97 to 1.46) at 2 years and 1.14 (95% CI: 0.77 to 1.68) at 5 years. Similarly, cancer-specific survival progressively increased over time and became statistically significant at 5 years. However, the results are limited by the fact that only 2 studies reported 5-year results for progression-free and cancer-specific survival and both of these studies were positive [622, 623]. The pooled odds ratio of cancer-specific survival was 1.20 (95% CI: 0.92 to 1.57) at 1 year, 1.22 (95% CI: 0.86 to 1.73) at 2 years and 1.58 (95% CI: 1.05 to 2.37) at 5 years.

TOXICITY

1. Clinical trial results

The majority of side effects reported in clinical studies with the non-steroidal anti-androgens are associated with their pharmacological effects (Table 9). The pharmacological effects of the anti-androgen class are

TABLE 9. Incidence of Pharmacological Events of Non-Steroidal Anti-Androgens*

	FLUTAMIDE	NILUTAMIDE	BICALUTAMIDE
MONOTHERAPY	Incidence (%)	Incidence (%)	Incidence (%)
Gynecomastia	13-86	50	16-60
Breast Pain	36-47	26	24-76
Hot Flashes	2-3	24-54	5-28
CAB THERAPY	Incidence (%)	Incidence (%)	Incidence (%)
Gynecomastia	1-24	1-4	6
Breast Pain	4-20	–	4
Hot Flashes	14-74	28-77	49

*Adapted from McLeod et al[642]

those that result from the chemical activity of the blockade of the androgen receptor. Less common side effects result from non-pharmacological events, which are attributed to the chemical structure of the anti-androgens, and usually are associated with the metabolites that result from the breakdown of the anti-androgens (Table 10).

There appear to be no clinically relevant differences between the three non-steroidal anti-androgens with respect to the severity of pharmacological adverse events. Gynecomastia and breast pain, common pharmacological side effects of the anti-androgen class, are reported more frequently with anti-androgen monotherapy than with either combined androgen blockade (CAB) or castration alone[642]. Hot flashes, which are a common side effect of castration, are seen more regularly during the use of CAB or castration alone than during anti-androgen monotherapy[643]. In the only

TABLE 10. Incidence of Non-Pharmacological Events of Non-Steroidal Anti-Androgens*

	FLUTAMIDE	NILUTAMIDE	BICALUTAMIDE
GASTROINTESTINAL EVENTS	Incidence (%)	Incidence (%)	Incidence (%)
Nauseas, Vomiting, and Abdominal Discomfort (Monotherapy)	5-6	Up to 65	6
Diarrhea (Monotherapy)	10-20	2-4	2-5
Nauseas, Vomiting, and Abdominal Discomfort (CAB therapy)	3-13	4-20	8-10
Diarrhea (CAB therapy)	14-24	2-4	1-10
HEPATIC TOXICITY	Incidence (%)	Incidence (%)	Incidence (%)
Laboratory Test Abnormalities	10	2-33	6
Clinical Hepatoxicity Requiring Treatment Discontinuation	3	1-3	1
CARDIOVASCULAR EVENTS	Minimal	Minimal	Minimal
HEMATOLOGICAL TOXICITY	10	7	7
OCULAR EVENTS	0	11-50	0
INTERSTITIAL PNEUMONITIS	0.06-0.13	1-2	0.02–0.05
PULMONARY FIBROSIS	Rare	1	Rare

*Adapted from McLeod et al[642]

double-blind comparison of flutamide versus bicalutamide, each administered in combination with an LHRH-A, the incidences of gynecomastia and hot flashes were similar[640].

Non-pharmacological adverse events have been reported for all three anti-androgens. All three drugs appear to affect adversely the gastrointestinal system, although the three compounds affects differ with respect to the nature, frequency, and severity of these adverse events[642]. Whether used as monotherapy or part of CAB, the three non-steroidal anti-androgens cause slightly more nausea, vomiting, and abdominal pain than castration alone[617, 629]. In the double-blind study of flutamide plus LHRH-A versus bicalutamide plus LHRH-A, 7% of the former and 8% of the latter, experienced nausea related to the treatment, while nausea was reported in over 10% of both groups, regardless of the cause of the adverse event[640, 643]. The incidence and severity of diarrhea with flutamide is greater than with either bicalutamide or nilutamide. In monotherapy studies, a daily dosage of 750 mg flutamide was associated with diarrhea rates of 10%-20%, and resulted in 5%-20% of the group discontinuing therapy[644, 645]. In the randomized studies of non-steroidal anti-androgens as part of CAB, rates of diarrhea in the range of 14% to 24% with flutamide have been reported, versus 1% to 10% for bicalutamide and 2% to 4% for nilutamide (Table 10).

Abnormal liver function tests, such as elevated transaminases, have been seen during clinical trials with each of the three non-steroidal anti-androgens. While some of the abnormal test results are due to concomitant medications or preexisting diseases, treatment with the anti-androgens cannot be ruled out as a cause. This toxicity has been reported with all three non-steroidal anti-androgens although the three compounds differ with respect to the nature and severity of the reported adverse events. Hepatic failure has been reported as a not infrequent event with both flutamide and nilutamide, and in approximately 1% of patients treated with bicalutamide[629, 643, 646, 647].

The potential of hepatic toxicity during anti-androgen treatment necessitates the periodic monitoring of liver function. The prescribing information for all three anti-androgens advises that transaminase levels be measured prior to starting therapy, at regular intervals for the first four months of treatment, and periodically thereafter. Therapy with patients on anti-androgens should be discontinued immediately if liver function is persistently abnormal or accompanied by symptoms such as anorexia, nausea, vomiting, fatigue, discolored urine, pruritus, or jaundice. Discontinuation of the anti-androgen treatment usually reverses abnormalities.

While steroidal anti-androgens, such as cyproterone, have been associated with clinical cardiovascular toxicity, a similar finding has not been reported when non-steroidal anti-androgens have been used[629]. In the double-blind study of flutamide plus an LHRH-A versus bicalutamide plus an LHRH-A, the incidence of cardiovascular adverse events was comparable in both groups, when all adverse events were considered, regardless of the cause of the event[640]. Anti-androgens are expected to decrease hemoglobin during therapy. In one monotherapy study, treatment with nilutamide gave rise to significantly lower hemoglobin levels compared with pretreatment values[648]. The prescribing information for nilutamide suggests that periodic blood counts be ordered during the first three months of treatment, while that of flutamide advises monitoring of methemoglobin levels in patients who are susceptible to aniline toxicity and who smoke.

Delayed adaptation to darkness is an adverse event that is seen frequently with the use of nilutamide[617, 629, 648]. Interstitial pneumonitis has also been attributed to nilutamide. In a recent comparison of nilutamide as a part of CAB versus bicalutamide monotherapy, withdrawal of therapy in 4.5% of the nilutamide group was required due to interstitial pneumonitis[649]. The prescribing information for nilutamide suggests that a chest radiograph be performed prior to treatment, and warns that if any new or worsening shortness of breath is experienced by the patient during treatment, the drug should be discontinued immediately until it can be determined if the symptoms are drug related.

Only one study has assessed the effect of combined androgen blockade on quality of life[635]. After a 3-month follow-up patients receiving flutamide and orchiectomy reported more diarrhea (8.6% vs 2.7%) than those treated with orchiectomy alone. At both the 3-month and 6-month follow-up, patients receiving combined androgen blockade reported significantly worse emotional functioning.

2. MedWatch data

We have also investigated the occurrence of one serious drug-associated toxicity, pneumonitis, using MedWatch data obtained from the Food and Drug Administration. This toxicity occurs in 1% to 2% of nilutamide-treated patients. While no flutamide- or bicalutamide-associated cases have been observed among 8,000 patients treated on phase III clinical trials, two case reports describes one case of flutamide-associated and one of bicalutamide-associated interstitial pneumonitis[650, 651]. Consequently, because of concern that interstitial pneumonitis might represent a class effect, post-marketing surveillance data were reviewed.

We identified 12, 16, and 50 cases of bicalutamide-, flutamide-, or

8. COMBINED ANDROGEN BLOCKADE WITH NON-STEROIDAL ANTIOANDROGENS FOR ADVANCED PROSTATE CANCER

nilutamide-associated pneumonitis, respectively, from this data source. Death from respiratory failure occurred in 3 bicalutamide-treated (25%), 7 flutamide-treated (46%), and 4 nilutamide-treated patients (8%). Survivors and non-survivors were similar with respect to duration of symptoms prior to diagnosis (median of 14 days and 9 days, respectively), while non-survivors had taken non-steroidal antiandrogens for shorter periods of time prior to the onset of symptoms (median of 3.5 weeks versus 8 weeks, respectively, p<0.01) and had more frequent occurrences during the time in which non-steroidal antiandrogen monotherapy preceded initiation of LhRH treatment (35.7% vs 3.2%, respectively [p<0.01]). Drug associated pneumonitis was estimated to develop in 0.06% to 0.13% flutamide-treated patients and 0.02% to 0.05% bicalutamide-treated patients. In contrast, clinical trials with nilutamide report an incidence of 1% to 2%[642].

INTERPRETATION

We found that the pooled estimates of the odds ratios for survival increased in favor of combined androgen blockade over time and were small, but statistically significant, when evaluated at 5-years of follow-up, but were not significantly different at 1-year and 2-year followup periods. Progression-free survival appeared to be improved with combined androgen blockade at the end of the first year, based on positive findings reported for three of seven studies[466, 618, 622-624, 629, 632], but not at later follow-up. Quality of life data were reported in one study, thus limiting our ability to incorporate this outcome measure in the overview analyses. Toxicity data indicate that these drugs are generally well-tolerated, although pharmacologic and non-pharmacologic adverse events have been noted.

In summary, after 12 years of clinical experience, efficacy data based on 27 RCTs with CAB, and toxicity data based on marketing surveillance of hundreds of thousands or patients, this therapy is well understood when used for metastatic prostate cancer patients. The more important questions in the future pertain to CAB when used for neoadjuvant treatment for radiation therapy patients. As use in these settings increase, consideration needs to be given to toxicities identified in the metastatic disease

The limitations of this study must be addressed. First, the quality of the analyses in this literature based overview are dependent on the quality of the original data. Only seven of the trials included 5-year follow-up for overall survival data, with three of these studies being ones for which statistically significant increased survival with combined androgen blockade were noted. However, it is reassuring that the estimates of increased survival derived in this literature-based effort is about the same as that included in the Prostate Cancer Trialists overview (2.9% increase in 5-year survival, 2p=0.005). The follow-up by the Trialists was typically for five years[322]. Similarly, while progression-free survival was improved at 1-year of follow-up, this estimate was based on data included in only 7 clinical trials. Three of these 7 studies were the clinical trials which found statistically significant increases in survival with combined androgen blockade[466, 622, 623]. Second, randomized clinical trials have not addressed second line use of non-steroidal anti-androgen, after initial progression. This strategy is undoubtedly less costly. Third, class differences in non-steroidal anti-androgens exist, such that diarrhea, the most common toxicity of flutamide therapy may be less of a concern with agents such as bicalutamide[640]. Phase III studies with bicalutamide as combined androgen blockade versus monotherapy have not been reported.

In conclusion, the most recent overviews consistently indicate that there is about a 3% improvement in 5-year survival rates with combined androgen blockade. Uncertainty centers on whether this increase is clinically meaningful. We feel that clinicians and patients should discuss the likelihood of a small to modest benefit for some individuals, the likelihood of $3600 annually in out-of-pocket costs for most patients, and the potential for side effects. There is empirical evidence that these discussions are occurring in some health care settings. For example, the most common reason that Veterans with prostate cancer shift to the VA system is because of anti-androgen costs, reflecting gaps in the availability of insurance coverage for prescription drugs in this population[652]. We conclude that clinicians and patients should discuss costs, potential toxicities, and potential benefits when considering the addition of a non-steroidal anti-androgen to castration.

Pathologic Changes Induced by Hormone Therapy in Normal Prostate Carcinoma

By Bernard Têtu and Theodurus H. van der Kwast

Key words: Androgen blockade, prostate cancer, hormone therapy.

ABSTRACT

Pathologists are increasingly aware of the changes induced by androgen ablation on prostatic tissue. Maximal Androgen Blockade (MAB), combining an LHRH agonist and a pure anti-androgen, induces significant downsizing of prostate cancer, especially in organ-confined disease. Indeed, tumor volume or density are reduced by approximately 40% after 3 months of MAB and by an additional 60% after 6 months. This is translated by an average 20% decrease in capsular penetration and 25% reduction in surgical margin involvement. On histology, normal prostate tissue and tumor undergo marked atrophy and shrinkage. Residual cancer cells may be very sparse and no cancer is found in up to 8% of cases. More significant is the apparent increased Gleason score induced by MAB which current knowledge relates to marked reduction of cancer cell number. Under MAB, residual cancer cells show evidence of lower activity and increased apoptosis. Such therapy-induced changes may be reversible, supporting the need for prolonged therapy. Furthermore, certain cases contain clones of tumor cells lacking therapy-induced changes, which most likely developed resistance to hormone therapy. Finally, the extent

9. PATHOLOGIC CHANGES INDUCED BY HORMONE THERAPY IN NORMAL PROSTATE CARCINOMA

of prostatic intraepithelial neoplasia (PIN) is markedly reduced under MAB and its morphology is strongly modified. Again, such changes may be reversible and may show evidence of resistance to therapy.

INTRODUCTION

For several decades, orchiectomy or high doses of estrogens were the only available forms of hormone therapy for prostate cancer[653, 654] and histologic changes induced by such treatments have been thoroughly described and are well recognized by most pathologists. However, in the last few decades, new drugs, such as Luteinizing Hormone-Releasing Hormone (LHRH) agonist and anti-androgens, have been introduced and increasingly used not only for advanced but also for localized disease. Pathologists can thus expect to see an increasing number of prostates with changes induced by such forms of treatment in radical prostatectomy specimens or on prostate biopsies.

LHRH AGONIST AND PURE ANTI-ANDROGEN

Changes to normal prostatic tissue

Maximal Androgen Blockade (MAB), combining an LHRH agonist and a pure antiandrogen, induces marked changes to benign prostatic tissue. Prostatic atrophy is present in more than 70% of cases whereas basal cell prominence, basal cell hyperplasia and epithelial cell vacuolization are found in more than 80% of cases and are very uncommon in prostates not exposed to MAB[655] (Figure 23). Furthermore, there is flattening and rupture of the epithelium of a variable number of benign prostatic glands with possible extravasation of prostatic secretion into the stroma[656]. The relative lack of androgen receptors in basal cells as opposed to epithelial and mesenchymal cells[657] may explain, at least in part, basal cell hyperplasia. It may be argued that basal cells do not respond to endocrine manipulation and therefore proliferate to compensate for the decrease of other cell types. However, we[658] recently demonstrated that, while basal cells proliferate more rapidly than luminal cells in normal conditions, following MAB, luminal cells show far more cycling activity than basal cells, more likely compensating for the rapid loss of androgen-responsive cells. Consequently, basal cell hyperplasia may reflect an imbalance between cell proliferation and cell death in both cell compartments.

9. Pathologic Changes Induced by Hormone Therapy in Normal Prostate Carcinoma

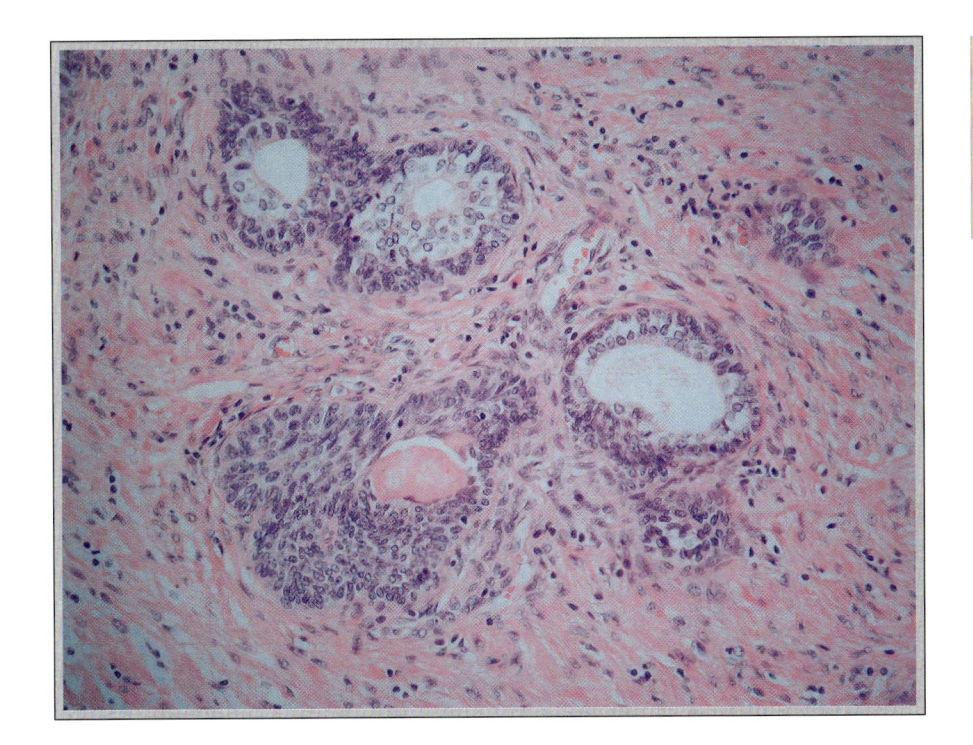

FIGURE 23. LHRH agonist and pure antiandrogen: epithelial cell vacuolization and basal cell hyperplasia (Hematoxylin and eosin, X200).

MAB leads to several characteristic changes that have been extensively described in the recent literature. Particularly striking is the significant downsizing of prostatic cancer volume, compared to prostates not exposed to MAB. By image analysis on histologic sections, after 3 months of MAB, we reported a 44% decrease in tumor volume compared to prostates not exposed to MAB ($p<0.007$)[655]. We found an additional 60% reduction in tumor volume following 3 additional months (6 months) of MAB[659]. Others reported decreased tumor size and density in 92% of patients with increased stroma in 88%[660]. There was a 40%[661] reduction of gland density and the area occupied by cancer cells was decreased by 50%[662]. A net downstaging of 10%[663], 20%[664] or 54%[665] has been achieved with MAB among stage B and C prostate cancers. However, in general, the effect seems to be more beneficial for stage B tumors[664]. The number of patients with pathologic stage D1 disease in the group exposed to MAB is usually not significantly different from that of patients who underwent surgery alone[664, 666, 667]. Furthermore, in our experience, the use of step sections and immunohistochemistry with cytokeratin stain does not improve the detection of lymph node micrometastases in MAB treated patients.

Downsizing of prostate cancer

Decreased margin invasion and capsular penetration

Table 11 summarizes data from the literature with respect to margin invasion and capsular penetration in prostate cancer under MAB. In stage B and C cancer, capsular penetration dropped from as high as 79%[663] or 81%[667] (average: 66%) in surgically-treated cases to as low as 19%[666] or 22%[665] (average: 41%) of cases only following MAB. Comparing data from the literature, there is thus a net improvement of capsular permeation of 25% and most studies found a statistically significant difference between both treatment groups. Margin involvement was also significantly decreased following MAB[660, 663, 665, 668, 669] and ranged from as high as 48%[669] in stage B to 74%[664] (average: 51%) in stage C surgically treated patients to as low as 8%[665] or 10%[666] (average: 28%) in those exposed to neoadjuvant MAB. The net improvement was also around 23%. Again, the advantage was found to be more significant for stage T2 (B) than for stage T3 (C) tumors[663, 664]. Certain authors claim that the use of immunostaining to cytokeratins, PSA and prostatic acid phosphatase were helpful at improving the detection of extracapsular extension and margin involvement[670] while others did not identify more cases with margin involvement than those detected by simple histologic examination[668]. After 6 months of MAB, capsular penetration[659] and margin involvement[659, 664] remained low but were not significantly different from the 3 month regimen. Comparing 3 and 8 months of therapy, Gleave et al[671] found a significant decrease of positive margins (17% at 3 months and 5% at 8 months) and organ-confinement remained high (71% at 3 months and 91% at 8 months). It is thus clear from those data that, under MAB, the total tumor burden is reduced and that a large proportion of tumor cells is destroyed.

TABLE 11. Influence of androgen blockade by monotherapy on margin invasion and capsular penetration.

Author	Number of patients Surgery/MAB	Stage	Margin invasion Surgery	MAB	Capsular penetration Surgery	MAB
Van Poppel et al, 1995[696] [1]	62/65	T2b, T3	46%	19%s[2]		
Dalkin et al, 1996[698] [3]	28/28	T1C, 2A, 2B	18%	18%	39%	43%
Goldenberg et al, 1996[699] [4]	101/112	T1bc, T2abc	65%	28%s	80%	58%s

Abbreviation: S: statistically significant;
Notes: [1] Estramustine phosphate only; [2] T2, posterolateral aspect of the prostate; for T3, positive margins were increased with the neoadjuvant therapy (40%/48%); [3] LHRH agonist only; [4] 12 weeks of cyproterone acetate only

Residual tumor

Residual tumor is often minimal after MAB and its detection needs a careful search. Occasional cases in the literature were found to lack residual cancer cells. Residual tumor was only present as a small focus of single cells in 8% of cases[655] or was reported to be "extremely focal" in 26%[672]. Occasionally, tumor cells were floating within branching spaces or "branching clefts"[660] that we designated as a "hemangiopericytoma-like pattern"[655, 656]. Furthermore, of patients treated by MAB for 3 months prior to surgery and whose prostate was totally embedded, certain studies failed to find residual tumor in 2%[663], 4%[666], 7%[665] and 8%[668] of cases. Additional step sections[673] and immunostaining for cytokeratins[668, 673] or Prostate Acid Phosphatase (PAP)[668] were successful at finding single microscopic foci of cancer in only part of those cases. After 3 additional months of therapy, again, no residual tumor was found in 10% of cases despite a thorough search[659]. Although others found cancer cells in all cases[660], those data clearly emphasize the dramatic decrease in tumor burden following MAB.

Those findings are important since smaller tumor size, organ confinement, lower margin involvement[674, 675], stage[676] and capsular penetration[420] are predictive of a better disease control and of better prognosis in patients not exposed to MAB. However, it is not clear whether the prognosis of prostate cancer depends on the status of the tumor at the time of diagnosis or at the time of surgery, after several months of neoadjuvant therapy. It has however been demonstrated that patients who receive prolonged MAB for more than 3 months[677] or 120 days[678] have a statistically significant biochemical survival advantage over those who are exposed to a similar treatment for a shorter time. This suggests that not only reduced tumor burden but also some form of irreversible biologic changes are necessary to improve the overall prognosis of those patients.

Morphologic changes to cancer cells

The histologic features and biologic characteristics of cancer tissue are strongly influenced by MAB. Overall, cancer glands undergo strong shrinkage with marked reduction in cell size[655, 672]. Ruptured adenocarcinomatous glands with mucin extravasation, comparable to pseudomyxoma ovariilike, has also been seen in 77% of cases, with mucin lakes occupying from less than 5% to as much as 100% of the tumor[679]. However, the most striking consequence of cancer cell shrinkage following MAB is the apparent increased Gleason score observed in most cases. Well-formed acinar structures are uncommon under MAB and cancer cells are mostly arranged in diffuse sheets, small glands or as single cells[655, 661, 672, 680, 681], features reminiscent of Gleason patterns 3 to 5 (Figure 24). In fact,

9. PATHOLOGIC CHANGES INDUCED BY HORMONE THERAPY IN NORMAL PROSTATE CARCINOMA

FIGURE 24. LHRH agonist and antiandrogen: increased Gleason score (Hematoxylin and eosin, X200).

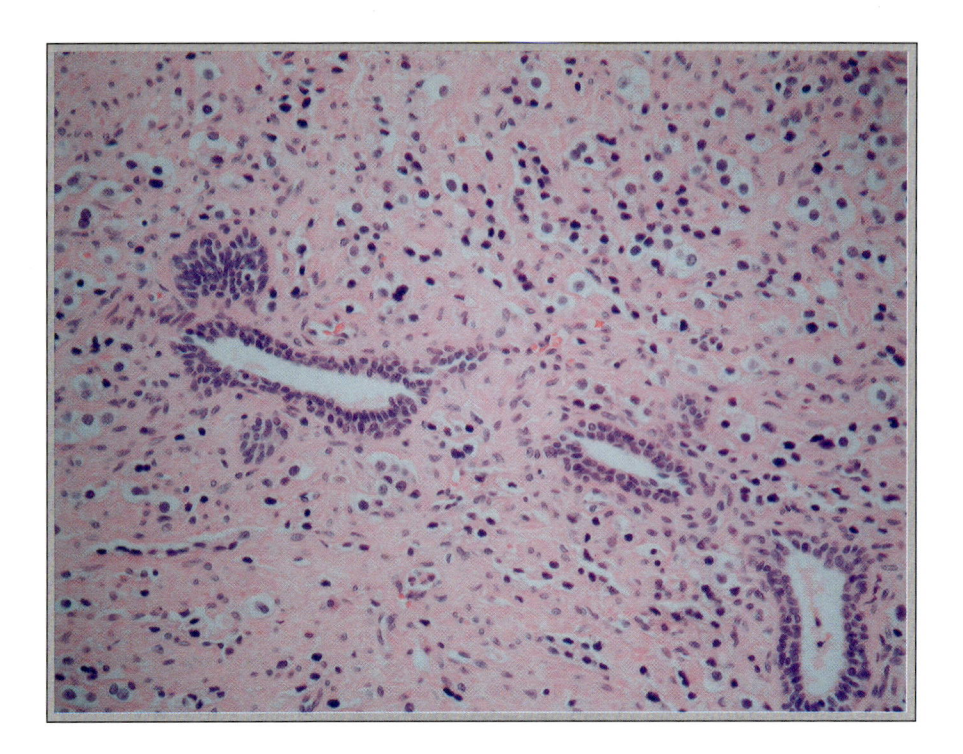

Armas et al[672] reported Gleason scores 7 to 10 in 94% of prostate cancers after MAB compared to only 26% in pre-treatment biopsies of the patients.

There are two possible explanations for these findings. On one hand, most of the tumor bulk may be destroyed by therapy, leaving only single viable or non-viable residual cancer cells with lower cell activity and undergoing apoptosis. On the other hand, as a result of the disappearance of most part of lower grade neoplasm, only the resistant higher grade component may persist which might suggest that MAB favors a selection of cancer cells with increased aggressiveness. In support to this latter hypothesis, Fair et al[666] reported that MAB-treated patients with persistence of disease beyond the prostate did significantly worse than those with comparable features treated by surgery alone. Furthermore, after androgen deprivation, there is increased loss of RB gene and erbB2 amplification[682] or overexpression[683-685], features of increased aggressiveness[684, 686], and AR expression by immunohistochemistry is markedly decreased[657], which could suggest a selection of androgen independant cells. However, most additional studies, as reported below, rather showed features of decreased activity by cancer cells following MAB and the bulk

9. PATHOLOGIC CHANGES INDUCED BY HORMONE THERAPY IN NORMAL PROSTATE CARCINOMA

of evidence rather supports the first hypothesis. Consequently, most authors now recommend not to use the Gleason score following MAB because of the lack of adapted criteria to grade those tumors, the poor reproducibility and the lack of biologic and clinical relevance of the grading after hormone manipulation[660, 672, 673].

Biologic changes in cancer cells

Several publications emphasized the small nucleolar size of prostate cancer cells exposed to MAB[655, 659, 672, 680, 687]. In fact, nucleolar diameter, as measured by image analysis, was reduced by close to 26% ($p<0.001$) after 3 months of MAB compared to surgery alone[655] and was further but not significantly reduced by 12% ($p=0.07$) after 6 months of MAB compared to a 3 month regimen[659]. Large nucleoli are generally regarded as a feature of high cell activity and is a major criterion in the diagnosis of prostate cancer. Decreased nucleolar size after MAB thus suggests decreased cellular activity. Furthermore, cell proliferation, as measured by Ki-67 (MIB-1) immunostaining is reduced by 46% after 3 months of MAB, compared to surgery alone, and by 33% after 6 months MAB compared to 3 months ($p<0.01$)[659]. Cancer cell proliferation, by Ki-67, was also reported to be markedly decreased in prostates exposed to 8 months of MAB compared to surgery alone[668]. Comparable data, using different technologies, have been reported by others. Armas et al[672] found that, of prostate cancers exposed to MAB, 67% had a PCNA (proliferating cell nuclear antigen) proliferation score of less than 10% whereas 90% of prostates not exposed to MAB had more than 10% proliferating cells. Similarly, 75% of cases exposed to MAB were diploid, by image analysis using Feulgen stains, and 80% of prostates from patients treated by surgery alone were nondiploid[672]. Finally, decreased mitotic activity has been reported in cancer cells of prostate exposed to MAB[687]. Overall, our data and those of the literature reveal that, following MAB, although cancer cells present apparent features of increased aggressiveness, most biologic parameters rather indicate lower cell activity compared to prostates not exposed to hormone manipulation. Similarly, the decreased expression of androgen receptors following MAB does not necessarily reflect a selection of androgen-independent cells since over 80% of endocrine-therapy-resistant human prostate cancers rather express intense levels of androgen receptors[496]. Furthermore, studies on apoptosis show that, not only cell activity is lower under MAB, but that also cell death is increased. Indeed, apoptic bodies are significantly more abundant in cancer cells under MAB[688]. Considering that those cancer cells have lower proliferative activity, the balance is clearly against cancer cells.

9. Pathologic Changes Induced by Hormone Therapy in Normal Prostate Carcinoma

Modified marker expression

Along with decreased biologic activity, the prevalence of expression of certain markers was also decreased following MAB. All patients submitted to MAB in our studies experienced a drastic reduction of serum PSA as well as a marked decrease of PSA staining by immunohistochemistry[656]. While 100% of cases had strong (+++) staining of both normal glands and cancer cells in prostatic tissue not submitted to MAB, merely 25% had such strong staining after 3 months of MAB. Comparable results were reported by others[689]. Similarly, as mentioned above, marked decrease of AR expression by immunohistochemistry was seen following MAB[657] in both normal glands ($p<0.001$) and cancer cells ($p=0.048$). Certain receptors were however upregulated following MAB. For instance, while Estrogen Receptors (ER) are virtually absent from prostatic tissue in patients treated by surgery alone, they were frequently overexpressed following MAB [690], but this expression was limited to stromal cells around prostatic glands and the significance of this finding is not clear.

Reversibility and resistance to therapy

Such changes are however reversible, at least under short term therapy. After 3 months of therapy, when MAB is discontinued for more than 19 days, nucleolar size tend to return to normal, suggesting a reactivation of cell activity[659]. Those findings are in keeping with the report that the cessation of short-term MAB is followed by an early rise in PSA[348]. Furthermore, certain cases show signs of possible resistance to treatment. In one of the very first studies on histologic changes under MAB, Murphy et al[661] reported therapy-induced changes of more than 25% of neoplastic glands in no more than 60% of cases, suggesting the presence of clones of resistant cancer cells in a fair subset of patients. Those patients have however received MAB for an average of 3 to 4 months[661]. This overall short term therapy may explain the relatively low rate of therapy-induced changes. However, more recently, we[659] found clones of cancer cells lacking typical regressive changes and high MIB-1 levels in approximately 10% of patients treated for more than 6 months and no significant delay before surgery (Figure 25). It is thus clear that cancer cells may develop resistance to MAB and that the delay between the cessation of MAB and surgery may be associated with signs of reactivation of cancer cells without evidence or resistance.

Changes on prostatic intraepithelial neoplasia

A significant reduction in the frequency[655, 660, 691] or extent of high grade prostatic intraepithelial neoplasia (PIN) as well as a more focal distribution[672] have been reported following MAB. Such findings have raised

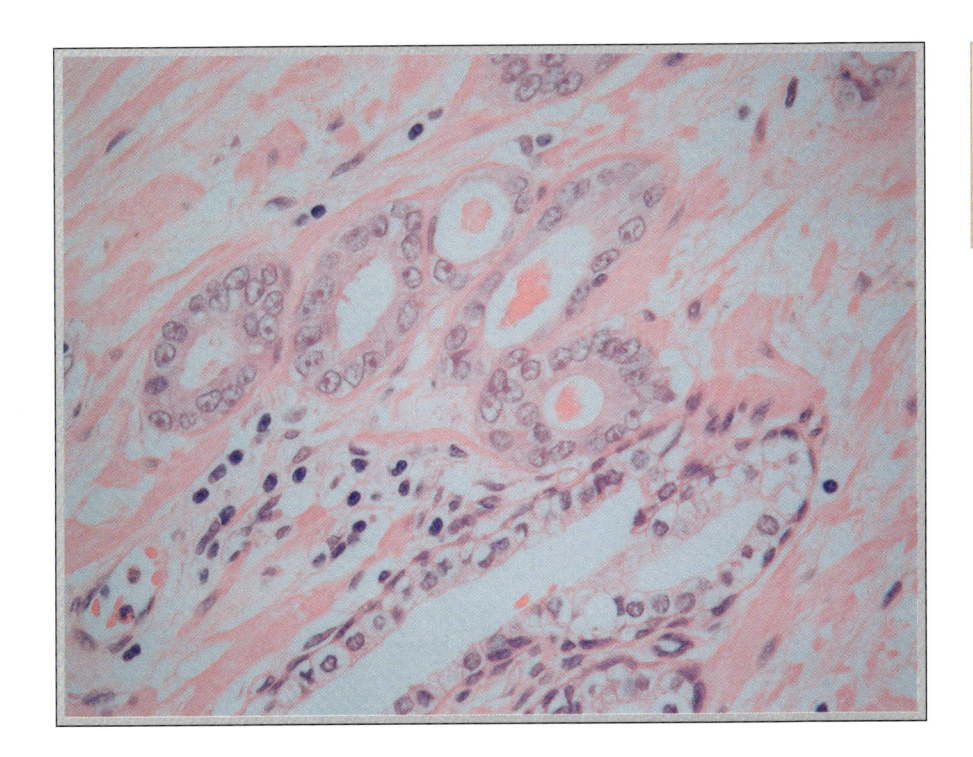

9. PATHOLOGIC CHANGES INDUCED BY HORMONE THERAPY IN NORMAL PROSTATE CARCINOMA

FIGURE 25. LHRH agonist and antiandrogen for 6 months: group of cancer cells lacking typical regressive changes (Hematoxylin and eosin, X400).

strong interest at using hormone therapy as a chemopreventive agent for prostate cancer. However, it is becoming clear that the criteria used to identify high grade PIN following MAB should be adapted because of the marked changes of cell morphology and it seems that persistent high grade PIN is more prevalent after MAB than initially reported. Indeed, nucleolar prominence, which is a hallmark of high grade PIN, is much less evident following MAB than in prostates not exposed to hormone therapy[655, 672, 692]. Using standard criteria, including nucleolar prominence as a key diagnostic criterion, we found high grade PIN in less than 10% of prostates exposed to MAB[655]. In order to be applicable for patients exposed to hormone manipulation, adapted criteria have been defined to distinguish high grade PIN from normal glands. They disregard nucleolar prominence and include increased nuclear size, nuclear crowding, anisonucleosis and disordered nuclear arrangement[693]. Using these adapted criteria, we showed that high grade PIN is present in 72% of cases after 3 months of MAB and in 59% at 6 months[693]. In the literature, high grade PIN was reported to range from 35%[660] to 83%[692] of cases following MAB. It is now clear that the tufted pattern, which is predominant in

9. Pathologic Changes Induced by Hormone Therapy in Normal Prostate Carcinoma

untreated prostates and, to a lesser extent in prostates exposed to 3 months of MAB, is virtually absent in prostates exposed to 6 months of MAB in which the flat pattern is predominant[693] (Figure 26a). Although the clinical significance of all those changes is unclear, they reflect a marked reduction of preneoplastic cell activity under MAB. However, it has also been found that when endocrine therapy is stopped more than one week before prostatectomy, even after 6 months of MAB, characteristic prominent nucleoli and MIB-1 positive cells reappear in most cases of high grade PIN[693] (Figure 26b), suggesting that those changes are reversible and that their eradication would need lifelong endocrine therapy[693]. Furthermore, the persistence of high grade PIN distant to cancer in 70% of cases and within the tumor in 20% and persistence of MIB-1 positive dysplastic cells even after 6 months of MAB suggest that, in certain cases, as for prostate cancer, residual high grade PIN may develop resistance to endocrine therapy[693].

Monotherapy

Estrogens are known to produce a number of well characterized morphological and immunohistochemical changes (Figure 27). In most cases, estrogens induce acinar atrophy, nuclear pyknosis, karyolysis of nuclei, decreased tumor size, vacuolation of cell cytoplasm, and squamous

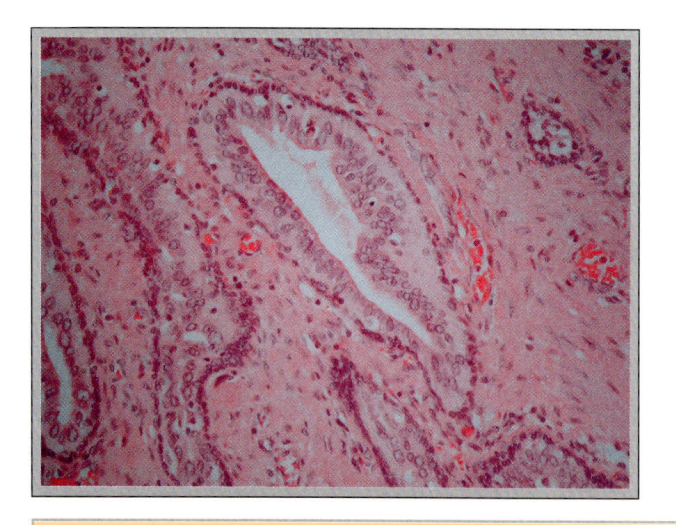

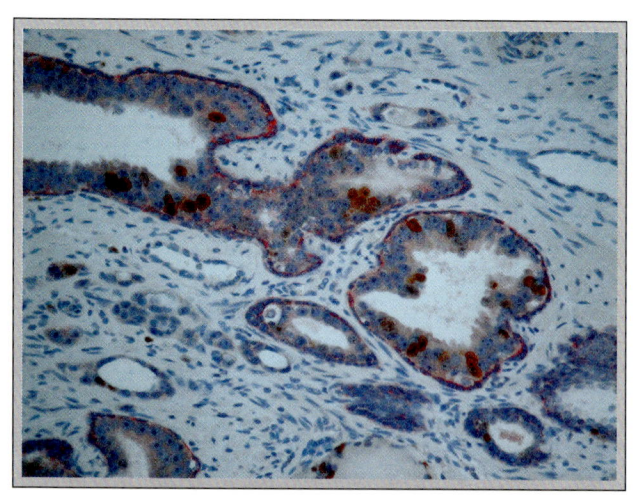

FIGURE 26. LHRH agonist and antiandrogen: **a)** prominence of flat PIN (Hematoxylin and eosin, X400); **b)** high grade PIN with characteristic prominent nucleoli and MIB-1 positive cells after interruption of endocrine therapy more than one week before prostatectomy (MIB-1 and 34βE12 immunohistochemistry, X400).

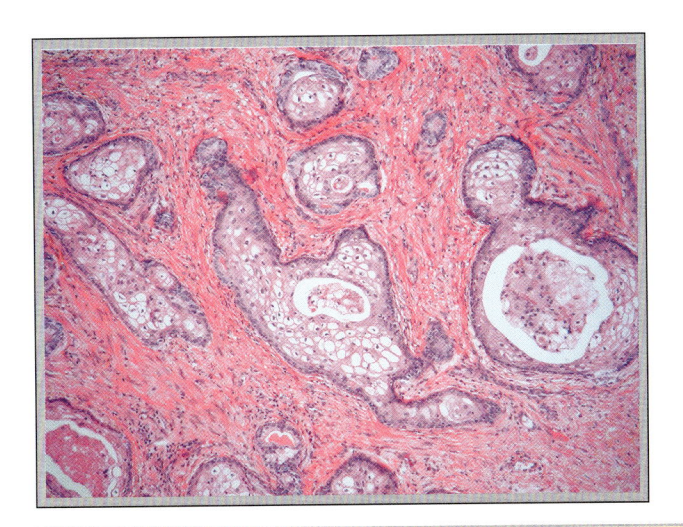

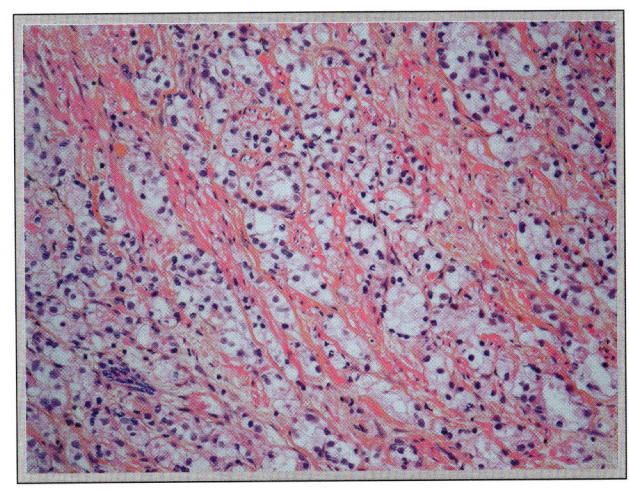

FIGURE 27. Estrogen therapy: changes induced to **a)** benign glands and **b)** cancer.

metaplasia in both benign and malignant components[694, 695]. Tumor size is also decreased. After 6 weeks of estramustine phosphate, a cytotoxic agent combining the effects of estrogens and an antimitotic spindle blocker effect, ultrasound showed that the tumor size decreased by 30% in T2b tumors and by 15% in T3 and that 48% of stage T3 tumors were clinically dowstaged to a stage T2 disease[696]. Furthermore, the Gleason score was increased in 70%[689] of cases. The staining for PAP and PSA was uniformly reduced in cancer following estrogen therapy[694]. Finally, there is also evidence that histologic regressive changes (vacuolization, pyknosis) under estrogen therapy are more pronounced in lower grade (acinar patterns) than in higher grade (cribriform and solid patterns) carcinomas[697].

Rare reports mention morphologic changes induced by antiandrogens only. Changes observed after 1 to 3 months of this treatment show similar changes but of smaller amplitude in normal prostatic tissue, whereas tumor cells are slightly modified[656]. Dalkin et al [698] using LHRH agonists only reported no improvement to margin invasion or organ-confinement compared to patients submitted to surgery alone (Table 12). Goldenberg et al[699], using cyproterone acetate alone, reported significant reduction in margin invasion and extra-prostatic extension. Marked atrophy and increased Gleason score, as found with MAB, were also observed[699]. Finasteride is a common agent used to treat benign prostatic hyperplasia and inhibits 5-alpha-reductase which converts testosterone to the more potent dihydrotestosterone. A recent study in which finasteride has been used in patients with prostate cancer and compared to prostates

9. PATHOLOGIC CHANGES INDUCED BY HORMONE THERAPY IN NORMAL PROSTATE CARCINOMA

TABLE 12. Influence of androgen blockage by monotherapy on margin invasion and capsular penetration.

Author	Number of patients Surgery/MAB	Stage	Margin invasion Surgery	MAB	Capsular penetration Surgery	MAB
Van Poppel et al, 1995[696] [1]	62/65	T2b, T3	46%	19%s[2]		
Dalkin et al, 1996[698] [3]	28/28	T1C, 2A, 2B	18%	18%	39%	43%
Goldenberg et al, 1996[699] [4]	101/112	T1bc, T2abc	65%	28%s	80%	58%s

Abbreviation: S: statistically significant;
Notes: [1] Estramustine phosphate only; [2] T2, posterolateral aspect of the prostate; for T3, positive margins were increased with the neoadjuvant therapy (40%/48%); [3] LHRH agonist only; [4] 12 weeks of cyproterone acetate only

of patients receiving a placebo, showed that cancer is morphologically unaltered and that the use of this drug should not cause difficulties at diagnosing prostate cancer in patients receiving this therapy for benign conditions[700].

Status of Androgen Blockade in Prostate Cancer in 2003

By Fernard Labrie

SUMMARY

The last 20 years have witnessed major advances in the field of prostate cancer, both in terms of diagnosis and treatment. This progress has resulted in a significant decrease of prostate cancer deaths in the population. In fact, using screening, practically 100% of prostate cancers can be diagnosed at a clinically localized or potentially curable stage, thus practically eliminating the diagnosis of metastatic and non curable disease. In fact, in the countries where screening is widely used, the diagnosis of advanced metastatic disease has become rare.

In addition to screening, the most important advance in the field of prostate cancer is androgen blockade, namely medical castration with LHRH agonists and combined androgen blockade. Despite the demonstrated benefits observed with combined androgen blockade in advanced metastatic disease, cure is a rare finding and treatment of localized disease should thus be the objective. Radical prostatectomy, external beam radiotherapy and brachytherapy can theoretically cure 50% to 60% of cases when the cancer is truly organ-confined. In 40% to 50% of cases, the cancer has already migrated outside the prostate, thus requiring systemic or endocrine therapy. Most importantly, taking mainly advantage of the extremely well tolerated castration with LHRH agonists, all the prospective randomized trials performed so far have demonstrated an important

10. STATUS OF ANDROGEN BLOCKADE IN PROSTATE CANCER IN 2002

prolongation of life in patients with localized prostate cancer treated with androgen blockade. In fact, in the six studies mentioned above, the improved survival ranges between 20% and 81% at 5 years of follow-up for patients who received androgen blockade for localized or locally advanced disease. While the very important benefits obtained so far in localized prostate cancer have been achieved with monotherapy (medical or surgical castration), there are good reasons to believe that even better results should be obtained with more complete androgen blockade or combined androgen blockade (CAB).

Detailed analysis of 57 patients who received combined androgen blockade (CAB) continuously for various time periods shows a 50% probability of no rise of PSA after cessation of CAB estimated at approximately 5 years of continuous CAB while a 90% probability of long term control or possible "cure" is obtained after a duration of treatment longer than 6.5 years. Long term control or possible cure is defined as the absence of PSA rise for at least 5 years after stopping androgen blockade.

The available data show that long term and continuous (not intermittent) androgen blockade is highly efficient and even curative in localized prostate cancer. Such treatment should be used without delay at the time of PSA rise in patients failing surgery or radiotherapy. The same treatment used alone should be considered for patients not candidates for other approaches due to poor general health, age or personal choice.

INTRODUCTION

Prostate cancer is the most frequently diagnosed cancer and the second cause of cancer death in men in North America. In fact, one out of nine men will be diagnosed with prostate cancer during his lifetime. At the present rate, prostate cancer will kill more than 3,000,000 men among the male population presently living in the United States. The medical and social consequences of prostate cancer in men are comparable to those of breast cancer in women.

The major source of controversy concerning early diagnosis and treatment of prostate cancer has been that, until recently, no prospective and randomized trial had shown statistically significant benefits of treatment of localized prostate cancer on survival[701, 702]. Such an absence of studies has been erroneously interpreted as being equivalent to the availability of negative data while, in fact, negative data have never been obtained in studies on the treatment of localized prostate cancer.

Most fortunately, six prospective randomized trials have recently demonstrated for the first time that an important prolongation of life was achieved in localized prostate cancer treated with androgen blockade[146, 342-345, 703]. In fact, the first prospective and randomized studies that have shown statistically significant benefits on survival in localized or locally advanced disease are those using androgen blockade. Quite remarkably, in various studies, the improved survival ranges between 20% and 81% at 5 years of follow-up.

IMPORTANCE OF DIAGNOSIS AT A LOCALIZED STAGE BY SCREENING

Since prostate cancer almost invariably develops insidiously without signs or symptoms until the non curable stage of bone metastases is reached, early treatment cannot be achieved without screening in asymptomatic men.

An important observation based on overwhelming scientific evidence is that prostate-specific antigen (PSA) can be efficiently used as a pre-screening test for prostate cancer, thus keeping the more costly and less well-tolerated digital rectal examination (DRE) and transrectal ultrasonography (TRUS) as second step procedures[323, 324, 704, 705]. Using this approach, practically 100% of prostate cancers can be diagnosed at a clinically localized or potentially curable stage, therefore practically eliminating the diagnosis of metastatic disease[323, 324, 706].

High Efficacy of Prescreening with PSA

The most important impact of screening, however, is on survival. Over a 10-year period starting in 1988 in the Quebec screening study, the annual cause-specific death rate incidences have been found at 16.0 and 50.5 per 100,000 man-years in the invited screened and control unscreened groups, respectively (p0.01)[188]. An update of these data obtained from this study is available in chapter 4[706]. The present data are in agreement with the 42% decrease observed in 1998 in the prostate cancer death rate in the Tyrol area where PSA screening had been made available since 1993 compared to the rest of Austria where PSA screening was not offered[361]. Since about two thirds of men were screened in Tyrol during that period, the 42% decreased death rate observed is comparable to the 68% value observed for the men who were screened in our study.

Major impact on survival

Medical castration with LHRH agonists

The discovery by our research group at the Laval University Medical Research Center in Quebec City that luteinizing hormone-releasing hormone (LHRH) agonists very efficiently achieve medical castration men[707-710] has eliminated the previous limitations associated with the blockade of testicular androgens, especially the psychological problems of surgical castration and the serious and even life-threatening side effects of estrogens[711-713]. The availability of medical castration with LHRH agonists[707] has thus opened the way to a much more acceptable treatment of localized disease.

DOUBLE SOURCE OF ANDROGENS IN THE HUMAN PROSTATE

Following the discovery of the castration effect of LHRH agonists[707], the next most important advance made in our understanding of the biology and endocrinology of prostate cancer and its impact on treatment is probably the observation that humans and some other primates are unique among animal species in having adrenals that secrete large amounts of the inactive precursor steroids dehydroepiandrosterone (DHEA), its sulfate DHEA-S, and some androstenedione (4-dione), which are converted into potent androgens in a large series of peripheral tissues, including the prostate (Figure 28). In fact, the plasma concentration of DHEA-S secreted by the adrenals in adult men is 100 to 500 times higher than that of testosterone[474], the main secretory product of the testicles. Such high circulating levels of DHEA-S (and also DHEA) provide high amounts of the prehormones or precursors required for conversion into active androgens in the prostate as well as in other peripheral intracrine tissues.

The local synthesis of active steroids in peripheral target tissues has been called intracrinology[478, 714]. The active androgens made locally in the prostate exert their action by interacting with the androgen receptor in the same cells where their synthesis takes place without being released in the extracellular environment or the general circulation. Contrary to the previous belief that the testes are responsible for 90 to 95% of total androgen production in men (as suggested by simple measurement of circulating serum testosterone following castration), it is now well recognized that the prostatic tissue efficiently transforms the inactive steroid precursors DHEA-S, DHEA, and 4-dione into the active androgens testosterone and DHT. In fact, the prostate synthesizes its own androgens to a level comparable to the androgens of testicular origin.

10. Status of Androgen Blockade in Prostate Cancer in 2002

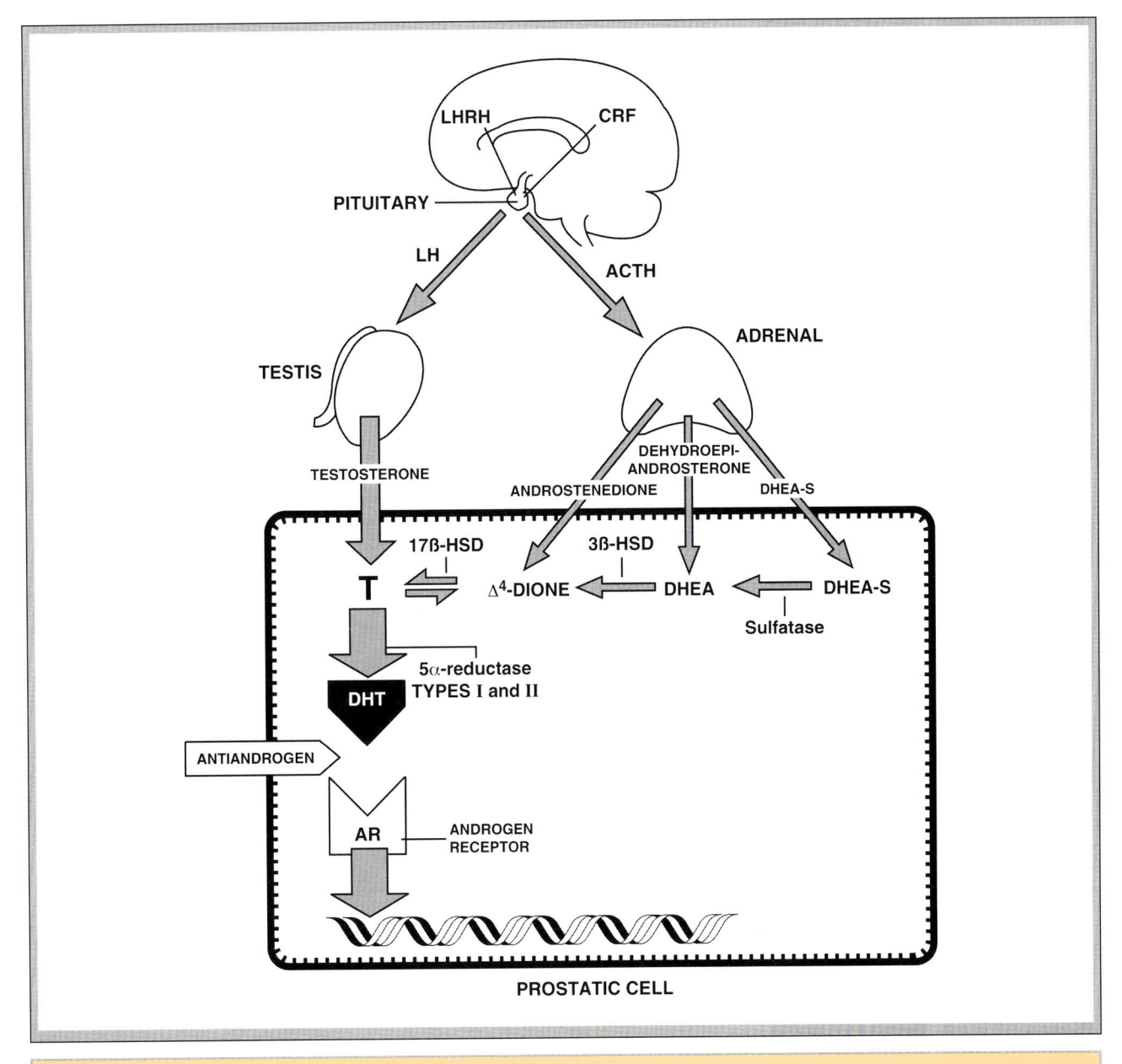

FIGURE 28. Intracrine activity of the human prostate or biosynthetic steps involved in the formation of the active androgen dihydrotestosterone (DHT) from testicular testosterone as well as from the inactive adrenal precursors dehydroepiandrosterone (DHEA), DHEA-sulfate (DHEA-S), and androstenedione (4-dione) in human prostatic tissue. 17-HSD = 17-hydroxysteroid dehydrogenase; 3-HSD = 3-hydroxysteroid dehydrogenase/Δ^5-Δ^4-isomerase. The widths of the arrows indicate the relative importance of the sources of DHT in the human prostate: 60% originating from the testes and 40% from the adrenals in 65-year old men. The testis secretes testosterone (T) which is transformed into the more potent androgen DHT by 5-reductase in the prostate. Instead of secreting T or DHT directly, the adrenal secretes very large amounts of DHEA, DHEA-sulfate (DHEA-S) and (4-dione), which are transported in the blood to the prostate and other peripheral tissues. These inactive precursors are then transformed locally into the active androgens T and DHT. The enzymatic complexes DHEA sulfatase, 3-HSD, 17-HSD and 5-reductase are all present in the prostatic cells, thus providing 40% of total DHT in this tissue.

Combined androgen blockade fist studied in advanced prostate cancer

The first treatment shown to prolong life in prostate cancer is combined androgen blockade (CAB) or the combination of an LHRH agonist (blocker of androgen secretion by the testes)[707] and a pure antiandrogen, a drug that blocks the action of the androgens produced locally in the prostate without exerting any androgenic activity by itself[466, 474, 641, 709, 715].

An interesting observation is that the demonstration of the benefits of CAB has been obtained in the most difficult group of patients to treat, namely those suffering from metastatic or advanced disease. Although there is no reason to believe that similar results should be obtained with bicalutamide, the two antiandrogens flutamide and nilutamide have both been shown, in prospective and randomized studies, to prolong life, to increase the number of complete and partial responses, to delay progression, and to provide better pain control (thus improving quality of life) in metastatic prostate cancer when added to surgical or medical castration compared to castration alone[322, 466, 622, 623, 715-718]. In the first large scale randomized study, patients who were treated with flutamide and Lupron lived, on average, 7.3 months longer than those who received Lupron plus placebo[466].

Analysis of all the studies performed with flutamide and nilutamide associated with medical or surgical castration compared to castration plus placebo shows that overall survival is increased by an average of 3 to 6 months[322, 466, 622, 623, 637, 715-718]. Since about 50% of patients at that age die from causes other than prostate cancer, this difference in overall survival translates into an average of 6 to 12 months of life gained for cancer-specific survival. These additional months, or sometimes, years of life can be obtained by simply adding a pure antiandrogen (flutamide, bicalutamide or nilutamide) to castration. These data demonstrate the particularly high level of sensitivity of prostate cancer to androgen deprivation, even at the very advanced stage of metastatic disease.

Bennett et al.[715] have performed a meta-analysis of all peer-reviewed published randomized controlled trials comparing treatment with flutamide in association with medical (LHRH agonist) or surgical castration with castration alone in advanced prostate cancer. Nine studies with 4,128 patients were included in the analysis which demonstrated a statistically significant 10% improvement in overall survival with the combination therapy using flutamide compared to castration alone. As shown in Table 13, similar benefits have been calculated in favor of flutamide plus castration versus castration alone in the meta-analysis of Bennett et al.[715] and that of the Prostate Cancer Trialist's Collaborative Group (PTCTG) (Figure 29).

With the clinical data summarized above, the controversy concerning

10. Status of Androgen Blockade in Prostate Cancer in 2002

TABLE 13. Hazard Ratios (RR) and 95% of confidence intervals (CIs) using alternative methods for estimating hazard ratios for survival data[715] and comparison with results from the 2000 PCTCG analysis

Year of Analysis	Method of metaanalysis	RR	95%	CI	Number of studies	
Bennett et al.[715]	Literature-based	0.90	0.79	1.00	9	
PCTCG[322]	Patient-level	0.92	0.89	0.95	12	2p = 0.02
	In favor of Flutamide + castration versus castration alone					

Mortality results from the 12 randomised trials of CAB (Castration + FLUTAMIDE) versus Castration alone in advanced prostate cancer

Year and Study Name	Deaths/Patients Allocated CX+Anti-A.	Deaths/Patients Adjusted* CX alone	CX + Anti-A. deaths Obs. -Exp.	Variance of O-E.	Ratio of death rates CX + Anti-A. : CX alone	Ratio (& SD)
85 NC/INT-0036/SWOG	274/311	276/306	-15.5	136.2		
85 118,630/1511/WPSG	45/59	39/51	-2.9	18.5		
86 118,630/1509/IPCSG	215/293	222/293	-12.3	104.8		
86 EORTC 30853	134/164	139/163	-18.7	64.7		
86 DAPROCA	119/129	127/133	0.5	58.8		
86 118,630/1507	86/120	92/125	-0.3	43.8		
86 M85712	81/113	75/110	9.2	38.6		
86 M85713	95/168	92/162	0.5	46.6		
87 PONCAP	91/159	106/160	-6.6	43.2		
87 Modena	51/60	54/62	0.4	21.3		
88 NCI/INT-0105/SWOG	468/698	480/687	-22.7	235.9		
89 Varese	56/137	51/140	-1.2	25.1		
subtotal *	1715/2411 (71.1%)	1753/2392 (73.3%)	-69.6	837.5		0.92 ± 0.03 (2p = 0.02)

■ 99% or ◇ 95% confidence intervals

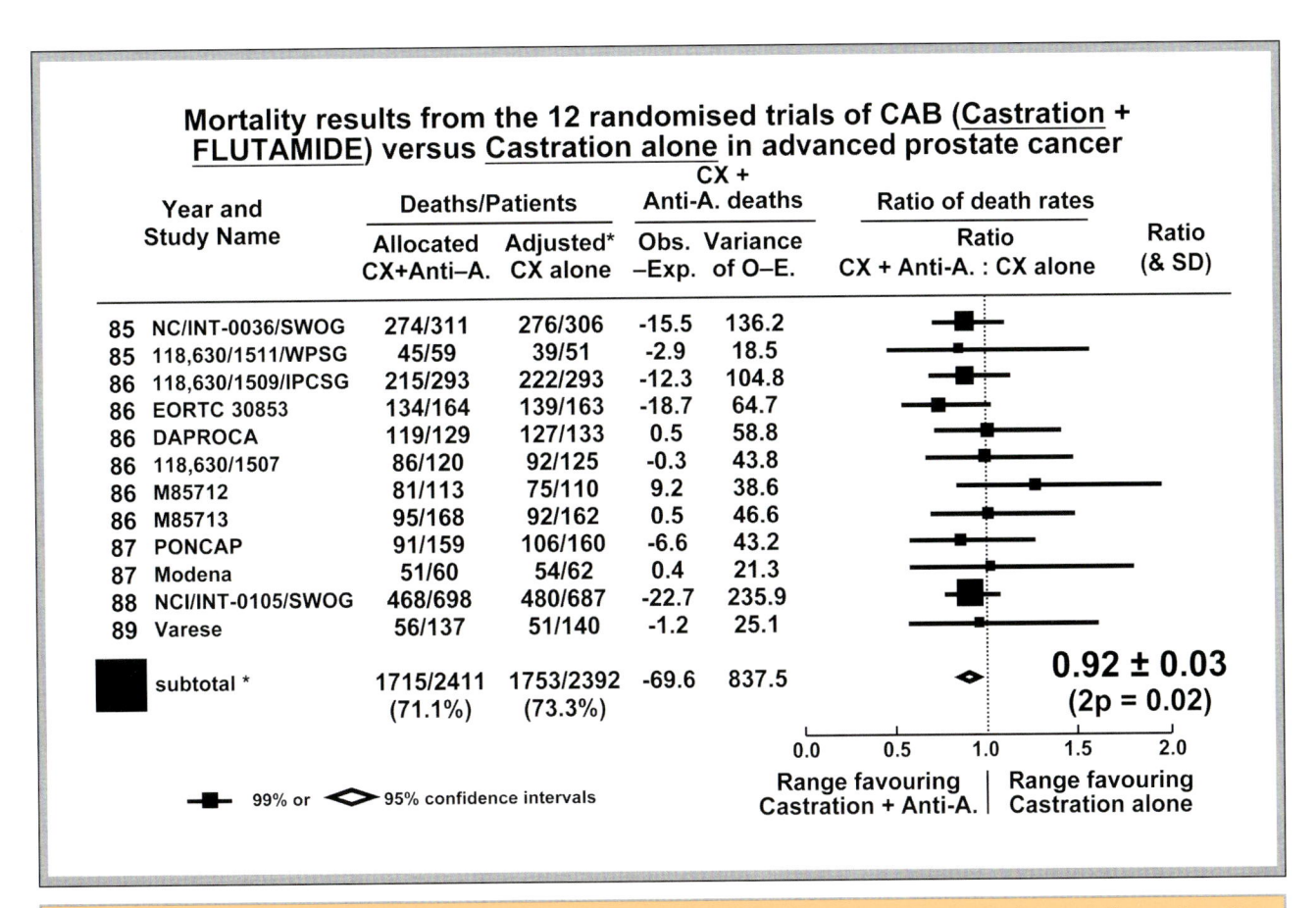

Range favouring Castration + Anti-A. | Range favouring Castration alone

FIGURE 29. Mortality results from the 12 randomized trials of CAB (Castration + Flutamide) versus Castration alone in advanced prostate cancer (PCTCG 2000).

CAB should be part of history and the addition of a pure antiandrogen should be recognized by all as providing an advantage of 3 to 6 months of life in metastatic disease or at a time when no alternative treatment even exists. When considering cancer-specific survival, the data show that 6 to 12 additional months of life are obtained by the simple addition of a pure antiandrogen[322, 623, 715, 719] to medical or surgical castration.

Greater Benefits of Androgen blockade in localized disease

Despite the recent advances in the treatment of metastatic prostate cancer using LHRH agonists and a pure antiandrogen[475, 707, 466, 623, 709, 715, 718, 322] it is well recognized that the only means of achieving an important reduction in prostate cancer mortality is treatment of localized disease[348, 720]. It is reasonable to suggest that the recently observed decline in prostate cancer mortality is due to earlier diagnosis with serum PSA and transrectal ultrasound[346], as well as improved treatment of localized disease by surgery, radiotherapy, brachytherapy and endocrine therapy[348, 350, 351, 720].

Most fortunately, six prospective randomized trials have recently demonstrated for the first time that an important prolongation of life was achieved in localized prostate cancer patients treated with androgen blockade (Table 14). In the EORTC (European Organization for Research and Treatment of Cancer) trial performed in stage T3 patients, overall survival at 5 years was increased from 62% in the group of patients who received radiation therapy alone to 79% (45% difference) in the group of patients who received androgen blockade using an LHRH agonist for 3 years and an antiandrogen for one month in association with radiotherapy[342]. Death from prostate cancer at 5 years was thus decreased by 77% by androgen blockade (Table 14). On the other hand, a 20% improvement in overall survival at five years has been found in RTOG trial 08351 in the subgroup of high Gleason score patients who received androgen blockade (LHRH agonist) indefinitely or until progression[343]. In another study, a 54% decrease in cancer-specific death has been found in patients with an 8-10 Gleason score who had androgen blockade in association with radiotherapy compared to radiotherapy alone[344], while a 39% decrease in cancer-specific death when castration was added to radiotherapy versus radiotherapy alone[345].

The results of another recent study are of particular interest. In that study, of 98 men who had stage T2 prostate cancer at diagnosis but who were found to have pelvic lymph node metastases at radical prostatectomy, 47 had immediate hormonal therapy while 51 were followed until progression[146]. After a median follow-up of 7.1 years, 16 have died from

TABLE 14. Randomized studies showing survival benefits following treatment of localized or asymptomatic metastatic prostate cancer.

Study	Benefits
EORTC[342]	77% decrease in cancer-specific death (p = 0.01)
RTOG trial[343]	37% decrease for Gleason score 8 to 10 (p = 0.03)
Quebec Screening Trial[188]	64% decrease in cancer-specific death (p = 0.0002)
Messing et al.[146]	81% decrease (p = 0.001)
Granfors et al.[345]	39% decrease in cancer-specific death (p = 0.06)
Hanks et al.[344]	59% decrease for Gleason score 8-10 (p = 0.007)

prostate cancer in the observation group compared to only 3 in the immediate therapy group for a 81% decrease in deaths from prostate cancer (p=0.001), for men who had immediate androgen blockade. The 64% decrease in the incidence of death from prostate cancer observed during the first 11 years of our randomized and prospective study on prostate cancer screening [706] can only be due to the treatments used, the majority of patients having received CAB.

It is of interest to mention that in a study of 3603 men with localized or locally advanced prostate cancer, monotherapy with bicalutamide (150 mg daily) reduced objective progression by 43% (p0.0001)[721]. Prior therapy with a curative intent had been given to 64% of patients (44% prostatectomy, 18% radiotherapy and 2% prostatectomy + radiotherapy), while 36% had been followed by watchful waiting. These results were obtained after a median follow-up of 2.6 years. A similar benefit was obtained for patients who received treatment with a curative intent or those followed by watchful waiting.

It is thus not surprising that hormone therapy alone is more and more recognized as highly efficient in localized or locally advanced prostate cancer[722]. In fact, prostate cancer growing in the prostate or in the tissue surrounding the prostate is very different from cancer growing in the bones. Localized disease is much easier to treat by androgen blockade because it does not contain androgen-insensitive clones. Moreover, androgen insensitivity does not (or very rarely) develop in localized prostate cancer under androgen blockade, contrary to the situation in metastatic disease where resistance to treatment is the usual outcome.

POSSIBILITY OF CURE WITH LONG TERM COMBINED ANDROGEN BLOCKADE

A word of caution is extremely important concerning the 20% increase in cancer-specific survival achieved in advanced metastatic disease with CAB compared to monotherapy. The benefits demonstrated with CAB in patients suffering from advanced disease should not be transferred as such to localized disease where the situation is much more favorable and better results are expected. In fact, in analogy with the treatment of any other cancer, the beneficial effects of androgen blockade are much greater when the same treatment is applied at an earlier stage of the disease. In this respect, as discussed later, recent data indicate that CAB might well be the best treatment for localized prostate cancer (as already recognized for advanced disease). Moreover, with long-term treatment of localized prostate cancer with CAB, the evidence obtained even suggests that cure of the disease can be obtained in the large majority of patients[720].

While the majority of studies performed so far in localized prostate cancer have used monotherapy (medical or surgical castration), there are good reasons to believe that even better results will be obtained with more complete androgen blockade or CAB. Since we had already obtained evidence for the high efficacy of CAB in localized prostate cancer[349], it was felt important to examine the outcome of these patients following cessation of continuous CAB administered continuously for periods up to 11.3 years. The data obtained indicate that cure of the disease can be obtained in the majority of patients with localized prostate cancer treated continuously with CAB for more than 6.5 years.

It is of major interest to see how PSA failure is inversely correlated with the duration of continuous CAB administration before cessation of treatment. In fact, of the 57 patients with B2/T2 or C/T3 disease treated continuously with CAB for various time intervals up to 11.7 years, only two PSA rises have occurred in the 33 patients who had received CAB for more than 6.5 years before stopping treatment. When taking 5 years with no PSA rise after cessation of CAB as parameter of long term control or possible cure of the cancer, the no failure rate is 90% (18/20) in this group of patients (Figure 30). When looking in more detail at this group of patients, the no failure rate is 87,5% (7/8) for patients previously treated with CAB for 6.5 to 10 years before stopping treatment, while it is 91% (11/12) for those previously treated for 10 to 11.7 years.

Based upon the above-described data, it can be estimated that a period of more than 6 years of continuous CAB is required to efficiently control localized prostate cancer. At approximately 6 years of treatment, long-term control or possible cure of the cancer appears to be achieved in approximately 50% of cases. However, as shown in Figure 30, when CAB is continued further, a much higher rate of success is achieved with an approximately 90% cure rate at treatment durations ranging from 6.5 to 11.7 years. In clinical practice, one possibility is to stop treatment at 6 years, thus achieving the required long term control of cancer in approxi-

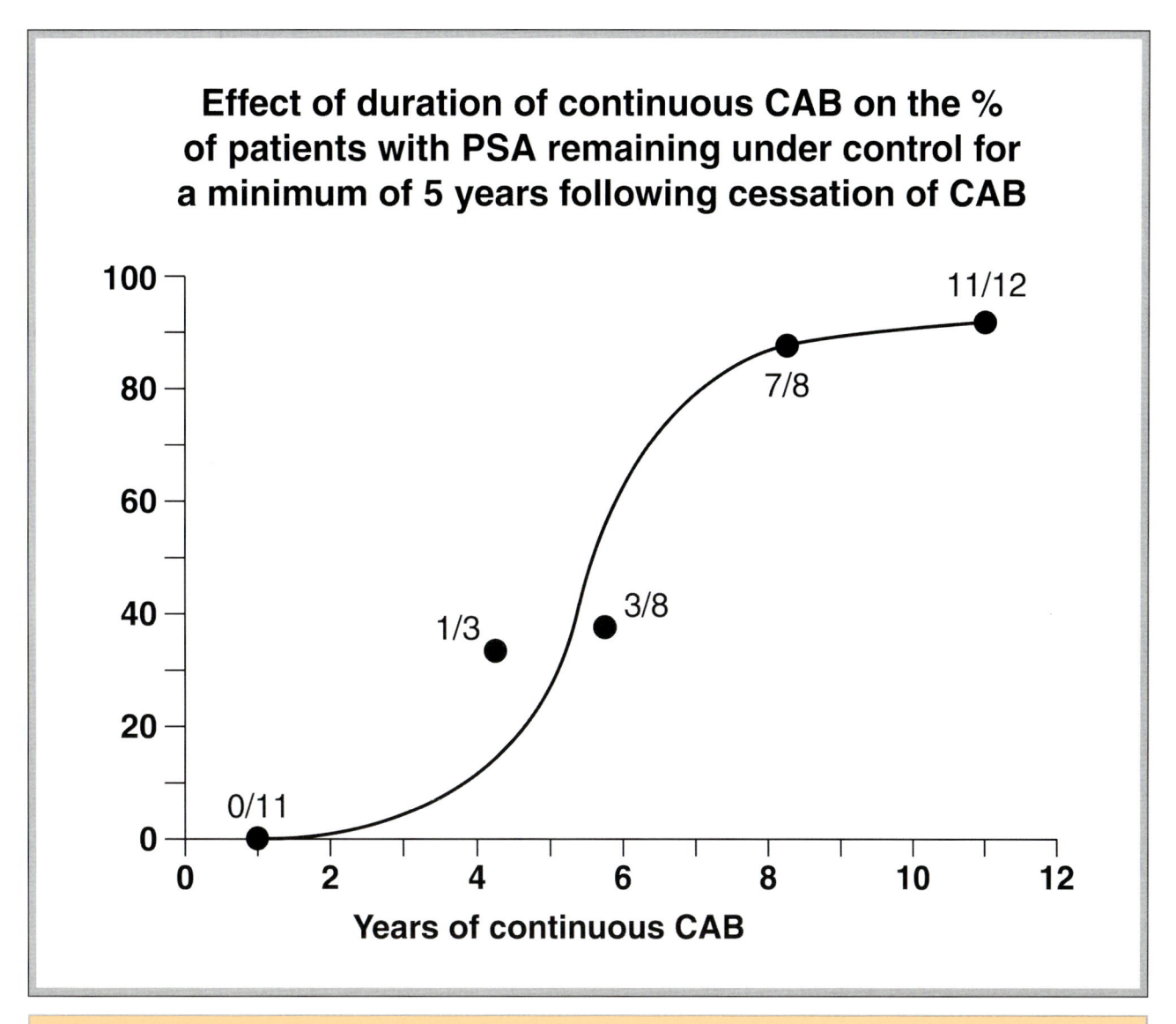

FIGURE 30. Effect of duration of treatment of localized prostate cancer with continuous CAB on the probability of "long term control or cure of the disease" as illustrated by a no increase of PSA for at least 5 years after cessation of CAB.

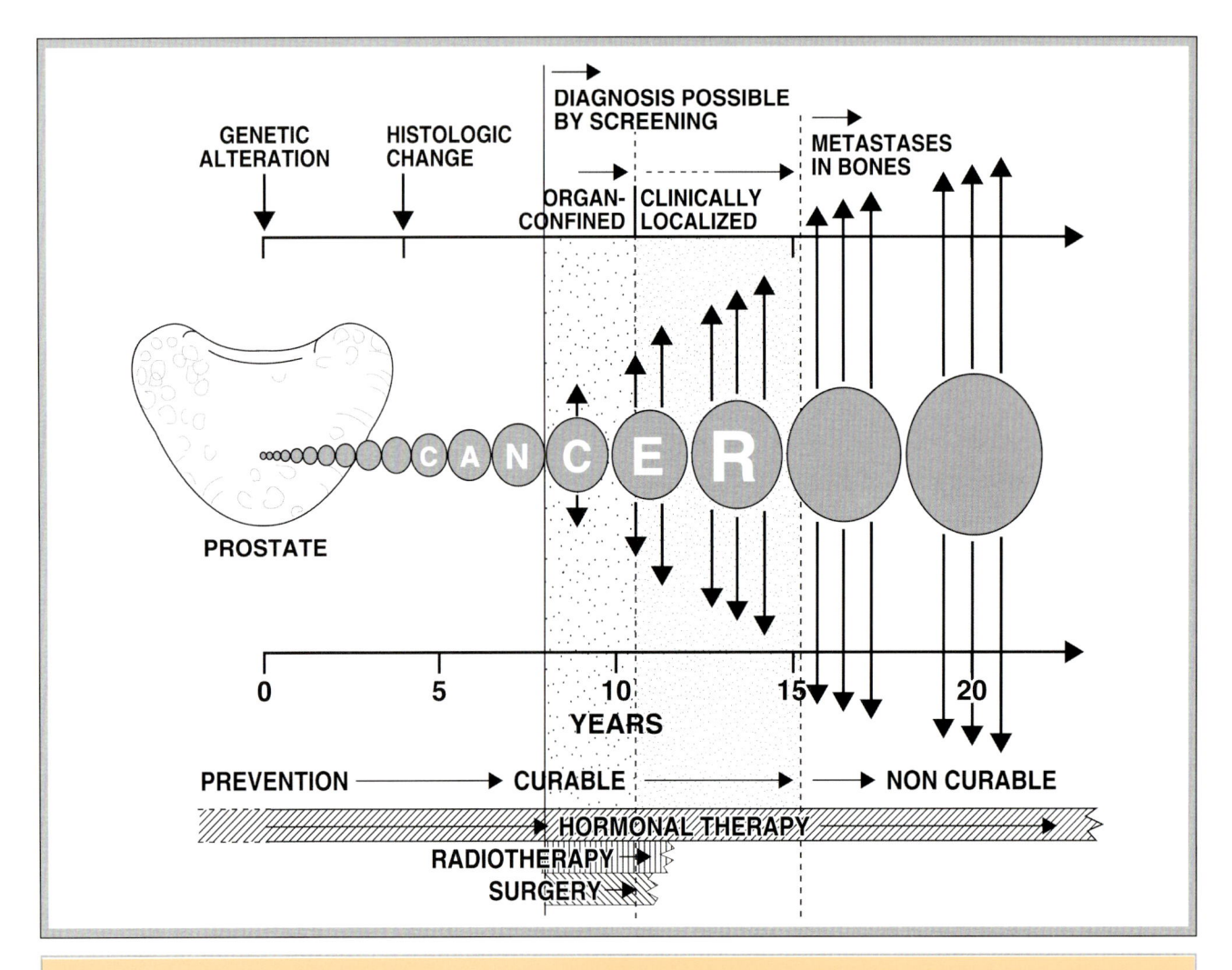

10. Status of Androgen Blockade in Prostate Cancer in 2002

FIGURE 31. Schematic representation of the evolution of prostate cancer from the time of appearance of the first genetic change which is followed by a series of cell divisions and other mutations, thus eventually resulting in a cancer cell. During the following years, the cancer cells can only be seen by gene markers and then, histological changes become visible. However, it is only after many years of evolution that the tumor reaches a relatively large volume (0.3 cc) which becomes detectable by screening with PSA, digital rectal examination and/or transrectal echography of the prostate. Depending upon the genes involved, the rate of cancer growth is variable between individuals and the scale shown is an estimated average. It is important to mention that when diagnosis has become possible by screening, approximately 60% of the cancers have already migrated outside the prostate and are no longer organ-confined.

The diagram also indicates the time when each treatment can be most efficiently used. Radical prostatectomy can cure the disease when the cancer is organ-confined and no cancer cell has migrated outside the prostate. Radiotherapy and brachytherapy (seed implants) are believed to have an efficacy comparable to that of surgery. Hormonal therapy, more specifically combined androgen blockade offers a high possibility of cure of the disease when treatment is started before the cancer migrates to the bones, even if it has migrated in the area surrounding the prostate. Hormonal therapy, however, must be continuous and long-term but not intermittent. At the advanced stage of bone metastases, only combined androgen blockade has been shown to prolong life compared to monotherapy but the possibility of a cure is minimal. Data obtained in localized disease show that long term combined androgen blockade can cure the disease in the majority of cases Much remains to be understood about the treatment of localized disease but this diagram is drawn according to the best knowledge available.

mately 50% of cases. In the event of a PSA rise expected in the other 50% of patients, the same CAB should be re-administered without delay for another 3 years. A major mistake made so far, starting with our own neoadjuvant trial started in 1988[351], is that CAB has generally been administered for much too short periods of time.

With the knowledge of the above-described data, is seems reasonable to suggest that the minimal duration of continuous CAB should be 6 years, thus providing on approximately 50% probability of long-term or possible cure of the cancer. With longer duration of CAB, the probability increases to about 90% at 8 to 10 years of treatment. The present data indicate that possible cure of the disease can be obtained in the majority of patients with localized prostate cancer treated continuously with CAB for more than 6 years, thus raising hopes for the treatment of patients who fail after surgery, radiotherapy or brachytherapy where no or minimally effective alternative therapeutic approaches exist. Such data clearly indicate the interest of a large scale randomized study comparing monotherapy versus CAB in the group of patients showing biochemical failure after first therapy with a curative intent. Care should be taken, however, to start treatment early after the rise of PSA in order to use androgen blockade at its maximal level of efficacy, namely when the cancer is still localized to the prostate or the prostatic area and before metastases reach the bones when cure has become an exception.

CONCLUSION

While showing the high efficacy of combined hormonal therapy in localized prostate cancer, the present data clearly indicate that long-term treatment, somewhat analogous to the 5 years of Tamoxifen in breast cancer, is required for optimal control of prostate cancer. Great caution should be taken, however, when using serum PSA as surrogate marker. In fact, serum PSA rapidly decreases to undetectable levels under androgen blockade although the cancer remains present for much longer periods of time, usually many years. Intermittent therapy should not be recommended outside prospective and randomized clinical trials.

Figure 31 is a schematic representation of the evolution of prostate cancer through its various stages of progression. This figure also indicates the timing of efficient screening and the corresponding treatment alternatives. It is clear that the impact of screening and early diagnosis of prostate cancer is entirely dependent upon the timing and the choice of the treatment used. Since the majority of cancers can now be diagnosed at the clinically localized stage with the available screening tests[323], the priority should focus on the choice of the best treatment for each patient.

With early diagnosis and treatment, as clearly demonstrated in the first randomized screening study[188], death from prostate cancer should decrease dramatically and should even become rare. Since prostate cancer is expected to be the cause of death of 3 million men presently living in the United States, a 64% decrease in prostate cancer death[188] corresponds to a saving of approximately 2 million lives in the United States alone. Further progress in the diagnosis and treatment of localized prostate cancer should improve these figures even further.

With the present knowledge, it is clear that all available means should be taken to prevent prostate cancer from migrating to the bones where treatment becomes extremely difficult and cure or even long-term control of the disease is an exception. The only way to prevent prostate cancer from migrating to the bones and thus becoming incurable, is efficient treatment of localized disease. It is also clear from the data summarized above that CAB could well be the most efficient therapy of localized prostate cancer while it was already recognized as the best therapy for metastatic disease.

Clearly, the rational use of the presently available diagnostic and therapeutic approaches could decrease prostate cancer death by at least 50%[188, 323]. As an example, between 1991 and 1999, the death rate from prostate cancer has decreased by 38% in Quebec City and its metropolitan area[320] while the death rate has decreased by 68% in the group of men who were screened[188]. The strategy used is available to all and the key to its success is immediate androgen blockade as soon as other therapies of localized prostate cancer fail.

STRATEGIES FOR PROSTATE CANCER PREVENTION

By Gary J. Kelloff, M.D., Howard R. Highley, Ph.D., DABT, Caroline C. Sigman, Ph.D.

INTRODUCTION

The prevention of prostate cancer is one of the most important goals of cancer prevention research. The documented prostate cancer incidence has been increasing in the US and internationally, due in part to aging populations as well as increasingly widespread use of screening techniques such as PSA testing. In the US alone it was estimated that about 180,400 men will be newly diagnosed with prostate cancer in 2001 and about 32,000 would die of the disease, presenting a significant public health challenge[192]. Strategies for reducing the occurrence of prostate cancers will be critical in limiting the morbidity and mortality of this disease. One valuable approach involves the development of chemopreventive drugs to slow the progression, reverse or inhibit carcinogenesis and thereby lower the risk of developing invasive or clinically significant disease. With its long latency and high incidence, prostate cancer is an important target for chemoprevention[723]. However, successful implementation of a prostate cancer chemoprevention strategy will require an understanding of the mechanisms whereby normal prostate tissues become malignant as well as improvements in the techniques to detect and diagnose early stage prostate cancers that will be amenable to chemopreventive intervention, leading to optimization of clinical trial designs that can provide a complete pathway from proof-of principle studies to pivotal trials that are sufficient to be granted regulatory agency approval for prostate cancer chemoprevention/risk reduction indications[723-725]. The following chapter will review the current status of chemoprevention research in prostate cancer focusing on: 1) methods for selection of chemopreventive agents for development as inhibitors of prostate carcinogenesis and the evaluation of their efficacy; 2) the identification of intermediate endpoints that may best serve as surrogates for cancer incidence reduction in prostate cancer chemoprevention trials; and 3) the principal clinical trial study cohorts at risk for development or progression of prostate neoplasia that will serve as the most efficient settings for the evaluation of novel chemopreventive pharmaceuticals, micronutrients or dietary supplements.

SELECTION OF CANDIDATE CHEMOPREVENTIVE AGENTS FOR THE CONTROL OF PROSTATE CARCINOGENESIS AND THE EVALUATION OF EFFICACY

Epidemiology and clinical experience from the use of neoadjuvant therapies in more advanced prostate cancer, as well as data from preclinical experimental, and basic mechanistic carcinogenesis studies can all provide rationales for pursuing the development of a candidate chemopreventive agent[723, 726, 727]. In addition, secondary analyses from completed chemoprevention trials examining the efficacy of agents in other organ systems can suggest re-examination in a prostate cancer cohort.

For example, the interest in both soy isoflavones and lycopene for the control of prostate cancer originated with epidemiologic studies. Four to five times more men die of prostate cancer in the US than in Japan, and the onset of prostate cancer occurs later in life. That these cancers grow more slowly in Japanese populations has been associated with the traditional utilization of more soy products in the diet than in the West[728]. Soy isoflavones possess antiproliferative properties through such mechanisms as inhibition of growth factor receptor tyrosine kinases (reviewed in 729) and inhibition of NF6B [730]. There is also increasing evidence that these agents may alter the plasma concentration and metabolism of testosterone, and possess weak estrogenic activity that exert significant effects on target tissues such as the prostate[731, 732]. Similarly, consumption of dietary tomato products was one of the few discernible food use patterns to be strongly associated with a decreased risk of prostate cancer in the Health Professional's Follow-up Study[733]. Further studies confirmed that increased serum levels of lycopene, the carotenoid pigment present in large amounts in tomatoes, were more highly correlated to decreased prostate cancer risk than were levels of other circulating, diet-derived nutrients[734]. From a mechanistic standpoint, it has been shown that lycopene is the most potent antioxidant carotenoid and that the free-radical scavenging activity of these compounds may protect prostate cells against oxidative mutagenesis[735]. Augmentation of both soy isoflavone and lycopene serum levels by dietary administration in animal models have been associated with chemopreventive efficacy in several tumor types[736-738]. Currently, there are a number of clinical studies planned or in progress to examine these agents in various prostate cancer cohorts (See Table 15).

A fundamental and universal feature of prostate cancer regulation is hormone dependence[739]. Many ongoing chemoprevention trials are investigating the use of pharmaceutical agents that either inhibit testosterone production (e.g., finasteride (Proscar®), block the androgen receptor (e.g., flutamide, bicalutamide (Casodex®) or short-circuit endocrine signaling (e.g., leuprolide)[740]. Although many of these agents are routinely used as initial or adjunctive therapies in individuals with more advanced prostate disease, the safety requirements for a chemopreventive agent are more stringent than for therapeutic agents, and chronic administration to at-risk normal or asymptomatic individuals may be needed to demonstrate chemopreventive efficacy. The first large scale trial to test the hypothesis that modulation of androgen levels can have a chemopreventive effect is the Prostate Cancer Prevention Trial (PCPT) started in 1993. This ten-year, two-arm Phase III trial has successfully accrued its full complement of more than 18,000 average risk men randomized to finasteride or placebo. Results of the study are expected in 2003. Additional evidence that androgen deprivation may be chemopreventive is provided by the observation that three or six months treatment with the combination of an antiandrogen (e.g., flutamide) and LHRH agonist (e.g., leuprolide) reduces the incidence of a prostatic adenocarcinoma precursor, prostatic intraepithelial neoplasia (PIN)[741].

Further, it has also been shown that estrogen derived from testosterone by aromatase action can also play a role in prostate carcinogenesis and that androgen blockade is insufficient to prevent estrogen-driven cell proliferation[742]. Animal models have shown that tamoxifen treatment is effective in suppressing prostate carcinogenesis[743]. Therefore, co-administration of antiestrogens such as toremifene, tamoxifen, or new selective estrogen modulators (SERMs)[744] may be complementary to current androgen modulation chemopreventive study designs.

Even secondary analyses of results from clinical trials designed to test chemoprevention hypotheses in other cancers can suggest new directions for clinical testing. Although ineffective in reducing lung cancer incidence,

TABLE 15. Phase I/II/III Clinical Chemoprevention Trials in Prostate Cancer[1]

Agent	Cohort (Treatment Period)	Endpoint(s)
Phase I Lycopene (food-based or vitamin supplement)	Normal Volunteers (Single Dose)	Pharmacokinetic Assessment
	African Americans with Elevated PSA but Cancer Negative Prostate Biopsy (PIN Allowed) (3 Months)	Pharmacokinetic Assessment. Tissue Distribution of Lycopene/Levels. Oxidative Stress Measurements Blood and Tissue, PSA, IGF-I, PCNA, TUNEL and PIN Histopathology Modulation
Soy Isoflavones	Stage C and D Prostate Cancer Patients (84 Days)	Pharmacokinetics, Genetic Biomarkers: DNA Topoisomerase II, Micronucleated Cell Frequency, tk/hprt (Lymphocytes)
Phase II DFMO	Scheduled for Prostatectomy (Stage A or B Prostatic Carcinoma or Bladder Cancer without Prostatic Carcinoma and Scheduled for Cystoprostatectomy) (14 Days)	Drug Effect Measurements: ODC Activity (Skin and Prostate), Polyamine Levels (Prostate). Histopathology (TRUS-Guided Biopsies). Biochemical Biomarkers: PSA, PAP, Testosterone
	Serum PSA 3–10 ng/ml (Includes Patients with Prostatic Carcinoma and PIN) (14 Days–1 Year)	Drug Effect Measurements: ODC Activity (Skin and Prostate), Polyamine Levels (Prostate). Histopathology (TRUS-Guided Biopsies). Biochemical Biomarkers: PSA, PAP, Testosterone
	Unaffected Brothers or Male First Cousins of Early Onset (<70 years old) Prostate Cancer Patients with Family History (One or More First Degree Affected Relatives) (1 Year)	Proliferation Biomarker: Spermine: Spermidine Ratio (Prostate); Biochemical Biomarkers: PSA, PSA Density; Differentiation Biomarkers: Matrilysin, Metalloproteinases, Gelatinase A, Cathepsin D, Laminins, Cytokeratins; Clinical: Bladder Outlet Obstruction
DFMO + Bicalutamide	Scheduled for Prostatectomy or Brachytherapy (28 Days)	Drug Effect Measurements: Polyamine Levels (Prostate); Biochemical Biomarkers: PSA; Proliferation Biomarkers: PCNA; Genetic/Regulatory Biomarkers: p53, EGFR, TGF
Soy Isoflavones	Scheduled For Radical Prostatectomy (Localized Prostate Cancer) (3 Weeks)	Histopathology (PIN Grade, Nuclear Polymorphism, Nucleolar Polymorphism, Ploidy). Proliferation Biomarkers (PCNA, Ki-67), Genetic/Regulatory Biomarkers (p53, bcl-2, pc-1, Chromosome 8p Loss)

Table continuous on next page

TABLE 15. *Cont'nue* Phase I/II/III Clinical Chemoprevention Trials in Prostate Cancer[1]		
Agent	**Cohort (Treatment Period)**	**Endpoint(s)**
Flutamide	Patients with HGPIN (12 Months)	PIN Grade and Incidence, Cancer Incidence, Nuclear Polymorphism, Nucleolar Size, Ploidy. Other Endpoints: PCNA, Angiogenesis, Apoptosis, LOH Chromosome 8, Growth Factors, PSA
Flutamide ± Toremifene	Scheduled for Radical Prostatectomy (4–8 weeks)	PIN Grade and Incidence, Nuclear Polymorphism, Nuclear Size, Ploidy.
Fenretinide	Scheduled For Prostate Cancer Surgery (4–8 Weeks)	Histopathology: PIN Grade, Nuclear Polymorphism, Nucleolar Polymorphism, Ploidy. Proliferation Biomarkers: PCNA, Ki-67. Differentiation Biomarkers: Lewis Y Antigen. Genetic/Regulatory Biomarkers: p53, EGFR, TGF?
Vitamin D Analog (1?-Hydroxy vitamin D2)	Scheduled for Radical Prostatectomy (4–8 weeks)	Nuclear Morphometry, Proliferation Biomarkers: Ki-67, Apoptotic Index. Differentiation Biomarkers: Androgen Receptor. Microvessel Density: Factor 8 Staining, Vitamin D Receptor and Metabolite Assay, Serum PSA and PSMA Levels, Plasma TGF? Level
NSAID (Celecoxib)	Scheduled for Radical Prostatectomy (4–8 Weeks)	Histopathology, Proliferation Biomarkers: PCNA, Ki-67, p27, p21, Apoptotic Index. DNA Adducts. Microvessel Density: Factor 8 staining, Serum PSA Levels, Prostaglandin Assays, COX-1,2 Expression.
Exisulind (Sulindac Sulfone)	Scheduled for Radical Prostatectomy (4–8 Weeks)	Apoptotic Index (TUNEL, bcl-2, Bax, Par-4, M30, PTEN) Histopathology (PIN Grade), Proliferation Biomarker (Ki-67, DNA Ploidy), PSA
	Increasing PSA after Radical Prostatectomy (12 Months)	PSA (from Baseline, Doubling Time)
Phase III Finasteride	≥55 Years of Age with Normal DRE and PSA <3.0 ng/ml (7 Years)	Prostate Cancer Incidence (Grade and Stage), BPH Incidence and Severity, Overall and Prostate-Specific Mortality, TURP, PSA Levels

Table continuous on next page

11. Strategies for Prostate Cancer Prevention

TABLE 15. *Cont'nue* Phase I/II/III Clinical Chemoprevention Trials in Prostate Cancer[1]

Agent	Cohort (Treatment Period)	Endpoint(s)
Phase III *(cont'ue)*		
l-Seleno-methionine + Vitamin E	Men ≥55 Years of Age (≥50 for African-Americans) with Normal DRE and PSA <3.0 ng/ml (7 Years)	Prostate Cancer Incidence, PSA and IGF-1 Levels, Blood Serum and Cell Samples for Micronutrients, Steroid Hormones, DNA and Hemoglobin adducts, polymorphic Gene Analysis (Androgen Receptor, 5-Reductase Type, CYP17, CYP1A1, -Hydroxysteroid Dehydrogenase, DNA Repair Proteins, GSMT)
l-Seleno-methionine	HGPIN (3 Years)	Prostate Cancer Incidence (Grade and Stage), PIN Grade, Other Histopathology and Proliferation Biomarkers

[1]See text for references to publications describing these studies.

one of the arms of the Finnish -tocopherol (vitamin E), -carotene trial showed a significant reduction in prostate cancer incidence and prostate cancer specific mortality in smokers taking vitamin E supplementation (50 mg/day) compared with controls (32% reduction in 14,564 men receiving -tocopherol *versus* 14,569 not receiving it) (Heinonen et al. 1998). Similarly, although selenium (200 μg Se/day) in the form of selenized brewer's yeast had no effect on non-melanoma skin cancer incidence in a placebo-controlled intervention study with 1312 patients, post-hoc analysis showed that selenium treatment was associated with a 63% reduction in prostate cancer in this skin cancer-risk cohort (13 cases in the selenium-treated group *versus* 35 cases in the placebo group of 974 total men) (Clark et al. 1998). Together these observations have been persuasive in the decision to start the current large randomized, placebo-controlled SELECT (SELenium, vitamin E Cancer prevention Trial) study in 32,400 men at average risk of prostate cancer (≥55 years of age; >50 years of age for African-Americans). More than 400 study sites are expected to participate in this 12- year duration study, and with rapid recruitment, the expectation is that most participants can be followed for at least 7 years. This will permit the assessment of the impact of treatment on a projected 1,500–2,000 cases of prostate cancer[745] that are expected to occur within this time interval. Specific molecular studies are also planned that are anticipated to provide information on factors that contribute to prostate cancer risk, including blood sample analysis of micronutrients, hormones, cytokines and other proteins.

Finally, chemopreventive drug candidates that have been shown to be efficacious and of limited toxicity in both *in vitro* and *in vivo* preclinical experimental models of carcinogenesis may then be considered for further testing in a clinical setting. There are a variety of animal models for prostate cancer that appear to be suitable for preclinical chemoprevention studies[746]. Human prostate xenografts in mice can be used to assess tumor growth inhibition, combined chronic treatment of Noble rats with testosterone and estradiol produces prostatic intraepithelial neoplasia (PIN), a cancer precursor, and sequential treatment of rats with carcinogens such as N-methyl-N-nitrosourea (MNU) and chronic testosterone treatment leads to a high incidence of prostatic adenocarcinoma. Recently, transgenic mouse models for prostate cancer were developed by targeting expression of the simian virus 40 (SV40) large tumor T antigen (TAg) to the mouse prostate epithelium using either the flanking region of the rat C3(1) gene, a prostatic steroid binding globulin gene[747], or using a prostate-specific rat probasin (PB) gene promoter to drive expression of the T antigen coding region (TRAMP)[748]. Mice expressing high levels of the transgenes specifically display progressive forms of prostatic cancer that histologically resemble human prostate cancer. Potential chemopreventive agents tested in these systems include antiproliferation or differentiation-inducing agents such as 2–difluoromethylornithine (DFMO) or retinoids. DFMO, an inhibitor of ornithine decarboxylase[749] has shown chemopreventive activity in the TRAMP model of prostate cancer[750] and is currently being tested in a familial prostate cancer cohort. The combination of an antiandrogen (bicalutamide) with DFMO is also under evaluation in the clinic (See Table 15). Recently, the FDA approved retinoid 9-*cis*-retinoic acid[751] was shown to modulate the growth of prostate cancer cells *in vitro* and to retard the development of prostate tumors in the Noble rat animal model. Other natural product-based or micronutrient-related substances under investigation as potential prostate chemopreventive agents include: vitamin D and its analogs[752, 753], and green tea components[754, 755]. A vitamin D analog is already under study in a Phase II chemoprevention setting; the effects of 1-hydroxyvitamin D2 on biomarkers of carcinogenesis are under evaluation in patients scheduled for radical prostatectomy (See Table 15).

Inhibition of cyclooxygenase (COX) by traditional NSAIDs and selective inhibitors of the pro-inflammatory COX-2 isoform may also prove to have chemopreventive efficacy in prostate. Limited epidemiological study results suggest that NSAID use is associated with reduced risk of prostate cancer[756-759]. Elevated levels of prostaglandin (PG) E_2 and arachidonic acid metabolism are seen in benign and malignant human prostate tumor cells, and NSAIDs inhibit prostate tumor cell growth[750, 760-763] The selective COX-2 inhibitors, NS-398 and celecoxib, were found to induce apoptosis in LNCaP and PC-3 prostate cancer cells[764, 765]. Besides apoptosis, suppression of angiogenesis is another possible chemopreventive mechanism associated with COX inhibition. COX is expressed in angiogenic vasculature within tumors and pre-existing vasculature nearby tumors in prostate (Koki et al. 1999). The effects of celecoxib on biomarkers of prostate carcinogenesis are under evaluation in a Phase II clinical study in patients scheduled to undergo radical prostatectomy (See Table 15).

Two other NSAID derivatives which have lost COX inhibitory but retained pro-apoptotic activity are also promising chemopreventive agents in prostate. Exisulind, the sulfone metabolite of sulindac, most probably stimulates apoptosis via inhibition of cyclic GMP phosphodiesterase. This drug was found to inhibit the rise of PSA in patients with recurring prostate cancer after radical prostatectomy[766]. The R-isomer of the traditional NSAID flurbiprofen showed chemopreventive activity in the TRAMP mouse model[767].

IDENTIFICATION OF INTERMEDIATE ENDPOINT BIOMARKERS FOR CANCER PREVENTION TRIALS

A major objective of prostate cancer prevention research is the identification of morphologic, molecular and biochemical markers that are causally related or correlated to the transition from normal prostatic epithelium to premalignant status to invasive adenocarcinoma. The most established marker of premalignant dysplasia or atypia is high grade PIN. Although this precursor lesion is observed in a small but significant number of prostate needle biopsies, it usually predicts a high likelihood of coexistent cancer or subsequent progression to cancer[768]. PIN has high prevalence, shown by the 40–50% PIN incidence in autopsy results from men in the 4th and 5th decades of age. However, because of the long latency and indolence of PIN progression to cancer, 40–50% prostate cancer incidence does not occur until the 8th decade[769, 770]. A wide spectrum of markers has been examined in PIN and the coincidence of their abnormal expression or modulation further confirms that PIN pathology is on the pathway to clinically significant prostate cancer. For example, PIN lesions have been shown to underexpress glutathione-S-transferase (GST), a detoxifying enzyme and overexpress markers of proliferation, such as Ki-67, when compared with benign prostate tissues[771, 772]. Genetic abnormalities such as 8p, 10q, 18p chromosomal loss and 7q31, 8p and c-myc gain, along with changes in chromatin texture and telomerase activation have all be detected in PIN lesions and adenocarcinoma, while these changes are absent in normal gland tissues[773]. Therapeutic androgen-deprivation therapy has been shown to induce apoptosis-driven histopathologic involution of PIN lesions along with regions of normal gland and cancer, suggesting hormone-dependence of the PIN lesion. However, other androgen-deprevation strategies such as 5-reductase inhibition by finasteride had no effect on PIN[700]. PIN is also not usually associated with significantly elevated PSA, and it is rarely if ever detected by ultrasonography, which is also consistent with its placement at an early step in the prostate cancer progression sequence. Most of these data suggest alterations of carcinogenesis biomarkers in high-grade PIN may be an important method of assessing the efficacy of a chemopreventive regimen, and the World Health Organization has recommended that PIN should be reported by pathologists as a practice standard[774].

PSA continues to be the foundation of early detection and monitoring of prostate cancer. Refinements in the use of PSA measurements (free *vs* bound values; velocity and doubling time parameters) have been used to improve the predictive value of this biochemical assay. Several recent studies have suggested that other serologic markers may have some promise as complementary markers of increased prostate cancer risk, such as IGF/IGF-BP3 or HK-2 and that these markers may be modulatable by chemopreventive intervention.

The development of DNA microarray technology now permits the simultaneous analysis of the expression of hundreds or thousands of gene transcripts. These techniques can be used to assess the differential patterns of expression that help distinguish features of prostate cancer carcinogenesis that are beyond the sensitivity of histopathologic evaluation or the monitoring of single molecular or biochemical markers. Indeed, unique prostate cancer "chips" and databases have been used to identify overexpressed genes strongly associated with cDNA libraries derived from cancer foci and high-grade PIN lesions that are not found in normal prostate tissues[775]. A number of these genes turn out to be novel uncharacterized genes or genes that have not previously been described in association with the physiology of prostate cells. Many of these genes may prove to be starting points for the further investigation of sensitive new diagnostic markers for staging, preventing or treating prostate cancer. The NCI Cancer Genome Anatomy Project (see http://www.ncbi.nlm.nih.gov/CGAP/hTGI/sumtab/cgapba/cgi) is building an index of all genes that are expressed in tumors and is developing web-based access to these informatics tools. The tumor type with the highest representation in the early versions of the CGAP database is prostate cancer and this increasingly used resource is now available to the prostate cancer research community.

Other technologies are being explored which should facilitate identification of new biomarkers and potential chemopreventive agents. These include quantitative computer-assisted morphometric analysis of histopathologic samples and *in vivo* imaging instrumentation. Three-dimensional ultrasonographic image analysis tools developed for brachytherapy will be increasingly valuable in directing the optimal biopsy sampling efforts required for definitive chemoprevention studies. New magnetic resonance imaging technologies[374, 776] and enhancing agents[777] with high sensitivity hold the potential for the remote detection of metabolic differences between malignant and premalignant structures in real time. Application of these technologies to chemoprevention may both aid in the identification of prospective cohorts for trial participation and permit easy monitoring of the effects of intervention.

STUDY POPULATIONS FOR PROSTATE CANCER PREVENTION STUDIES AND CLINICAL TRIAL DESIGN: MATCHING THE AGENT WITH THE COHORT

Because of the variable spectrum of toxicities exhibited with potential chemopreventive agents, a major consideration in prostate prevention clinical trial design is to match the therapeutic index of a particular agent to a target population in order to maximize both chemopreventive efficacy and quality of life[727]. Potential populations at points of intervention corresponding to increasing risk categories include 1) Asymptomatic men in the general population that are ≥55 years of age (or >50 years of age for African-American men) with normal PSA; 2) Subjects/kindreds with a strong family history of early-onset prostate cancer; 3) Men with elevated PSA but negative biopsy for cancer and 4) Subjects with suspicious histological changes such as high-grade PIN but no cancer detected even after re-biopsy; and 5) Individuals with minimal volume, low Gleason score, localized prostate cancer that have opted for watchful waiting or prostatectomy.

The two large definitive Phase III trials, PCPT and SELECT, conducted in the general population will clearly present opportunities to assess chemoprevention concepts using "gold standard" cancer-incidence endpoints. However, these kinds of trials are expensive, protracted and, because of their scale, can result in design commitments many years in advance of complete understanding of an agent's activities. For example, potential biopsy sample bias associated with finasteride treatment-associated prostate gland shrinkage and potential PSA detection bias due to inhibition of PSA required careful trial design considerations to minimize. However, this agent may not provide chemopreventive benefit in all cohorts. Recently a smaller study of finasteride in a different cohort (men with elevated PSA but negative pretreatment biopsy) who underwent treatment for a shorter duration (12 months) showed no evidence of chemoprevention and some risk of progression in patients with preexisting PIN[778]. Chemoprevention trials designed to reverse high-grade PIN may be confounded by the presence of underlying but undetected cancer. This problem might be addressed by requiring a second biopsy without cancer before entry into the study and by including a large enough sample size to ensure comparable coexistent cancer in both study and control groups[779]. The SELECT trial clinical design includes a repeat biopsy (sextant or greater) at an interval after initial high-grade PIN diagnosis to exclude individuals with coexistent cancer who might confound the findings. All patients will be followed for at least 7 years from randomization to provide long-term outcomes information.

There is obvious complementary value to designing smaller, shorter duration Phase II studies using cohorts and agents with different risk/benefit ratios than can be examined in large Phase III studies. For instance, recent studies indicate that the familial/genetic contribution to prostate cancer may be significant. Brothers and male first-cousins of individuals who develop early-onset (at <60 years of age) prostate cancer have a significantly increased risk of developing disease (odds ratios of approximately 5–6 and 3–4, respectively). Linkage analyses in families with multiple cases of prostate cancer have lead to the search for a putative hereditary prostate cancer gene (HPC-1)[14]. Susceptibility loci on several chromosomes are being explored. Conflicting evidence associating risk with polymorphisms in steroid reductase *(SRAD5A2)*, 17-hydroxylase cytochrome P450 *(CYP17)*, and androgen receptor genes has also been reported[111, 780]. Confirmation results from these studies may eventually provide diagnostic tests for the detection of genetic high-risk cohorts that might benefit from chemopreventive intervention. Until such time, several studies are proceeding with the evaluation of low toxicity agents in populations of unaffected relatives of high risk families that have been contacted through prostate cancer registries. Similar investigations are focused on dietary supplement intervention in higher-risk ethnic groups like African-Americans[781].

Other cohorts proposed for Phase II trials are patients with localized cancers or those with premalignant lesions or no-evidence of disease but rising PSA. For such patients, the trials are conducted within the context of standard treatment which may be prostatectomy or watchful waiting. For example, the prototypical pre-surgical Phase II study provides a valuable setting to examine biomarker modulation. These patients are treated with the chemopreventive drug during the four- to eight-week interval between diagnostic biopsy and prostatectomy. As shown in Table 15, changes in various biomarkers between the diagnostic biopsy tissue and resected tissue taken by prostatectomy are then evaluated. Several trials sponsored by the National Cancer Institute, Division of Cancer Prevention (NCI, DCP) following this paradigm are currently in progress or are completed, including studies with flutamide in combination with toremifene; DFMO monotherapy or DFMO in combination with bicalutamide; soy isoflavones; the retinoid fenretinide; a vitamin D analog; the NSAID celecoxib; and the selective apoptosis inducer exisulind. In patients with PIN followed by watchful waiting, the primary endpoint is PIN regression and cancer incidence reduction, and the treatment period can be for up to three years. A trial with flutamide monotherapy has been performed in this PIN cohort and an early Phase III trial of selenomethionine intervention is now underway. In patients under watch for recurrence of prostatic carcinoma, exisulind was found to delay the rise in PSA associated with disease recurrence[766].

CONCLUSIONS AND FUTURE DIRECTIONS

The treatment and prevention of prostate cancer is an enormous healthcare challenge. In prevention and treatment of early disease, the challenge will be met by the identification and careful characterization of efficacious drugs, accompanied by technological advances in molecular risk assessment, diagnostics, and imaging. Both initial diagnosis of prostate cancer and early assessment of chemopreventive efficacy have traditionally relied on biopsy as the standard by which other diagnostic methods are judged. However, biopsy sampling issues can complicate the interpretation of chemopreventive outcomes in certain clinical trial designs. In this regard, advances in imaging science hold the prospect of improving both diagnosis of the prostate cancer and analysis of carcinogenesis biomarkers. These tools will be increasingly valuable in directing the optimal biopsy sampling efforts required for definitive chemoprevention studies. they will also improve resolution for staging and biopsy sampling and lead to non-invasive molecular spectroscopic evaluation of an individual lesion's risk of progression.

11. STRATEGIES FOR PROSTATE CANCER PREVENTION

In 1998, the NCI convened a panel of experts, the Prostate Cancer Progress Review Group, to review progress against this particular cancer and to develop recommendations for strengthening resources and addressing problems and opportunities in this field[782] see http:/wwwosp.nci.nih.gov/planning/prg/toc htm). The recommendations put forth by these scientists are essentially the implementation of strategies described in this chapter. In order to increase the rate of which discoveries are translated into more effective programs of detection, diagnosis and prevention, the following areas of increased emphasis for prevention research were highlighted [see http:/www.nci/nih/gov/prostate.html]: 1) The importance of understanding the critical molecular genetic and cellular events underlying the etiology of prostate cancer will guide the development of cancer prevention strategies and the selection of relevant forms of chemopreventive agents for testing: 2) The value of being able to identify men at increased risk for the development of prostate due to hereditary, dietary or other environmental risk factors will help shape the design of trials that can demonstrate chemopreventive efficacy; 3) Advances in the development of technology and tools that help validate and permit the application of surrogate endpoints, providing reliable prognostic and outcomes measurement, will ultimately accelerate the regulatory approval of prostate cancer prevention drugs or supplements.

REFERENCES

1. Hsing, A.W., Y.T. Gao, G. Wu, X. Wang, J. Deng, Y.L. Chen, I.A. Sesterhenn, F.K. Mostofi, J. Benichou and C. Chang, Polymorphic CAG and GGN repeat lengths in the androgen receptor gene and prostate cancer risk: a population-based case-control studyh in China. Cancer Res, 2000. 60: p. 5111-5116.
2. Labrie, F., Cancer of the Prostate, in The UICC Manual of Clinical Oncology (8th edition), R. Pollock, Editor. in press.
3. Morganti, G., L. Gianferrari, A. Cresseri, G. Arrigoni and G. Lovati, Recherches clinico-statistiques et ginitiques sur les nιoplasies de la prostate. Acta Genet, 1956. 6: p. 304-305.
4. Eeles, R., The UK Familial Prostate Study Co-ordinating Group & The CRC/BPG UK Familial Prostate Study Collaborators. Prostate Cancer and Prostatic Diseases, 1999. 2: p. 9-15.
5. Ostrander, E.A. and J.L. Stanford, Genetics of prostate cancer: too many loci, too few genes. Am J Hum Genet, 2000. 67: p. 1367-1375.
6. Singh, R.E.R., F. Durocher, J. Simard, S. Edwards, M. Badzioch, Z. Kote-Jarai, D. Teare, D. Ford, D. Dearnaley, A. Ardern-Jones, A. Murkin, A. Dowe, R. Shearer, J. Kelly, T.C.B.U.F.P.C.S. Collaborators, F. Labrie, D. Easton, S.A. Narod, P.N. Tonin, and W.D. Foulkes, High risk genes predisposing to prostate cancer - Do they exist? Prostate cancer and prostatic diseases, 2000. 3: p. 241-247.
7. Nwosu, V., J. Carpten, J.M. Trent and R. Sheridan, Heterogeneity of genetic alterations in prostate cancer: evidence of the complex nature of the disease. Hum Mol Genet, 2001. 10: p. 2313-2318.
8. Eeles, R., L.A. Cannon-Albright, S.A.J. Ponder, D.F. Easton and A. Horwich, Familial Prostate Cancer and it's Management, in Genetic Predisposition to Cancer. 1996. p. 320-332.
9. Cannon, L., D.T. Bishop, M. Skolnick, S. Hunt, J.L. Lyon and C.R. Smart, Genetic Epidemiology of Prostate Cancer in the Utah Mormon Genealogy. Cancer Surv, 1982. 1: p. 47-69.
10. Carter, B.S., T.H. Beaty and G.D. Steinberg, Mendelian inheritance of familial prostate cancer. Proc Natl Acad Sci, 1993. 89: p. 3367-3371.
11. Steinberg, G.D., B.S. Carter, T.H. Beaty, B. Childs and P.C. Walsh, Family history and the risk of prostate cancer. Prostate, 1990. 17: p. 337-347.
12. Lichtenstein, P., N.V. Holm, P.K. Verkasalo, A. Iliadou, J. Kaprio, M. Koskenvuo, E. Pukkala, A. Skytthe and K. Hemminki, Environmental and heritable factors in the causation of cancer — analyses of cohorts of twins from Sweden, Denmark and Finland. N Engl J Med, 2000. 343: p. 78-85.
13. Schaid, D.J., S.K. McDonnell and S.N. Thibodeau, Regression models for linkage heterogeneity applied to familial prostate cancer. Am J Hum Genet, 2001. 68: p. 1189-1196.
14. Gronberg, H., S.D. Isaacs, J.R. Smith, J.D. Carpten, G.S. Bova, D. Freije, J. Xu, D.A. Meyers, F.S.

REFERENCES

Collins, J.M. Trent, P.C. Walsh, and W.B. Isaacs, Characteristics of prostate cancer in families potentially linked to the hereditary prostate cancer 1 (HPC1) locus. JAMA, 1997. 278: p. 1251-1255.

15. Narod, S., A. Dupont, L. Cusan, P. Diamond, J.L. Gomez, R.E. Suburu and F. Labrie, The impact of family history on early detection of prostate cancer. Nat. Med., 1995. 1: p. 99-101.

16. Monroe, K.R., M.C. Yu, L.N. Kolonel, G.A. Coetzee, L.R. Wilkens, R.K. Ross and B. Henderson, Evidence of an X-linked or recessive component to prostate cancer risk. Nat Med, 1995. 1: p. 827-829.

17. Cui, J., M.P. Staples, J.L. Hopper, D.R. English, M.R. McCredie and G.G. Giles, Segregation analyses of 1,476 population-based Australian families affected by prostate cancer. Am J Hum Genet, 2001. 68: p. 1207-1218.

18. Smith, J.R., D. Freije, J.D. Carpten, H. Gronberg, J. Xu, S.D. Isaacs, M.J. Brownstein, G.S. Bova, H. Guo, P. Bujnovsky, D.R. Nusskern, J.E. Damber, A. Bergh, M. Emanuelsson, O.P. Kallioniemi, J. Walker-Daniels, J.E. Bailey-Wilson, B. T.H., D.A. Meyers, P.C. Walsh, F.S. Collins, J.M. Trent, and W.B. Isaacs, Major susceptibility locus for prostate cancer on chromosome 1 suggested by a genome-wide search. Science, 1996. 274: p. 1371-1374.

19. Gibbs, M., J.L. Stanford, R.A. McIndoe, G.P. Jarvik, S. Kolb, E.L. Goode, L. Chakrabarti, E.F. Schuster, V.A. Buckley, E.L. Miller, S. Brandzel, S. Li, L. Hood, and E.A. Ostrander, Evidence for a rare prostate cancer-susceptibility locus at chromosome 1p36. Am J Hum Genet, 1999. 64: p. 776-787.

20. Gibbs, M., J.L. Stanford, G.P. Jarvik, M. Janer, M. Badzioch, M.A. Peters, E.L. Goode, S. Kolb, L. Chakrabarti, M. Shook, R. Basom, E.A. Ostrander, and L. Hood, A genomic scan of families with prostate cancer identifies multiple regions of interest. Am J Hum Gen, 2000. 67: p. 100-109.

21. Goddard, K.A., J.S. Witte, B.K. Suarez, W.J. Catalona and J.M. Olson, Model-free linkage analysis with covariates confirms linkage of prostate cancer to chromosomes 1 and 4. Am J Hum Genet, 2001. 68: p. 1197-1206.

22. Suarez, B.K., J. Lin, J.K. Burmester, K.W. Broman, J.L. Weber, T.K. Banerjee, K.A. Goddard, J.S. Witte, R.C. Elston and W.J. Catalona, A genome screen of multiplex sibships with prostate cancer. Am J Hum Genet, 2000. 66: p. 933-944.

23. Witte, J.S., K.A. Goddard, D.V. Conti, R.C. Elston, J. Lin, B.K. Suarez, K.W. Broman, J.K. Burmester, J.L. Weber and W.J. Catalona, Genomewide scan for prostate cancer aggressiveness loci. Am J Hum Genet, 2000. 67: p. 92-99.

24. Hsieh, C.L., I. Oakley-Girvan, R.R. Balise, J. Halpern, R.P. Gallagher, A.H. Wu, L.N. Kolonel, L.E. O'Brien, I.G. Lin, D.J. Van Den Berg, C.Z. Teh, D.W. West, and A.S. Whittenmore, A genome screen of families with multiple cases of prostate cancer: evidence of genetic heterogeneity. Am J Hum Genet, 2001. 69: p. 148-158.

25. Neuhausen, S.L., J.M. Farnham, E. Kort, S.V. Tavtigian, M.H. Skolnick and L.A. Cannon-Albright, Prostate cancer susceptibility locus HPC1 in Utah high-risk pedigrees. Hum Mol Genet, 1999. 8: p. 2437-2442.

26. Tavtigian, S.V., J. Simard, D.H.F. Teng, V. Abtin, M. Baumgard, A. Beck, N.J.C.A.R. Carillo, Y. Chen, P. Dayananth, M. Desrochers, M. Dumont, J.M. Farnham, D. Frank, C. Frye, S. Ghaffari, J.S. Gupte, R.Hu, D. Iliev, T. Janecki, E.N. Kort, K.E. Laity, A.Leavitt, G. Leblanc, J. McArthur-Morrison, A. Pederson, B. Penn, K.T. Peterson, J.E. Reid, S. Richard, M. Schroeder, R. Smith, S.C. Snyder, B. Swedlund, J. Swensen, A. Thomas, M. Tranchant, A. Woodhland, F. Labrie, M.H. Skolnick, S. Neuhausen, J. Rommens, and L.A. Cannon-Albright, A candidate prostate cancer susceptibility gene at chromosome 17p. Nature Genetics, 2001. 27: p. 172-180.

27. Berry, R., D.J. Schaid, J.R. Smith, A.J. French, J.J. Schroeder, S.K. McDonnell, B.J. Peterson, Z.Y. Wang, J.D. Carpten, S.G. Roberts, D.J. Tester, M.L. Blute, J.M. Trent, and S.N. Thibodeau, Linkage analyses at the chromosome 1 loci 1q24=25 (HPC1), 1q42.2-43(PCAP), and 1p36(CAPB) in families with hereditary prostate cancer. American Journal of Human Genetics, 2000. 66: p. 539-546.

28. Berthon, P., A. Valeri, A. Cohen-Akenine, E. Drelon, T. Paiss, G. Wohr, A. Latil, P. Millasseau, I. Mellah, N. Cohen, H. Blanche, C. Bellane-Chantelot, F. Demenais, P. Teillac, A. Le Duc, R. de Petriconi, R. Hautmann, I. Chumakov, L. Bachner, N.J. Maitland, R. Lidereau, W. Vogel, G. Fournier, P. Mangin, and O. Cussenot, Predisposing gene for early-onset prostate cancer, localized on chromosome 1q42.2-43. Am J Hum Genet, 1998(1416-1424).

29. Xu, J., S.L. Zheng, J.D. Carpten, N.N. Nupponen, C.M. Robbins, J. Mestre, T.Y. Moses, D.A. Faith, B.D. Kelly, S.D. Isaacs, K.E. Wiley, C.M. Ewing, P. Bujnovskzky, B. Chang, J. Bailey-Wilson, E.R. Bleecker, P.C. Walsh, J.M. Trent, D.A. Meyers, and W.B. Isaacs, Evaluation of linkage and association of HPC2/ELAC2 in patients with familial or sporadic prostate cancer. Am J Hum Genet, 2001. 68: p. 901-911.

30. Xu, J., D. Meyers, D. Freije, S. Isaacs, K. Wiley, D. Nusskern, C. Ewing, E. Wilkens, P. Bujnovszky, G.S. Bova, P. Walsh, W. Isaacs, J. Schleutker, M. Matikainen, T. Tammela, T. Visakorpi, O.P. Kallioniemi, R. Berry, D. Schaid, A. French, S. McDonnell, J. Schroeder, M. Blute, S. Thibodeau, and J. Trent, Evidence for a prostate cancer susceptibility locus on the X chromosome. Nat Genet, 1998. 20: p. 175-179.

31. McIndoe, R.A., J.L. Stanford, M. Gibbs, G.P. Jarvik, S. Brandzel, C.L. Neal, S. Li, J.T. Gammack, A.A. Gay, E.L. Goode, L. Hood, and E.A. Ostrander, Linkage analysis of 49 high-risk families does not support a common familial prostate cancer-susceptibility gene at 1q24-25. Am J Hum Genet, 1997. 61: p. 347-353.

32. Eeles, A.R., F. Durocher, S. Edwards, D. Teare, M. Badzioch, R. Hamoudi, S. Gill, P. Biggs, D. Dearnaley, A. Ardern-Jones, A. Dowe, R. Shearer, D.L. McLennan, R.L. Norman, P. Ghadirian, A. Aprikian, D. Ford, C. Amos, T.M. King, The Cancer Research Campaign/British Prostate Group UK Familial Prostate Cancer Study Collaborators, F. Labrie, J. Simard, S.A. Narod, D. Easton, and W.D. Foulkes, Linkage analysis of chromosome 1q markers in 136 prostate cancer families. Am. J. Hum. Genet., 1998. 62: p. 653-658.

33. Goode, E.L., J.L. Stanford, M.A. Peters, M. Janer, M. Gibbs, S. Kolb, M.D. Badzioch, L. Hood, E.A. Ostrander and G.P. Jarvik, Clinical characteristics of prostate cancer in an analysis of linkage to four putative susceptibility loci. Clin Cancer Res, 2001. 7: p. 2739-2749.

34. Xu, J. and the International Consortium for Prostate Cancer Genetics, Combined analysis of hereditary prostate cancer linkage to 1q24-25: Results from 772 hereditary prostate cancer families from the International Consortium for Prostate Cancer Genetics. Am. J. Hum. Genet., 2000. 66: p. 945-957.

35. Cancel-Tassin, G., A. Latil, A. Valeri, P. Mangin, G. Fournier, P. Berthon and O. Cussenot, PCAP is the major known prostate cancer predisposing locus in families from south and west Europe. Eur J Hum Genet, 2001. 9: p. 135-142.

36. Schleutker, J., M. Matikainen, J. Smith, P. Koivisto, A. Baffoe-Bonnie, T. Kainu, E. Gillanders, R. Sankila, E. Pukkala, J. Carpten, D. Stephan, T. Tammela, M. Brownstein, J. Bailey-Wilson, J. Trent, and O.P. Kallioniemi, A genetic epidemiological study of hereditary prostate cancer (HPC) in Finland: frequent HPCX linkage in families with late-onset disease. Clin Cancer Res, 2000. 6(4810-4815).

37. Lange, E.M., H. Chen, K. Brierley, E.E. Perrone, C.H. Bock, E. Gillanders, M.E. Ray and K.A. Cooney, Linkage analysis of 153 prostate cancer families over a 30-cM region containing the putative susceptibility locus HPCX. Clin Cancer Res, 1999. 5: p. 4013-4020.

38. Bochum, S., T. Paiss, W. Vogel, K. Herkommer, R. Hautmann and J. Haeussler, Confirmation of the prostate cancer susceptibility locus HPCX in a set of 104 German prostate cancer families. Prostate, 2002. 52: p. 12-19.

39. Berry, R., J.J. Schroeder, A.J. French, S.K. McDonnell, B.J. Peterson, J.M. Cunningham, S.N. Thibodeau and D.J. Schaid, Evidence for a prostate cancer-susceptibility locus on chromosome 20. Am J Hum Genet, 2000. 67(82-91).

40. Zheng, S.L., S.D. Isaacs, K. Wiley, B. Chang, E.R. Bleecker, P.C. Walsh, J.M. Trent, D.A. Meyers and W.B. Isaacs, Evidence for a prostate cancer linkage to chromosome 20 in 159 hereditary prostate cancer families. Hum Gent, 2001. 108: p. 430-435.

41. Bock, C.H., J.M. Cunningham, S.K. McDonnell, D.J. Schaid, B.J. Peterson, R.J. Pavlic, J.J. Schroeder, J. Klein, A.J. French, A. Marks, S.N. Thibodeau, E.M. Lange, and D.A. Cooney, Analysis of the prostate cancer-susceptibility locus HPC20 in 172 families affected by prostate cancer. Am J Hum Genet, 2001. 68: p. 795-801.

42. Badzioch, M., R. Eeles, G. Leblanc, W.D. Foulkes, G. Giles, S. Edwards, D. Goldgar, J.L. Hopper, D.T. Bishop, P. Moller, K. Heimdal, D. Easton, and J. Simard, Suggestive evidence for a site specific prostate cancer gene on chromosome 1p36. The CRC/BPG UK Familial Prostate Cancer Study

Coordinators and Collaborators. J Med Genet, 2000. 37: p. 947-949.

43. Abate-Shen, C. and M.M. Shen, Molecular genetics of prostate cancer. Genes Dev, 2000. 14: p. 2410-2434.

44. Xu, J., M. Kalos, J.A. Stolk, E.J. Zasloff, X. Zhang, R.L. Houghton, A.M. Filho, M. Nolasco, R. Badaro and S.G. Reed, Identification and characterization of prostein, a novel prostate-specific protein. Cancer Res, 2001. 61: p. 1563-1568.

45. Abkevich, V., N.J. Camp, A. Gutin, J.M. Farnham, L. Cannon-Albright and A. Thomas, A robust multi-point linkage statistic (tlod) for mapping complex trait loci. Genet Epidemiol, 2001. 21: p. S492-S497.

46. Xu, J., S.L. Zheng, G.A. Hawkins, D.A. Faith, B. Kelly, S.D. Isaacs, K.E. Wiley, B. Chang, C.M. Ewing, P. Bujnovszky, J.D. Carpten, E.R. Bleecker, P.C. Walsh, J.M. Trent, D.A. Meyers, and W.B. Isaacs, Linkage and association studies of prostate cancer susceptibility: evidence for linkage at 8p22-23. Am J Hum Genet, 2001. 69: p. 341-350.

47. Suarez, B.K., D.S. Gerhard, J. Lin, B. Haberer, L. Nguyen, N.K. Kesterson and W.J. Catalona, Polymorphisms in the prostate cancer susceptibility gene HPC2/ELAC2 in multiplex families and healthy controls. Cancer Res, 2001. 61: p. 4982-4984.

48. Slager, S.L., D.J. Schaid, J.M. Cunningham, S.K. McDonnell, A. French, B.J. Peterson, A.F. Marks, S. Hebbring, B. Koch, S. Anderson, and S.N. Thibodeau, Linkage analysis on prostate cancer agressiveness. Am J Genet, 2002. 71(S): p. S247.

49. Carpten, J., N. Nupponen, S. Isaacs, R. Sood, C. Robbins, J. Xu, M. Faruque, T. Moses, C. Ewing, E. Guillanders, P. Hu, P. Bujnovsky, I. Makalowska, A. Baffoe-Bonnie, D. Faith, J. Smith, D. Stephan, K. Wiley, M. Brownstein, D. Gildea, B. Kelly, R. Jenkins, H. G., M. Matikainen, J. Schleutker, K. Klinger, T. Connors, Y. Xiang, Z. Wang, A. De Marzo, N. Papadopoulos, O.P. Kallioniemi, R. Burk, D. Meyers, H. Gronberg, P. Meltzer, R. Silverman, J. Bailey-Wilson, P. Walsh, W. Isaacs, and J. Trent, Germline mutations in the ribonuclease L gene in families showing linkage with HPC1. Nat Genet, 2002. 30: p. 181-184.

50. Xu, J., S.L. Zheng, A. Komiya, J.C. Mychaleckyj, S.D. Isaacs, J.J. Hu, D. Sterling, E.M. Lange, G.A. Hawkins, A. Turner, C.M. Ewing, D.A. Faith, J.R. Johnson, H. Suzuki, P. Bujnovszky, K.E. Wiley, A.M. DeMarzo, G.S. Bova, B. Chang, M.C. Hall, D.L. McCullough, A.W. Partin, V.S. Kassabian, J.D. Carpten, J.E. Bailey-Wilson, J.M. Trent, J. Ohar, E.R. Bleecker, P.C. Walsh, W.B. Isaacs, and D.A. Meyers, Germline mutations and sequence variants of the macrophage scavenger receptor 1 gene are associated with prostate cancer risk. Nat Genet, 2002. 32: p. 321-325.

51. Cannon-Albright, L.A., D.E. Goldgar, L.J. Meyer, C.M. Lewis, D.E. Anderson, J.W. Fountain, M.E. Hegi, R.W. Wiseman, E.M. Petty and A.E. Bale, Assignment of a locus for familial melanoma, MLM, to chromosome 9p13-p22. Science, 1992. 258: p. 1148-1152.

52. Miki, Y., J. Swensen, D. Shattuck-Eidens, P.A. Futreal, K. Harshman, S. Tavtigian, Q. Liu, C. Cochran, L.M. Bennett, W. Ding, R. Bell, J. Rosenthal, C. Hussey, T. Tran, M. McClure, C. Frye, T. Hattier, R. Phelps, A. Haugen-Strano, H. Katcher, K. Yakumo, Z. Gholami, D. Shaffer, S. Stone, S. Bayer, C. Wray, R. Bogden, P. Dayananth, J. Ward, P. Tonin, S. Narod, P.K. Bristow, F.H. Norris, L. Helvering, P. Morrison, P. Rosteck, M. Lai, J.C. Barrett, C. Lewis, S. Neuhausen, L. Cannon-Albright, D. Goldgar, R. Wiseman, A. Kamb, and M.H. Skolnick, A strong candidate for the breast and ovarian susceptibility gene BRCA1. Science, 1994. 266: p. 66-71.

53. Wooster, R., S.L. Neuhausen, J. Mangion, Y. Quirk, D. Ford, N. Collins, K. Nguyen, S. Seal, T. Tran, D. Averill, P. Fields, G. Marshall, S. Narod, G.M. Lenoir, H. Lynch, J. Feunteun, P. Devilee, C.J. Cornelisse, F.H. Menko, P.A. Daly, W. Orminston, R. McManus, C. Pye, C.M. Lewis, L.A. Cannon-Albright, B. Peto, Ponder, M.H. Skolnick, D.F. Easton, D. Goldgar, and M. Stratton, Localization of a breast cancer susceptibility gene, BRCA2, to chromosome 13q12-13. Science, 1994. 265: p. 2088-2090.

54. Vogel, A., O. Schilling, M. Niecke, J. Bettmer and W. Meyer-Klaucke, ElaC encodes a novel binuclear zinc phosphodiesterase. J Biol Chem, 2002. 277: p. 29078-29085.

55. Schiffer, S., S. Rosch and A. Marchfelder, Assigning a function to a conserved group of proteins: the tRNA 3'-processing enzymes. Embo J, 2002(2769-2777).

56. Rebbeck, T.R., A.H. Walker, C. Zeigler-Johnson, S. Weisburg, A.M. Martin, K.L. Nathanson, A.J. Wein

and S.B. Malkowicz, Association of HPC2/ELAC2 genotypes and prostate cancer. Am J Genet, 2000. 67: p. 1014-1019.

57. Vesprini, D., R.K. Nam, J. Trachtenberg, M.A. Jewett, S.V. Tavtigian, M. Emami, M. Ho, A. Toi and S.A. Narod, HPC2 variants and screen-detected prostate cancer. Am J Hum Genet, 2001. 68: p. 912-917.

58. Wang, L., S.K. McDonnell, D.A. Elkins, S.L. Slager, E. Christensen, A.F. Marks, J.M. Cunningham, B.J. Peterson, S.J. Jacobsen, J.R. Cerhan, M.L. Blute, D.J. Schaid, and S.N. Thibodeau, Role of HPC2/ELAC2 in hereditary prostate cancer. Cancer Res, 2001. 61: p. 6494-6499.

59. Rokman, A., T. Ikonen, N. Mononen, V. Autio, M.P. Matikainen, P.A. Koivisto, T.L. Tammela, O.P. Kallioniemi and J. Schleutker, ELAC2/HPC2 involvement in hereditary and sporadic prostate cancer. Cancer Res, 2001. 61: p. 6038-6041.

60. Meitz, J.C., S.M. Edwards, D.F. Easton, A. Murkin, A. Ardern-Jones, R.A. Jackson, S. Williams, D.P. Dearnaley, M.R. Stratton, R.S. Houlston, and R.A. Eeles, HPC2/ELAC2 polymorphisms and prostate cancer risk: analysis by age and onset of disease. Br J Cancer, 2002. 87: p. 905-908.

61. Shea, P.R., R.E. Ferrell, A.L. Patrick, L.H. Kuller and C.H. Bunker, ELAC2 and prostate cancer risk in Afro-Caribbeans of Tobago. Hum Genet, 2002. 111: p. 398-400.

62. Camp, N.J. and S.V. Tavtigian, Meta Analysis of Associations of the Ser217Leu and Ala541Thr variants in ELAC2(HPC2) and Prostate Cancer. Am J Hum Genet, 2002. 71: p. 1475-1478.

63. Rokman, A., T. Ikonen, E.H. Seppala, N. Nupponen, V. Autio, N. Mononen, J. Bailey-Wilson, J. Trent, J. Carpten, M.P. Matikainen, P.A. Koivisto, T.L. Tammela, O.P. Kallioniemi, and J. Schleutker, Germline alterations of the RNASEL gene, a candidate HPC1 gene at 1q25, in patients and families with prostate cancer. Am J Hum Genet, 2002. 70: p. 1299-1304.

64. Rennert, H., D. Bercovich, A. Hubert, D. Abeliovich, U. Rozovsky, A. Bar-Shira, S. Soloviov, L. Schrieber, H. Matzkin, G. Rennert, L. Kadouri, T. Peretz, Y. Yaron, and A. Orr-Urtreger, A novel founder mutation in the RNASEL gene, 471delAAAG, is associated with prostate cancer in Ashkenazi Jews. Am J Hum Genet, 2002. 71: p. 981-984.

65. Casey, G., P.J. Neville, S.J. Plummer, Y. Xiang, L.M. Krumroy, E.A. Klein, W.J. Catalona, N. Nupponen, J.D. Carpten, J.M. Trent, R.H. Silverman, and J.S. Witte, RNASEL Arg462Gln variant is implicated in up to 13% of prostate cancer cases. Nat Genet, 2002. 4: p. 4.

66. Wang, L., S.K. MdDonnell, D.A. Elkins, S.L. Slager, E. Christensen, A.F. Marks, J.M. Cunningham, B.J. Peterson, S.J. Jacobsen, J.R. Cerhan, M.L. Blute, D.J. Schaid, and S.N. Thibodeau, Analysis of the RNASEL gene in familial and sporadic prostate cancer. Am J Hum Genet, 2002. 71: p. 116-123.

67. Anderson, D.E. and M.D. Badzioch, Breast cancer risks in relatives of male breast cancer patients. J Natl Cancer Inst, 1992. 84: p. 1114-1117.

68. Tulinius, H., V. Egilsson, G.H. Olafsdottir and H. Sigvaldason, Risk of prostate, ovarian, and endometrial cancer among relatives of women with breast cancer. Bmj, 1992. 305: p. 855-857.

69. Ford, D., D.F. Easton, D.T. Bishop, S. Narod and D.E. Goldgar, Risks of cancer in BRCA1 mutation carriers. Lancet, 1994. 343: p. 692-695.

70. Consortium, T.B.C.L., Cancer risks in BRCA2 mutation carriers. The Breast Cancer Linkage Consortium. J Natl Cancer Inst, 1999. 91: p. 1310-1316.

71. Thorlacius, S., G. Olafsdottir, L. Tryggvadottir, S. Neuhausen, J.G. Jonassen, S.V. Tavtigian, H. Tulinius, H.M. Ogmundsdottir and J.E. Eyfjord, A single BRCA2 mutation in male and female breast cancer families from Iceland with varied cancer phenotypes. Nat Genet, 1996. 13: p. 117-119.

72. Sigurdsson, S., S. Thorlacius, J. Tomasson, L. Tryggvadottir, K. Benediktsdottir, J.E. Eyfjord and E. Jonsson, BRCA2 mutation in Icelandic prostate cancer patients. J Mol Med, 1997. 75: p. 758-761.

73. Thorlacius, S., J.P. Struewing, P. Hartge, G.H. Olafsdottir, H. Sigvaldason, L. Tryggvadottir, S. Wacholder, H. Tulinius and J.E. Eyfjord, Population-based study of risk of breast cancer in carriers of BRCA2 mutation. Lancet, 1998. 352: p. 1337-1339.

74. Lehrer, S., F. Fodor, R.G. Stock, N.N. Stone, C. Eng, H.K. Song and M. McGovern, Absence of 185delAG mutation of the BRCA1 gene and 617delT mutation of the BRCA2 gene in Ashkenazi Jewish men with prostate cancer. Br J Cancer, 1998. 78: p. 771-773.

75. Hubert, A., T. Peretz, O. Manor, L. Kaduri, N. Wienberg, I. Lerer, M. Sagi and D. Abeliovich, The

REFERENCES

Jewish Ashkenazi founder mutations in the BRCA1/BRCA2 genes are not found at an increased frequency in Ashkenazi patients with prostate cancer. Am J Hum Genet, 1999. 65: p. 921-924.

76. Wilkens, E.P., D. Freije, J. Xu, D.R. Nusskern, H. Suzuki, S.D. Isaacs, K. Wiley, P. Bujnovsky, D.A. Meyers, P.C. Walsh, and W.B. Isaacs, No evidence for a role of BRCA1 or BRCA2 mutations in Ashkenazi Jewish families with hereditary prostate cancer. Prostate, 1999. 39: p. 280-284.

77. Nastiuk, K.L., M. Mansukhani, M.B. Terry, P. Kularatne, M.A. Rubin, J. Melamed, M.D. Gammon, M. Ittmann and J.J. Krolewski, Common mutations in BRCA1 and BRCA2 do not contribute to early prostate cancer in Jewish men. Prostate, 1999. 40: p. 172-177.

78. Gayther, S.A., K.A. De Foy, P. Harrington, P. Pharoah, W.D. Dunsmuir, S.M. Edwards, C. Gillett, A. Ardern-Jones, D.P. Dearnaley, D.F. Easton, D. Ford, R.J. Shearer, R.S. Kirby, A.L. Dowe, J. Kelly, M.R. Stratton, B.A. Ponder, D. Barnes, and R.A. Eeles, The frequency of germ-line mutations in the breast cancer predisposition genes BRCA1 and BRCA2 in familial prostate cancer. The Cancer Research Campaign/British Prostate Group United Kingdom Familial Prostate Cancer Study Collaborators. Cancer Res, 2000. 60: p. 4513-4518.

79. Gronberg, H., A.K. Ahman, M. Emanuelsson, A. Bergh, J.E. Damber and A. Borg, BRCA2 mutation in a family with hereditary prostate cancer. Genes Chromosomes Cancer, 2001. 30: p. 299-301.

80. Sinclair, C.S., R. Berry, D. Schaid, S.N. Thibodeau and F.J. Couch, BRCA1 and BRCA2 have a limited role in familial prostate cancer. Cancer Res, 2000. 60: p. 1371-1375.

81. Ross, R.K., G.A. Coetzee, C.L. Pearce, J.K. Reichardt, P. Bretsky, L.N. Kolonel, B.E. Henderson, E. Lander, D. Altshuler and G. Daley, Androgen metabolism and prostate cancer: establishing a model of genetic susceptibility. Eur Urol, 1999. 35: p. 355-361.

82. Makridakis, N.M. and J.K. Reichardt, Molecular epidemiology of hormone-metabolic loci in prostate cancer. Epidemiol Rev, 2001. 23: p. 24-29.

83. Montgomery, J.S., D.K. Price and W.D. Figg, The androgen receptor gene and its influence on the development and progression of prostate cancer. J Pathol, 2001. 195: p. 138-146.

84. Grossman, M.E., H. Huang and D.J. Tindall, Androgen receptor signaling in androgen-refractory prostate cancer. J Natl Cancer Inst, 2001. 93: p. 1687-1697.

85. Henshall, S.M., D.I. Quinn, C.S. Lee, D.R. Head, D. Golovsky, P.C. Brenner, W. Delprado, P.D. Stricker, J.J. Grygiel and R.L. Sutherland, Altered expression of androgen receptor in the malignant epithelium and adjacent stroma is associated with early relapse in prostate cancer. Cancer Res, 2001. 61: p. 423-427.

86. Linja, M.J., K.J. Savinainen, O.R. Saramaki, T.L. Tammela, R.L. Vessella and T. Visakorpi, Amplification and overexpression of androgen receptor gene in hormone-refractory prostate cancer. Cancer Res, 2001. 61: p. 3550-3555.

87. Chamberlain, N.L., E.D. Driver and R.L. Miesfeld, The length and location of CAG trinucleotide repeats in the androgen receptor N-terminal domain affect transactivation function. Nucleic Acids Res, 1994. 22: p. 3181-3186.

88. Kazemi-Esfarjani, P., M.A. Trifiro and L. Pinsky, Evidence for a repressive function of the long polyglutamine tract in the human androgen receptor: possible pathogenetic relevance for the (CAG)n-expanded neuronopathies. Hum Mol Genet, 1995. 4: p. 523-527.

89. Beilin, J., E.M. Ball, J.M. Favaloro and J.D. Zajac, Effect of the androgen receptor CAG repeat polymorphism on transcriptional activity: specificity in prostate and non-prostate cell lines. J Mol Endocrinol, 2000. 25: p. 85-96.

90. U, M., T. Miyashita, Y. Ohtsuka, Y. Okamura-Oho, Y. Shikama and M. Yamada, Extended polyglutamine selectively interacts with caspase-8 and -10 in nuclear aggregates. Cell Death Differ, 2001. 8: p. 377-386.

91. Irvine, R.A., H. Ma, M.C. Yu, R.K. Ross, M.R. Stallcup and G.A. Coetzee, Inhibition of p160-mediated coactivation with increasing androgen receptor polyglutamine length. Hum Mol Genet, 2000. 9: p. 267-274.

92. Coetzee, G.A. and R.K. Ross, Re: Prostate cancer and the androgen receptor. J Natl Cancer Inst, 1994. 86: p. 872-873.

93. Chen, C., N. Lamharzi, N.S. Weiss, R. Etzioni, D.A. Dightman, M. Barnett, D. DiTommaso and G. Goodman, Androgen receptor polymorphisms and the incidence of prostate cancer. Cancer Epidemiol Biomarkers Prev, 2002. 11: p. 1033-1040.

94. Coughlin, S.S. and I.J. Hall, A review of genetic polymorphisms and prostate cancer risk. Ann Epidemiol, 2002. 12: p. 182-196.
95. Miller, E.A., J.L. Stanford, L. Hsu, E. Noonan and E.A. Ostrander, Polymorphic repeats in the androgen receptor gene in high-risk sibships. Prostate, 2001. 48: p. 200-205.
96. Stanford, J.L., J.J. Just, M. Gibbs, K.G. Wicklund, C.L. Neal, B.A. Blumenstein and E.A. Ostrander, Polymorphic repeats in the androgen receptor gene: molecular markers of prostate cancer risk. Cancer Res, 1997. 57: p. 1194-1198.
97. Chang, B.L., S.L. Zheng, G.A. Hawkins, S.D. Isaacs, K.E. Wiley, A. Turner, J.D. Carpten, E.R. Bleecker, P.C. Walsh, J.M. Trent, D.A. Meyers, W.B. Isaacs, and J. Xu, Joint effect of HSD3B1 and HSD3B2 genes is associated with hereditary and sporadic prostate cancer susceptibility. Cancer Res, 2002. 62: p. 1784-1789.
98. Morissette, J., F. Durocher, J.F. Leblanc, T. Normand, F. Labrie and J. Simard, Genetic linkage mapping of the steroid 5a-reductase type 2 (SRD5A2) gene close to D2S352 on chromosome 2p23-22 region. Cytogenet. Cell Genet., 1996. 73: p. 304-307.
99. Labrie, F., A. Bılanger, V. Luu-The, C. Labrie, J. Simard, L. Cusan, J.L. Gomez and B. Candas, DHEA and the intracrine formation of androgens and estrogens in peripheral target tissues: its role during aging. Steroids, 1998. 63: p. 322-328.
100. Ross, R.K., L. Berstein, R.A. Lobo, H. Shimizu, F.Z. Stanczyk, M.C. Pike and B.E. Henderson, 5alpha-reductase activity and risk of prostate cancer among Japanese and US white and black males. Lancet, 1992. 339: p. 887-889.
101. Reichardt, J.K.V., N. Makridakis, B.E. Henderson, M.C. Yu, M.C. Pike and P.K. Ross, Genetic variability of the human SRD5A2 gene: implications for prostate cancer risk. Cancer Res., 1995. 55: p. 3973-3975.
102. Makridakis, N., R.K. Ross, M.C. Pike, L. Chang, F.Z. Stanczyk, L.N. Kolonel, C.Y. Shi, M.C. Yu, B.E. Henderson and J.K. Reichardt, A prevalent missense substitution that modulates activity of prostatic steroid 5alpha-reductase. Cancer Res, 1997. 57: p. 1020-1022.
103. Makridakis, N.M., E. di Salle and J.K. Reichardt, Biochemical and pharmacogenetic dissection of human steroid 5 alpha-reductase type II. Pharmacogenetics, 2000. 10: p. 407-413.
104. Makridakis, N.M., R.K. Ross, M.C. Pike, L.E. Crocitto, L.N. Kolonel, C.L. Pearce, B.E. Henderson and J.K. Reachardt, Association of missense substitution in SRD5A2 gene with prostate cancer in African-American and Hispanic men in Los Angeles, USA. Lancet, 1999. 354: p. 975-978.
105. Jaffe, J.M., S.B. Malkowicz, A.H. Walker, S. MacBride, R. Peschel, J. Tomaszewski, K. Van Arsdalen, A.J. Wein and T.R. Rebbeck, Association of SRD5A2 genotype and pathological characteristics of prostate tumors. Cancer Res, 2000. 60: p. 1626-1630.
106. Margiotti, K., F. Sangiuolo, A. De Luca, F. Froio, C.L. Pearce, V. Ricci-Barbini, F. Micali, M. Bonafe, C. Franceschi, B. Dallapiccola, G. Novelli, and J.K. Reichardt, Evidence for an association between the SRD5A2 (type II steroid 5 alpha-reductase) locus and prostate cancer in Italian patients. Dis Markers, 2000. 16: p. 147-150.
107. Mononen, N., T. Ikonen, K. Syrjakoski, M. Matikainen, J. Schleutker, T.L. Tammela, P.A. Koivisto and O.P. Kallioniemi, A missense substitution A49T in the steroid 5-alpha-reductase gene (SRD5A2) is not associated with prostate cancer in Finland. Br J Cancer, 2001. 84: p. 1344-1347.
108. Hsing, A.W., C. Chen, A.P. Chokkalingam, Y.T. Gao, D.A. Dightman, H.T. Nguyen, J. Deng, J. Cheng, I.A. Sesterhenn, F.K. Mostofi, F.Z. Stanczyk, and J.K. Rechardt, Polymorphic markers in the SRD5A2 gene and prostate cancer risk: a population-based case-control study. Cancer Epidemiol Biomarkers Prev, 2001. 10: p. 1077-1082.
109. Nedelcheva Kristensen, V., E.K. Haraldsen, K.B. Anderson, P.E. Lonning, B. Erikstein, R. Karesen, O.S. Gabrielsen and A.L. Borresen-Dale, CPY17 and breast cancer risk: the polymorphism in the 5' flanking area of the gene does not influence binding to Sp-1. Cancer Res, 1999. 59: p. 2825-2828.
110. Lin, C. and W.L. Miller. The T/C allelic polymorphism at nucleotide +27 of the human CYP17 Gene is not associated with altered transcriptional activity. in The Endocrine Society's 83rd annual meeting. 2001. Denver, Colorado.
111. Lunn, R.M., D.A. Bell, J.L. Mohler and J.A. Taylor, Prostate cancer risk and polymorphism in 17

REFERENCES

hydroxylase (CYP17) and steroid reductase (SRDA2). Carcinogenesis, 1999. 20: p. 1727-1731.

112. Gsur, A., G. Bernhofer, S. Hinteregger, G. Haidinger, G. Schatzl, S. Madersbacher, M. Marberger, C. Vutuc and M. Micksche, A polymorphism in the CYP17 gene is associated with prostate cancer risk. Int J Cancer, 2000. 87: p. 434-437.

113. Yamada, Y., M. Watanabe, M. Murata, M. Yamanaka, Y. Kubota, H. Ito, T. Katoh, J. Kawamura, R. Yatani and T. Shiraishi, Impact of genetic polymorphisms of 17-hydroxylase cytochrome P-450 (CYP17) and steroid 5alpha-reductase type II (SRD5A2) genes on prostate-cancer risk among the Japanese population. Int J Cancer, 2001. 92: p. 683-686.

114. Wadelius, M., A.O. Andersson, J.E. Johansson, C. Wadelius and E. Rane, Prostate cancer associated with CYP17. Pharmacogenetics, 1999. 9: p. 635-639.

115. Habuchi, T., Z. Liqing, T. Suzuki, R. Sasaki, N. Tsuchiya, H. Tachiki, N. Shimoda, S. Satoh, K. Sato, Y. Kakehi, T. Kamoto, O. Ogawa, and T. Kato, Increased risk of prostate cancer and benign prostatic hyperplasia associated with a CYP17 gene polymorphism with a gene dosage effect. Cancer Res, 2000. 60: p. 5710-5713.

116. Chang, B., S.L. Zheng, S.D. Isaacs, K.E. Wiley, J.D. Carpten, G.A. Hawkins, E.R. Bleecker, P.C. Walsh, J.M. Trent, D.A. Meyers, W.B. Isaacs, and J. Xu, Linkage and association of CYP17 gene in hereditary and sporadic prostate cancer. Int J Cancer, 2001. 95: p. 354-359.

117. Simard, J., A.M. Moisan and Y. Morel, Congenital Adrenal Hyperplasia due to 3beta-Hydroxysteroid Dehydrogenase/Delta5-Delta4 Isomerase Deficiency. Semin Reprod Med, 2002. 20: p. 255-276.

118. van't Veer, L.J., H. Dai, M.J. van de Vijver, Y.D. He, A.A. Hart, M. Mao, H.L. Peterse, K. van der Kooy, M.J. Marton, A.T. Witteveen, G.J. Schrieber, R.M. Kerkhoven, C. Roberts, P.S. Linsley, R. Bernards, and S.H. Friend, Gene expression profiling predicts clinical outcome of breast cancer. Nature, 2002. 415: p. 530-536.

119. Blackshaw, S., R.E. Fraioli, T. Furukawa and C.L. Cepko, Comprehensive analysis of photoreceptor gene expression and the identification of candidate retinal disease genes. Cell, 2001. 107: p. 579-589.

120. Greenlee, R.T., T. Murray, S. Bolden and P.A. Wingo, Cancer statistics, 2000. CA Cancer J. Clin., 2000. 50(1): p. 7-33.

121. Thompson, I.M. and E.J. Zeidman, Presentation and clinical course of patients ultimately succumbing to carcinoma of the prostate. Scand J Urol Nephrol, 1991. 25(2): p. 111-4.

122. Nadji, M., S.Z. Tabei, A. Castro, T.M. Chu, G.P. Murphy, M.C. Wang and A.R. Morales, Prostatic-specific antigen: an immunohistologic marker for prostatic neoplasms. Cancer, 1981. 48(5): p. 1229-32.

123. Crawford, D. and S. Waxman, The history of prostate specific antigen, in Prostate Specific Antigen, M.K. Brawer, Editor. 2001, Marcel Dekker Inc.: New York. p. 3.

124. Abouelfadel, Z. and E.D. Crawford, Experience of Prostate Cancer Awareness Week in Current Clinical Urology, in Prostate Cancer Screening, R.M.a.K.E. Thompson IM, Editor. 2001, Humana Press Inc: Totowa, NJ. p. 239-254.

125. Bose, P. and J.S. Green, Does Prostate Cancer Screening Detect Potentially Curable Disease?, in Challenges in Prostate Cancer, W. Bowsher, Editor. 2000, Blackwell Science: London. p. 65-75.

126. Thompson, I., P. Caroll, C. Coley, G. Sweat, D. McLeod and P. Schellhammer, The PSA best practices policy of the American Urological Association. AUA Update Series, 2001. Lesson 9 Vol. XX(66-72).

127. Von Eschenbach, A., R. Ho, G.P. Murphy, M. Cunningham and N. Lins, American Cancer Society guideline for the early detection of prostate cancer: update 1997. CA Cancer J. Clin., 1997. 47(5): p. 261-264.

128. Research, A.A.o.F.P.C.o.C.P.a., Summary of Policy Recommendations for Periodic Health Examination. 1996.

129. Paper, A.o.I.M.P., Part III Screening for Prostate Cancer Part II Estimating the risks, benefits and costs. Clinical Guideline, 1997. 126: p. 480-484.

130. Chodak, G.W., R.A. Thisted, G.S. Gerber, J.-E. Johansson, J. Adolfsson, G.W. Jones, G.D. Chisholm, B. Moskovitz, P.M. Livne and J. Warner, Results of conservative management of clinically localized prostate cancer. N. Engl. J. Med., 1994. 330: p. 242-248.

131. Albertsen, P.C., J.A. Hanley, D.F. Gleason and

M.J. Barry, Competing risk analysis of men aged 55 to 74 years at diagnosis managed conservatively for clinically localized prostate cancer. Jama, 1998. 280(11): p. 975-80.

132. D'Amico, A.V., R. Whittington, S.B. Malkowicz, D. Schultz, K. Blank, G.A. Broderick, J.E. Tomaszewski, A.A. Renshaw, I. Kaplan, C.J. Beard, and A. Wein, Biochemical outcome after radical prostatectomy, external beam radiation therapy, or interstitial radiation therapy for clinically localized prostate cancer. Jama, 1998. 280(11): p. 969-74.

133. Gerber, G.S., R.A. Thisted, P.T. Scardino, H.G. Frohmuller, F.H. Schroeder, D.F. Paulson, A.W. Middleton Jr., D.B. Rukstalis, J.A. Smith Jr., P.F. Schellhammer, M. Ohori, and G.W. Chodak, Results of radical prostatectomy in men with clinically localized prostate cancer. Multi-institutional pooled analysis. JAMA, 1996. 276: p. 615-619.

134. Pound, C.R., A.W. Partin, M.A. Eisenberger, D.W. Chan, J.D. Pearson and P.C. Walsh, Natural history of progression after PSA elevation following radical prostatectomy. Jama, 1999. 281(17): p. 1591-7.

135. Catalona, W.J. and D.S. Smith, Cancer recurrence and survival rates after anatomic radical retropubic prostatectomy for prostate cancer: intermediate-term results. J Urol, 1998. 160(6 Pt 2): p. 2428-34.

136. Polascik, T.J., C.R. Pound, T.L. DeWeese and P.C. Walsh, Comparison of radical prostatectomy and iodine 125 interstitial radiotherapy for the treatment of clinically localized prostate cancer: a 7-year biochemical (PSA) progression analysis. Urology, 1998. 51(6): p. 884-9; discussion 889-90.

137. Ragde, H., L.J. Korb, A.A. Elgamal, G.L. Grado and B.S. Nadir, Modern prostate brachytherapy. Prostate specific antigen results in 219 patients with up to 12 years of observed follow-up. Cancer, 2000. 89(1): p. 135-41.

138. Blasko, J.C., P.D. Grimm, J.E. Sylvester, K.R. Badiozamani, D. Hoak and W. Cavanagh, Palladium-103 brachytherapy for prostate carcinoma. Int J Radiat Oncol Biol Phys, 2000. 46(4): p. 839-50.

139. Crook, J., H. Lukka, L. Klotz, N. Bestic and M. Johnston, Systematic overview of the evidence for brachytherapy in clinically localized prostate cancer. Cmaj, 2001. 164(7): p. 975-81.

140. Beyer, D.C. and J.B. Priestley, Jr., Biochemical disease-free survival following 125I prostate implantation. Int J Radiat Oncol Biol Phys, 1997. 37(3): p. 559-63.

141. Shipley, W.U., H.D. Thames, H.M. Sandler, G.E. Hanks, A.L. Zietman, C.A. Perez, D.A. Kuban, S.L. Hancock and C.D. Smith, Radiation therapy for clinically localized prostate cancer: a multi-institutional pooled analysis. Jama, 1999. 281(17): p. 1598-604.

142. Valicenti, R., J. Lu, M. Pilepich, S. Asbell and D. Grignon, Survival advantage from higher-dose radiation therapy for clinically localized prostate cancer treated on the Radiation Therapy Oncology Group trials. J Clin Oncol, 2000. 18(14): p. 2740-6.

143. Walsh, P.C., T.L. DeWeese and M.A. Eisenberger, A structured debate: immediate versus deferred androgen suppression in prostate cancer-evidence for deferred treatment. J Urol, 2001. 166(2): p. 508-15; discussion 515-6.

144. Byar, D.P. and D.K. Corle, Hormone therapy for prostate cancer: results of the Veterans Administration Cooperative Urological Research Group studies. NCI Monogr., 1988(7): p. 165-170.

145. Group, P.C.W.P.I., Immediate versus deferred treatment for advanced prostatic cancer: initial results of the Medical Research Council. Br J Urol, 1997. 79: p. 235.

146. Messing, E.M., J. Manola, M. Sarosdy, G. Wilding, E.D. Crawford and D. Trump, Immediate hormonal therapy compared with observation after radical prostatectomy and pelvic lymphadenectomy in men with node-positive prostate cancer. N. Engl. J. Med., 1999. 341: p. 1781-1788.

147. Ellis, W.J., M.P. Chetner, S.D. Preston and M.K. Brawer, Diagnosis of prostatic carcinoma: the yield of serum prostate specific antigen, digital rectal examination and transrectal ultrasonography. J Urol, 1994. 152(5 Pt 1): p. 1520-5.

148. Semjonow, A., G. De Angelis and H.P. Schmid, Variability of Immunoassays for PSA, in Prostate Specific Antigen, M.K. Brawer, Editor. 2001, Marcel Dekker Inc.: New York. p. 31-62.

149. Leewansangtong, S., S. Goktas, R. Lepoff, K. Holthaus and E.D. Crawford, Comparability of serum prostate-specific antigen measurement between the hybritech Tandem-R and Abbott AxSYM assays. Urology, 1998. 52(3): p. 467-9.

150. Carter, H.B., C.H. Morrell, J.D. Pearson, L.J. Brant, C.C. Plato, E.J. Metter, D.W. Chan, J.L.

REFERENCES

Fozard and P.C. Walsh, Estimation of prostatic growth using serial prostate-specific antigen measurements in men with and without prostate disease. Cancer Res, 1992. 52(12): p. 3323-8.

151. Djavan, B., A.R. Zlotta, G. Byttebier, S. Shariat, M. Omar, C.C. Schulman and M. Marberger, Prostate specific antigen density of the transition zone for early detection of prostate cancer. J Urol, 1998. 160(2): p. 411-8; discussion 418-9.

152. Djavan, B., A.R. Zlotta, M. Remzi, K. Ghawidel, B. Bursa, S. Hruby, R. Wolfram, C.C. Schulman and M. Marberger, Total and transition zone prostate volume and age: how do they affect the utility of PSA-based diagnostic parameters for early prostate cancer detection? Urology, 1999. 54(5): p. 846-52.

153. Ohori, M., J.K. Dunn and P.T. Scardino, Is prostate-specific antigen density more useful than prostate-specific antigen levels in the diagnosis of prostate cancer? Urology, 1995. 46(5): p. 666-71.

154. Oesterling, J.E., S.J. Jacobsen, C.G. Chute, H.A. Guess, C.J. Girman, L.A. Panser and M.M. Lieber, Serum prostat- specific antigen in a community-based population of healthy men. Establishment of age-specific reference ranges. JAMA, 1993. 270: p. 860-864.

155. Dalkin, B.L., F.R. Ahmann and J.B. Kopp, Prostate specific antigen levels in men older than 50 years without clinical evidence of prostatic carcinoma. J Urol, 1993. 150(6): p. 1837-9.

156. Catalona, W.J., J.A. Beiser and D.S. Smith, Serum free prostate specific antigen and prostate specific antigen density measurements for predicting cancer in men with prior negative prostatic biopsies. J Urol, 1997. 158(6): p. 2162-7.

157. Bangma, C.H., R. Kranse, B.G. Blijenberg and F.H. Schroder, The value of screening tests in the detection of prostate cancer. Part I: Results of a retrospective evaluation of 1726 men. Urology, 1995. 46(6): p. 773-8.

158. Crawford, E.D., S. Leewansangtong, S. Goktas, K. Holthaus and M. Baier, Efficiency of prostate-specific antigen and digital rectal examination in screening, using 4.0 ng/ml and age-specific reference range as a cutoff for abnormal values. Prostate, 1999. 38(4): p. 296-302.

159. Partin, A.W., S.R. Criley, E.P. Subong, H. Zincke, P.C. Walsh and J.E. Oesterling, Standard versus age-specific prostate specific antigen reference ranges among men with serum PSA concentration of 2.6 to 4.0 ng/ml and benign prostate examination. JAMA, 1997. 14: p. 1452-1455.

160. Borer, J.G., J. Sherman, M.C. Solomon, M.W. Plawker and R.J. Macchia, Age specific prostate specific antigen reference ranges: population specific. J Urol, 1998. 159(2): p. 444-8.

161. Benson, M.C., I.S. Whang, C.A. Olsson, D.J. McMahon and W.H. Cooner, The use of prostate specific antigen density to enhance the predictive value of intermediate levels of serum prostate specific antigen. J. Urol., 1992. 147(3 Pt 2): p. 817-821.

162. Noguchi, M., J. Yahara, H. Koga, O. Nakashima and S. Noda, Necessity of repeat biopsies in men for suspected prostate cancer. Int J Urol, 1999. 6(1): p. 7-12.

163. Fowler, J.E., Jr., S.A. Bigler, D. Miles and D.A. Yalkut, Predictors of first repeat biopsy cancer detection with suspected local stage prostate cancer. J Urol, 2000. 163(3): p. 813-8.

164. Mettlin, C., P.J. Littrup, R.A. Kane, G.P. Murphy, F. Lee, A. Chesley, R. Badalament and F.K. Mostofi, Relative sensitivity and specificity of serum prostate specific antigen (PSA) level compared with age-referenced PSA, PSA density, and PSA change. Data from the American Cancer Society National Prostate Cancer Detection Project. Cancer, 1994. 74(5): p. 1615-20.

165. Djavan, B., A. Zlotta, M. Remzi, K. Ghawidel, A. Basharkhah, C.C. Schulman and M. Marberger, Optimal predictors of prostate cancer on repeat prostate biopsy: a prospective study of 1,051 men. J Urol, 2000. 163(4): p. 1144-8; discussion 1148-9.

166. Knowles, D., E. Bagiella and M.C. Benson, PSA Density: Does it Still Have Utility?, in Prostate Specific Antigen, M.K. Brawer, Editor. 2001, Marcel Dekker Inc: New York. p. 51-62.

167. Lilja, H., A. Christensson, U. Dahlen, M.T. Matikainen, O. Nilsson, K. Pettersson and T. Lovgren, Prostate-specific antigen in serum occurs predominantly in complex with alpha 1-antichymotrypsin. Clin Chem, 1991. 37(9): p. 1618-25.

168. Stenman, U.H., J. Leinonen, H. Alfthan, S. Rannikko, K. Tuhkanen and O. Alfthan, A complex between prostate-specific antigen and alpha 1-antichymotrypsin is the major form of prostate-specific antigen in serum of patients with prostatic cancer: assay of the complex improves clinical sen-

sitivity for cancer. Cancer Res., 1991. 51(1): p. 222-226.
169. Kuriyama, M., P.A. Abrahamsson, K. Imai, S. Akimoto, N. Deguchi, Y. Shichiri, Y. Sugiyama, T. Niwa and T. Inoue, Determination of serum prostate-specific antigen-alpha1-antichymotrypsin complex for diagnosis of prostate cancer in Japanese cases. Scand J Urol Nephrol, 2001. 35(1): p. 5-10.
170. Zhang, W.M., P. Finne, J. Leinonen and U.H. Stenman, Characterization and determination of the complex between prostate-specific antigen and alpha 1-protease inhibitor in benign and malignant prostatic diseases. Scand J Clin Lab Invest Suppl, 2000(233): p. 51-8.
171. Matsumoto, K., N. Konishi, T. Samori, E. Kimura, M. Doi, S. Kato and Y. Yuki, ELISA for a complexed antigen with a monoclonal antibody blocking reaction with the free antigen-assay-specific for complexed prostate-specific antigen. J Immunol Methods, 2000. 234(1-2): p. 99-106.
172. Imai, K., H. Yamanaka, Y. Kubota, M. Miki, T. Ito, H. Akaza, K. Uchida, S. Egawa, M. Kuriyama, H. Watanabe, K. Okihara, T. Kotake, M. Usami, Y. Arai, H. Maeda, K. Sagiyama, Y. Saito, H. Sakai, and K. Shida, [Clinical utility of the free prostate specific antigen (PSA), alpha 1-antichymotrypsin-complexed PSA, and free/total PSA ratio using the specific and sensitive enzyme-linked immunosorbent assay "E-plate EIKEN PSA"]. Hinyokika Kiyo, 1998. 44(10): p. 755-63.
173. Hara, I., H. Miyake, S. Hara, N. Yamanaka, Y. Ono, H. Eto, Y. Takechi, S. Arakawa and S. Kamidono, Value of the serum prostate-specific antigen-alpha 1-antichymotrypsin complex and its density as a predictor for the extent of prostate cancer. BJU Int, 2001. 88(1): p. 53-7.
174. Bacquet, C.R., J.W. Horm, T. Gibbs and P. Greenwald, Socioeconomic factors and cancer incidence amongh blacks and whites. J Natl Cancer Inst, 1991. 83: p. 551-557.
175. Demers, R.Y., G.M. Swanson, L.K. Weiss and T.Y. Kau, Increasing incidence of cancer of the prostate. The experience of black and white men in the Detroit metropolitan area. Arch Intern Med, 1994. 154(11): p. 1211-6.
176. Cussenot, O., A. Valeri, P. Berthon, G. Fournier and P. Mangin, Hereditary prostate cancer and other genetic predispositions to prostate cancer (Review). Urol Int, 1998. Suppl 2(Discussion 35): p. 30-34.
177. Dember, L., H. Gronberg and D. J.E., Familial prostate cancer and possible associated malignancies: nation-wide register cohort study in Sweden. Int J Cancer, 1998. 78: p. 293-297.
178. Bolton, D.M., The role of genes and a family history of prostate cancer, in Challenges in Prostate Cancer, W. Bowsher, Editor. 2000, Blackwell Science: London. p. 19-28.
179. Carter, H.B., J.I. Epstein, D.W. Chan, J.L. Fozard and J.D. Pearson, Recommended prostate-specific antigen testing intervals for the detection of curable prostate cancer. JAMA, 1997. 277(18): p. 1456-1460.
180. Leewansangtong, S., E.D. Crawford and S.G. Gordon, Longitudinal followup for Prostate Cancer Awareness Week (PCAW): Screening intervals. J Urol, 1988: p. 159-177.
181. Smart, C.R., The results of prostate carcinoma screening in the U.S. as reflected in the surveillance, epidemiology, and end results program. Cancer, 1997. 80(9): p. 1835-44.
182. Catalona, W.J., D.S. Smith, T.L. Ratliff and J.W. Basler, Detection of organ-confined prostate cancer is increased through prostate-specific antigen-based screening. JAMA, 1993. 270: p. 948-954.
183. Newcomber Lam Stanford, J.L., B.A. Blumenstein and M.K. Brawer, Temporal trends in rates of prostate cancer: declining incidence of advanced stage disease, 1974 to 1994. J Urol, 1997. 158: p. 1427-1430.
184. Mettlin, C.J., G.P. Murphy, D.S. Rosenthal and H.R. Menck, The National Cancer Data Base report on prostate carcinoma after the peak in incidence rates in the U.S. The American College of Surgeons Commission on Cancer and the American Cancer Society. Cancer, 1998. 83(8): p. 1679-84.
185. Orenstein, D.K., A. Velasco and G.L. Andriole, PSA and early detection in PSA,, Brawer, Editor. p. 137-157.
186. Perotti, M., F. Rabbani, A. Farkas, W.S. Ward and K.B. Cummings, Trends in poorly differentiated prostate cancer 1973-1994: observations from the Surveillance, Epidemiology and End Results database. J Urol, 1998. 160: p. 811-815.
187. Roberts, R.O., E.J. Bergstralh, S.K. Katusic, M.M.

REFERENCES

Lieber and S.J. Jacobsen, Decline in prostate cancer mortality from 1980 to 1997, and an update on incidence trends in Olmsted County, Minnesota. J. Urol., 1999. 161: p. 529-533.

188. Labrie, F., B. Candas, A. Dupont, L. Cusan, J.L. Gomez, R.E. Suburu, P. Diamond, J. Lıvesque and A. Bılanger, Screening decreases prostate cancer death: first analysis of the 1988 Quebec prospective randomized controlled trial. Prostate, 1999. 38(2): p. 83-91.

189. Ablin, R.J., W.A. Soanes, P. Bronson and E. Witebsky, Precipitating antigens of the normal human prostate. J. Reprod. Fertil., 1970. 22(3): p. 573-574.

190. Wang, M.C., L.A. Valenzuela, G.P. Murphy and T.M. Chu, Purification of human prostate specific antigen. Invest. Urol., 1979. 17: p. 159-163.

191. Papsidero, L.D., M.C. Wang, L.A. Valenzuela, G.P. Murphy and T.M. Chu, A prostate antigen in sera of prostatic cancer patients. Cancer Res., 1980. 40(7): p. 2428-2432.

192. Greenlee, R.T., M.B. Hill-Harmon, T. Murray and M. Thun, Cancer Statistics, 2001. CA Cancer J. Clin., 2001. 51(1): p. 15-36.

193. Nixon, R.G. and M.K. Brawer, Enhancing the specificity of prostate-specific antigen (PSA): an overview of PSA density, velocity and age-specific reference ranges. Br J Urol, 1997. 79(Suppl 1): p. 61-7.

194. Polascik, T.J., J.E. Oesterling and A.W. Partin, Prostate specific antigen: a decade of discovery—what we have learned and where we are going. J. Urol., 1999. 162(2): p. 293-306.

195. McCormack, R.T., H.G. Rittenhouse, J.A. Finlay, R.L. Sokoloff, T.J. Wang, R.L. Wolfert, H. Lilja and J.E. Oesterling, Molecular forms of prostate-specific antigen and the human kallikrein gene family: a new era. Urology, 1995. 45(5): p. 729-44.

196. Rittenhouse, H.G., J.A. Finlay, S.D. Mikolajczyk and A.W. Partin, Human Kallikrein 2 (hK2) and prostate-specific antigen (PSA): two closely related, but distinct, kallikreins in the prostate. Crit Rev Clin Lab Sci, 1998. 35(4): p. 275-368.

197. Yousef, G.M. and E.P. Diamandis, The new human tissue kallikrein gene family: structure, function, and association to disease. Endocr Rev, 2001. 22(2): p. 184-204.

198. Diamandis, E.P., G.M. Yousef, J. Clements, L.K. Ashworth, S. Yoshida, T. Egelrud, P.S. Nelson, S. Shiosaka, S. Little, H. Lilja, U.H. Stenman, H.G. Rittenhouse, and H. Wain, New nomenclature for the human tissue kallikrein gene family. Clin Chem, 2000. 46(11): p. 1855-8.

199. Kwiatkowski, M.K., F. Recker, T. Piironen, K. Pettersson, T. Otto, M. Wernli and R. Tscholl, In prostatism patients the ratio of human glandular kallikrein to free PSA improves the discrimination between prostate cancer and benign hyperplasia within the diagnostic "gray zone" of total PSA 4 to 10 ng/mL. Urology, 1998. 52(3): p. 360-5.

200. Nam, R.K., E.P. Diamandis, A. Toi, J. Trachtenberg, A. Magklara, A. Scorilas, P.A. Papnastasiou, M.A. Jewett and S.A. Narod, Serum human glandular kallikrein-2 protease levels predict the presence of prostate cancer among men with elevated prostate-specific antigen. J Clin Oncol, 2000. 18(5): p. 1036-42.

201. Partin, A.W., W.J. Catalona, J.A. Finlay, C. Darte, D.J. Tindall, C.Y. Young, G.G. Klee, D.W. Chan, H.G. Rittenhouse, R.L. Wolfert, and D.L. Woodrum, Use of human glandular kallikrein 2 for the detection of prostate cancer: preliminary analysis. Urology, 1999. 54(5): p. 839-45.

202. Kumar, A., S.D. Mikolajczyk, A.S. Goel, L.S. Millar and M.S. Saedi, Expression of pro form of prostate-specific antigen by mammalian cells and its conversion to mature, active form by human kallikrein 2. Cancer Res, 1997. 57(15): p. 3111-4.

203. Lovgren, J., K. Rajakoski, M. Karp, a. Lundwall and H. Lilja, Activation of the zymogen form of prostate-specific antigen by human glandular kallikrein 2. Biochem Biophys Res Commun, 1997. 238(2): p. 549-55.

204. Takayama, T.K., K. Fujikawa and E.W. Davie, Characterization of the precursor of prostate-specific antigen. Activation by trypsin and by human glandular kallikrein. J Biol Chem, 1997. 272(34): p. 21582-8.

205. Diamandis, E.P., G.M. Yousef, C. Petraki and A.R. Soosaipillai, Human kallikrein 6 as a biomarker of alzheimer's disease. Clin Biochem, 2000. 33(8): p. 663-7.

206. Diamandis, E.P., G.M. Yousef, A.R. Soosaipillai and P. Bunting, Human kallikrein 6 (zyme/protease M/neurosin): a new serum biomarker of ovarian carcinoma. Clin Biochem, 2000. 33(7): p. 579-83.

207. Luo, L.Y., L. Grass, D.J. Howarth, P. Thibault, H. Ong and E.P. Diamandis, Immunofluorometric assay of human kallikrein 10 and its identification in biological fluids and tissues. Clin Chem, 2001. 47(2): p. 237-46.

208. Luo, L.Y., P. Bunting, A. Scorilas and E.P. Diamandis, Human kallikrein 10: a novel tumor marker for ovarian carcinoma? Clin Chim Acta, 2001. 306(1-2): p. 111-8.

209. Stenman and et al., Cancer Res., 1991. 51: p. 222.

210. Christensson, A., T. Bjork, O. Nilsson, U. Dahlen, M.T. Matikainen, A.T. Cockett, P.A. Abrahamsson and H. Lilja, Serum prostate specific antigen complexed to alpha 1-antichymotrypsin as an indicator of prostate cancer. J Urol, 1993. 150(1): p. 100-5.

211. Zhang, W.M., P. Finne, J. Leinonen, S. Vesalainen, S. Nordling, S. Rannikko and U.H. Stenman, Characterization and immunological determination of the complex between prostate-specific antigen and alpha2-macroglobulin. Clin Chem, 1998. 44(12): p. 2471-9.

212. Zhang, W.M., P. Finne, J. Leinonen, S. Vesalainen, S. Nordling and U.H. Stenman, Measurement of the complex between prostate-specific antigen and alpha1-protease inhibitor in serum. Clin Chem, 1999. 45(6 Pt 1): p. 814-21.

213. Lilja, H., A. Haese, T. Bjork, M.G. Friedrich, T. Piironen, K. Pettersson, E. Huland and H. Huland, Significance and metabolism of complexed and noncomplexed prostate specific antigen forms, and human glandular kallikrein 2 in clinically localized prostate cancer before and after radical prostatectomy. J Urol, 1999. 162(6): p. 2029-34; discussion 2034-5.

214. Brawer, M.K., G.E. Meyer, J.L. Letran, D.D. Bankson, D.L. Morris, K.K. Yeung and W.J. Allard, Measurement of complexed PSA improves specificity for early detection of prostate cancer. Urology, 1998. 52(3): p. 372-8.

215. Brawer, M.K., C.D. Cheli, I.E. Neaman, J. Goldblatt, C. Smith, M.K. Schwartz, D.J. Bruzek, D.L. Morris, L.J. Sokoll, D.W. Chan, K.K. Yeung, A.W. Partin, and W.J. Allard, Complexed prostate specific antigen provides significant enhancement of specificity compared with total prostate specific antigen for detecting prostate cancer. J Urol, 2000. 163(5): p. 1476-80.

216. Mitchell, I.D., B.L. Croal, A. Dickie, N.P. Cohen and I. Ross, A prospective study to evaluate the role of complexed prostate specific antigen and free/total prostate specific antigen ratio for the diagnosis of prostate cancer. J Urol, 2001. 165(5): p. 1549-53.

217. Stephan, C., K. Jung, M. Lein, P. Sinha, D. Schnorr and S.A. Loening, Molecular forms of prostate-specific antigen and human kallikrein 2 as promising tools for early diagnosis of prostate cancer. Cancer Epidemiol Biomarkers Prev, 2000. 9(11): p. 1133-47.

218. Mikolajczyk, S.D., L.S. Grauer, L.S. Millar, T.M. Hill, A. Kumar, H.G. Rittenhouse, R.L. Wolfert and M.S. Saedi, A precursor form of PSA (pPSA) is a component of the free PSA in prostate cancer serum. Urology, 1997. 50(5): p. 710-4.

219. Mikolajczyk, S.D., L.S. Millar, T.J. Wang, H.G. Rittenhouse, R.L. Wolfert, L.S. Marks, W. Song, T.M. Wheeler and K.M. Slawin, "BPSA," a specific molecular form of free prostate-specific antigen, is found predominantly in the transition zone of patients with nodular benign prostatic hyperplasia. Urology, 2000. 55(1): p. 41-5.

220. Nurmikko, P., K. Pettersson, T. Piironen, J. Hugosson and H. Lilja, Discrimination of prostate cancer from benign disease by plasma measurement of intact, free prostate-specific antigen lacking an internal cleavage site at Lys145-Lys146. Clin Chem, 2001. 47(8): p. 1415-23.

221. Stenman, U., P. Finne, W. Zhang and J. Leinonen, Prostate-specific antigen and other prostate cancer markers. Urology, 2000. 56(6): p. 893-8.

222. Leinonen, J., W.M. Zhang and U.H. Stenman, Complex formation between PSA isoenzymes and protease inhibitors. J Urol, 1996. 155(3): p. 1099-103.

223. Bjork, T., A. Bjartell, P.A. Abrahamsson, S. Hulkko, A. di Sant'Agnese and H. Lilja, Alpha 1-antichymotrypsin production in PSA-producing cells is common in prostate cancer but rare in benign prostatic hyperplasia. Urology, 1994. 43(4): p. 427-34.

224. Jung, K., B. Brux, M. Lein, B. Rudolph, G. Kristiansen, S. Hauptmann, D. Schnorr, S.A. Loening and P. Sinha, Molecular forms of prostate-specific antigen in malignant and benign prostatic tissue: biochemical and diagnostic implications. Clin Chem, 2000. 46(1): p. 47-54.

REFERENCES

225. Ornstein, D.K., C. Englert, J.W. Gillespie, C.P. Paweletz, W.M. Linehan, M.R. Emmert-Buck and E.F. Petricoin, 3rd, Characterization of intracellular prostate-specific antigen from laser capture microdissected benign and malignant prostatic epithelium. Clin Cancer Res, 2000. 6(2): p. 353-6.

226. Mikolajczyk, S.D., L.S. Millar, T.J. Wang, H.G. Rittenhouse, L.S. Marks, W. Song, T.M. Wheeler and K.M. Slawin, A precursor form of prostate-specific antigen is more highly elevated in prostate cancer compared with benign transition zone prostate tissue. Cancer Res, 2000. 60(3): p. 756-9.

227. Catalona, W.J., D.S. Smith, R.L. Wolfert, T.J. Wang, H.G. Rittenhouse, T.L. Ratliff and R.B. Nadler, Evaluation of percentage of free serum prostate-specific antigen to improve specificity of prostate cancer screening. Jama, 1995. 274(15): p. 1214-20.

228. Catalona, W.J., Clinical utility of measurements of free and total prostate-specific antigen (PSA): a review. Prostate Suppl, 1996. 7: p. 64-9.

229. Catalona, W.J., D.S. Smith and D.K. Ornstein, Prostate cancer detection in men with serum PSA concentrations of 2.6 to 4.0 ng/mL and benign prostate examination. Enhancement of specificity with free PSA measurements. JAMA, 1997. 277(18): p. 1452-1455.

230. Partin, A.W., W.J. Catalona, P.C. Southwick, E.N. Subong, G.H. Gasior and D.W. Chan, Analysis of percent free prostate-specific antigen (PSA) for prostate cancer detection: influence of total PSA, prostate volume, and age. Urology, 1996. 48(6A Suppl.): p. 55-61.

231. Catalona, W.J., A.W. Partin, K.M. Slawin, M.K. Brawer, R.C. Flanigan, A. Patel, J.P. Richie, J.B. deKernion, P.C. Walsh, P.T. Scardino, P.H. Lange, E.N. Subong, R.E. Parson, G.H. Gasior, K.G. Loveland, and P.C. Southwick, Use of the percentage of free prostate-specific antigen to enhance differentiation of prostate cancer from benign prostatic disease: a prospective multicenter clinical trial. Jama, 1998. 279(19): p. 1542-7.

232. Catalona, W.J., A.W. Partin, J.A. Finlay, D.W. Chan, H.G. Rittenhouse, R.L. Wolfert and D.L. Woodrum, Use of percentage of free prostate-specific antigen to identify men at high risk of prostate cancer when PSA levels are 2.51 to 4 ng/mL and digital rectal examination is not suspicious for prostate cancer: an alternative model. Urology, 1999. 54(2): p. 220-4.

233. Stephan, C., B. Vogel, K. Jung, H. Cammann, M. Lein, D. Schnorr and S.A. Leoning, A 5 year prospective evaluation of percent free PSA in combination with an artificial neural network (ANN) for detection of prostate cancer. J Urol, 2001. 165(Suppl): p. 313-314.

234. Mettlin, C., A.E. Chesley, G.P. Murphy, G. Bartsch, A. Toi, R. Bahnson and P. Church, Association of free PSA percent, total PSA, age, and gland volume in the detection of prostate cancer. Prostate, 1999. 39(3): p. 153-8.

235. Tornblom, M., U. Norming, C. Becker, H. Lilja and O. Gustafsson, Variation in percentage-free prostate-specific antigen (PSA) with prostate volume, age and total PSA level. BJU Int, 2001. 87(7): p. 638-42.

236. Haese, A., M. Graefen, J. Noldus, P. Hammerer, E. Huland and H. Huland, Prostatic volume and ratio of free-to-total prostate specific antigen in patients with prostatic cancer or benign prostatic hyperplasia. J Urol, 1997. 158(6): p. 2188-92.

237. Stephan, C., M. Lein, K. Jung, D. Schnorr and S.A. Loening, The influence of prostate volume on the ratio of free to total prostate specific antigen in serum of patients with prostate carcinoma and benign prostate hyperplasia. Cancer, 1997. 79(1): p. 104-9.

238. Ornstein, D.K., D.S. Smith, P.A. Humphrey and W.J. Catalona, The effect of prostate volume, age, total prostate specific antigen level and acute inflammation on the percentage of free serum prostate specific antigen levels in men without clinically detectable prostate cancer. J Urol, 1998. 159(4): p. 1234-7.

239. Arcangeli, C.G., P.A. Humphrey, D.S. Smith, T.J. Harmon, D.L. Shepherd, D.W. Keetch and W.J. Catalona, Percentage of free serum prostate-specific antigen as a predictor of pathologic features of prostate cancer in a screening population. Urology, 1998. 51(4): p. 558-64; discussion 564-5.

240. Elgamal, A.A., F.J. Cornillie, H.P. Van Poppel, W.M. Van de Voorde, R. McCabe and L.V. Baert, Free-to-total prostate specific antigen ratio as a single test for detection of significant stage T1c prostate cancer. J Urol, 1996. 156(3): p. 1042-7; discussion 1047-9.

241. Pannek, J., H.G. Rittenhouse, D.W. Chan, J.I. Epstein, P.C. Walsh and A.W. Partin, The use of percent free prostate specific antigen for staging clinically localized prostate cancer. J Urol, 1998. 159(4): p. 1238-42.

242. Bangma, C.H., R. Kranse, B.G. Blijenberg and F.H. Schroder, The free-to-total serum prostate specific antigen ratio for staging prostate carcinoma. J Urol, 1997. 157(2): p. 544-7.

243. Henricks, W.H., B.G. England, D.A. Giacherio, J.E. Oesterling and K.J. Wojno, Serum percent-free PSA does not predict extraprostatic spread of prostate cancer. Am J Clin Pathol, 1998. 109(5): p. 533-9.

244. Lerner, S.E., S.J. Jacobsen, H. Lilja, E.J. Bergstralh, J. Ransom, G.G. Klee, T. Piironen, M.L. Blute, M.M. Lieber, H. Zincke, K. Pettersson, D. Peterson, and J.E. Oesterling, Free, complexed, and total serum prostate-specific antigen concentrations and their proportions in predicting stage, grade, and deoxyribonucleic acid ploidy in patients with adenocarcinoma of the prostate. Urology, 1996. 48(2): p. 240-8.

245. Graefen, M., P.I. Karakiewicz, P.T. Scardino, M.W. Kattan, A. Haese, P.G. Hammerer, J. Palisaar, E. Huland and H. Huland, Percentage of free PSA (%PSA) is not an independent predictor of pathological stage or PSA recurrence in patients with localized prostate cancer treated with radical prostatectomy (RP). J Urol, 2001. 165(Suppl.): p. 281.

246. Li, W., Y. Ren, V. Mee and P.Y. Wong, Prostate-specific antigen ratio correlates with aggressiveness of histology grades of prostate cancer. Clin Biochem, 1999. 32: p. 31-37.

247. Morote, J., G. Encabo, M.A. Lopez and I.M. De Torres, The free-to-total serum prostatic specific antigen ratio as a predictor of the pathological features of prostate cancer. BJU Int, 1999. 83(9): p. 1003-6.

248. Southwick, P.C., W.J. Catalona, A.W. Partin, K.M. Slawin, M.K. Brawer, R.C. Flanigan, A. Patel, J.P. Richie, P.C. Walsh, P.T. Scardino, P.H. Lange, G.H. Gasior, R.E. Parson, and K.G. Loveland, Prediction of post-radical prostatectomy pathological outcome for stage T1c prostate cancer with percent free prostate specific antigen: a prospective multicenter clinical trial. J Urol, 1999. 162(4): p. 1346-51.

249. Carter, H.B., A.W. Partin, A.A. Luderer, E.J. Metter, P. Landis, D.W. Chan, J.L. Fozard and J.D. Pearson, Percentage of free prostate-specific antigen in sera predicts aggressiveness of prostate cancer a decade before diagnosis. Urology, 1997. 49: p. 379-384.

250. Horninger, W., H. Volgger, H. Rogatsch, D. Strohmeyer, H. Steiner, A. Hobisch, H. Klocker and G. Bartsch, Predictive value of total and percent free prostate specific antigen in high grade prostatic intraepithelial neoplasia lesions: results of the Tyrol Prostate Specific Antigen Screening Project. J Urol, 2001. 165(4): p. 1143-5.

251. Kilic, S., E. Kukul, A. Danisman, E. Guntekin and M. Sevuk, Ratio of free to total prostate-specific antigen in patients with prostatic intraepithelial neoplasia. Eur Urol, 1998. 34(3): p. 176-80.

252. Morote, J., G. Encabo, M. Lopez and I.M. de Torres, Influence of high-grade prostatic intraepithelial neoplasia on total and percentage free serum prostatic specific antigen. BJU Int, 1999. 84(6): p. 657-60.

253. Morote, J., C.X. Raventos, G. Encabo, M. Lopez and I.M. de Torres, Effect of high-grade prostatic intraepithelial neoplasia on total and percent free serum prostatic-specific antigen. Eur Urol, 2000. 37(4): p. 456-9.

254. Ramos, C.G., G.F. Carvahal, D.E. Mager, H. B. and W.J. Catalona, The effect of high grade prostatic intraepithelial neoplasia on serum total and percentage of free prostate specific antigen levels. J Urol, 1999. 162: p. 1587-1590.

255. Tarle, M. and I. Kraljic, Free and total serum PSA values in patients with prostatic intraepithelial neoplasia (PIN), prostate cancer and BPH. Is F/T PSA a potential probe for dormand and manifest cancer? Anticancer Res, 1997. 17: p. 1531-1534.

256. Stephan, C., M. Lein, K. Jung, D. Schnorr and S.A. Leoning, Can prostate specific antigen derivatives reduce the frenquency of unnecessary prostate biopsies? J Urol, 1997. 157: p. 1371.

257. Lee, C.T. and P.T. Scardino, Percent free Prostate-specific antigen for first-time prostate biopsy. Urology, 2001. 57: p. 594-598.

258. Horninger, W., G. Bartsch, P.B. Snow, J.M. Brandt and A.W. Partin, The problem of cutoff levels in a screened population. Cancer, 2001. 91: p. 1667-1672.

REFERENCES

259. Finne, P., R. Finne, A. Auvinen, H. Juusela, J. Aro, L. Maattanen, M. Hakama, S. Rannikko, T.L. Tammela and U. Stenman, Predicting the outcome of prostate biopsy in screen-positive men by a multilayer perceptron network. Urology, 2000. 56: p. 418-422.

260. Han, M., P.B. Snow, J.I. Epstein, T.Y. Chan, K.A. Jones, P.C. Walsh and A.W. Partin, A neutral network predicts progression for men with gleason score 3+4 versus 4+3 tumors after radical prostatectomy. Urology, 2000. 56: p. 994-999.

261. Han, M., P.B. Snow, J.M. Brandt and A.W. Partin, Evaluation of artificial neural networks for the prediction of pathologic stage in prostate carcinoma. Cancer, 2001. 91: p. 1661-1666.

262. Ziada, A.M., T.C. Lisle, P.B. Snow, R.F. Levine, G. Miller and E.D. Crawford, Impact of different variables on the outcome of patients with clinically confined prostate carcinoma. Cancer, 2001. 91: p. 1653-1660.

263. Montie, J.E. and J.T. Wei, Artificial neural networks for prostate carcinoma risk assessment. Cancer, 2001. 91: p. 1647-1652.

264. Catalona, W.J., K.A. Roehl and J.A.V. Antenor, Robustness of free PSA measurements to reduce unnecessary biopsies in the 2.6 to 4.0 ng/ml total PSA range. J Urol, 2001. 165(Suppl): p. 282-283.

265. Wu, J.T., P. Zhang, G.H. Liu and L. Wilson, Development of an immunoassay specific for the PSA-ACT complex without the problem of high background. J Clin Lab Anal, 1998. 12: p. 14-19.

266. Partin, A.W., M.K. Brawer, E.N.P. Subong, C.A. Kelley, J.L. Cox, D.J. Bruzek, J. Pannek, G.E. Meyer and D.W. Chan, Prospective evaluation of percent free-PSA and complexed-PSA for early detection of prostate cancer. Prostate Cancer Prostatic Diseases, 1998(1).

267. Wang, T.J., H.J. Linton, J. Payne, H.G. Rittenhouse, D.W. Chan, A.W. Partin, R.L. Wolfert and K. Kuus-Reichel, Generation of PSA-ACT-specific monoclonal antibodies and their application in a sandwich immunoassay. Hybridoma, 1999. 18: p. 535-541.

268. Stamey, T.A. and C.E. Yemoto, Examination of the 3 molecular forms of serum prostate specific antigen for distinguishing negative from positive biopsy: relationship to transition zone volume. J Urol, 2000. 163: p. 119-126.

269. Lein, M., K. Jung, P. Hammerer, M. Graefen, A. Semjonow, P. Stieber, M. Ossendorf, B. Brux, C. Stephan, D. Schnorr, and S.A. Leoning, A multicenter clinical trial on the use of alpha1-antichymotrypsin-prostate-specific antigen in prostate cancer diagnosis. Prostate, 2001. 47: p. 77-84.

270. Jung, K., B. Brux, M. Lein, A. Knabich, P. Sinha, B. Rudolph, D. Schnorr and S.A. Leoning, Determination of alpha1-antichymotrypsin-PSA complex in serum does not improve the differentiation between benign prostatic hyperplasia and prostate cancer compared with total PSA and percent free PSA. Urology, 1999. 53: p. 1160-1167.

271. Allard, W.J., Z. Zhou and K.K. Yeung, Novel immunoassay for the measurement of complexed prostate-specific antigen in serum. Clin Chem, 1998. 44: p. 1216-1223.

272. Jung, K., U. Elgeti, M. Lein, B. Brux, P. Sinha, B. Rudolph, S. Hauptmann, D. Schnorr and S.A. Leoning, Ratio of free or complexed prostate-specific antigen (PSA) to total PSA: which ratio improves differentiation between benign prostatic hyperplasia and prostate cancer? Clin Chem, 2000. 46: p. 55-62.

273. Lein, M., K. Jung, U. Elgeti, T. Petras, C. Stephan, B. Brux, P. Sinha, B. Winkelmann, D. Schnorr and S. Leoning, Comparison of the clinical validity of free prostate-specific antigen, alpha-1 antichymotrypsin-bound prostate-specific antigen and complexed prostate-specific antigen in prostate cancer diagnosis. Eur Urol, 2001. 39: p. 57-64.

274. Rittenhouse, H.G. and D.W. Chan, Can complexed PSA be used as a single test for detecting prostate cancer? Urology, 1999. 54: p. 4-5.

275. Stephan, C., K. Jung, M. Lein, D. Schnorr and S.A. Leoning, Complexed prostate specific antigen provides significant enhancement of specificity compared with total prostate specific antigen for detecting prostate cancer. J Urol, 2000. 164: p. 1671-1672.

276. Cheli, C.D., R.J. Babaian, H. Fritsche, H. Lepor, S. Taneja, S. Childs, T.A. Stamey, G. Bartsch, L.J. Sokoll, D.W. Chan, A.W. Partin, and M.K. Brawer, Preliminary results of a multicenter prospective evaluation of complexed PSA. J Urol, 2001. 165(Suppl): p. 205.

277. Jung, K., C. Stephan, U. Elgeti, M. Lein, B. Brux, G. Kristiansen, B. Rudolph, S. Hauptmann, D. Schnorr and S.A. Leoning, Molecular forms of

prostate-specific antigen in serum with concentrations of total prostate-specific antigen <4 migrograms/l - are they useful tools for early detection and screening of prostate cancer? Int J Cancer, 2001. 93: p. 759-765.

278. Okihara, K., H.A. Fritsche, A. Ayala, D.A. Johnston, W.J. Allard and R.J. Babnaian, Can complexed prostate specific antigen and prostatic volume enhance prostate cancer detection in men with total prostate specific antigen between 2.5 and 4.0 ng/ml. J Urol, 2001. 165: p. 1930-1936.

279. Zhang, W.M., P. Finne, J. Leinonen, J. Salo and U.H. Stenman, Determination of prostate-specific antigen complexed to alpha(2)-macroglobulin in serum increases the specificity of free to total PSA for prostate cancer. Urology, 2000. 56: p. 267-272.

280. Finne, P., W.M. Zhang, A. Auvinen, J. Leinonen, L. Maattanen, S. Rannikko, T.L. Tammela and U.H. Stenman, Use of the complex between prostate specific antigen and alpha 1-protease inhibitor for screening prostate cancer. J Urol, 2000. 164: p. 1956-1960.

281. Marks, L.S., A.S. Llanes, H.J. Linton, C.L. Gasior, L.S. Millar, S.D. Mikolajczyk, H.G. Rittenhouse, W.A. Munroe, L.J. Sokoll, A.W. Partin, and D.W. Chan, BPSA is a potential serum marker for benign prostatic hyperplasia (BPH). J Urol, 2001. Suppl(165): p. Suppl.

282. Peter, J., C. Unverzagt, T.N. Krogh, O. Vorm and W. Hoesel, Identification of precursor forms of free prostate-specific antigen in serum of prostate cancer patients by immunosorption and mass spectrometry. Cancer Res, 2001. 61: p. 957-962.

283. Becker, C., T. Piironen, J. Kiviniemi, H. Lilja and K. Pettersson, Sensitive and specific immunodetection of human glandular kallikrein 2 in serum. Clin Chem, 2000. 46: p. 198-206.

284. Black, M.H., A. Magklara, C.V. Obiezu, D.N. Melegos and E.P. Diamandis, Development of an ultrasensitive immunoassay for human glandular kallikrein with no cross-reactivity from prostate-specific antigen. Clin Chem, 1999. 45: p. 790-799.

285. Klee, G.G., M.K. Goddmanson, S.J. Jacobsen, C.Y. Young, J.A. Finlay, H.G. Rittenhouse, R.L. Wolfert and D.J. Tindall, Highly sensitive automated chemiluminometric assay for measuring free human glandular kallikrein-2. Clin Chem, 1999. 45: p. 800-806.

286. Becker, C., T. Piironen, K. Pettersson, T. Bjφrk, K.J. Wojno, J.E. Oesterling and H. Lilja, Discrimination of men with prostate cancer from those with benign disease by measurements of human glandular kallikrein 2 (HK2) in serum. J Urol, 2000. 163: p. 311-316.

287. Magklara, A., A. Scorilas, W.J. Catalona and E.P. Diamandis, The combination of human glandular kallikrein and free prostate-specific antigen (PSA) enhances discrimination between prostate cancer and benign prostatic hyperplasia in patients with moderately increased total PSA. Clin Chem, 1999. 45: p. 1960-1966.

288. Darson, M.F., A. Pacelli, P. Roche, H.G. Rittenhouse, R.L. Wolfert, C.Y. Young, G.G. Klee, D.J. Tindall and D.G. Bostwick, Human glandular kallikrein 2 (hK2) expression in prostatic intraepithelial neoplasia and adenocarcinoma: a novel prostate cancer marker. Urology, 1997. 49: p. 857-862.

289. Darson, M.F., A. Pacelli, P. Roche, H.G. Rittenhouse, R.L. Wolfert, M.S. Saedi, C.Y. Young, G.G. Klee, D.J. Tindall and D.G. Bostwick, Human glandular kallikrein 2 expression in prostate adenocarcinoma and lymph node metastases. Urology, 1999. 53: p. 939-944.

290. Magklara, A., A. Scorilas, C. Stephan, G.O. Kristiansen, S. Hauptmann, K. Jung and E.P. Diamandis, Decreased concentrations of prostate-specific antigen and human glandular kallikrein 2 in malignant versus nonmalignant prostatic tissue. Urology, 2000. 56: p. 527-532.

291. Haese, A., C. Becker, J. Noldus, M. Graefen, E. Huland, H. Huland and H. Lilja, Human glandular kallikrein 2: a potential serum marker for predicting the organ confined versus nonorgan confined growth of prostate cancer. J Urol, 2000. 163: p. 1491-1497.

292. Recker, F., M.K. Kwiatkowski, T. Piironen, K. Pettersson, A. Huber, G. Lómmen and R. Tscholl, Human glandular kallikrein as a tool to improve discrimination of poorly differentiated and non-organ-confined prostate cancer compared with prostate-specific antigen. Urology, 2000(55): p. 481-485.

293. Haese, A., J. Noldus, M. Graefen, T. Steuber, H. Huland, C. Becker and H. Lilja, Human glandular kallikrein 2 (hK2) is superior to total PSA in pre-

REFERENCES

dicting organ-confined disease and pathological stage of clinically localized prostate cancer with a total PSA <10ng/ml. J Urol, 2001. 165(Suppl): p. 234.

294. Nam, R.K., S.A. Narod, J. Trachtenberg, A. Magklara, E.P. Diamandis and M.A. Jewett, Use of human kallikrein-2 (hK2) levels in patient selection for prostate biopsy. J Urol, 2001. 165(Suppl): p. 204.

295. Haese, A., J. Noldus, R.P. Henke, E. Huland, H. Huland, K. Petterson, T. Piironen, C. Becker and H. Lilja, Correlation of human glandular kallikrein 2 (hK2) and total PSA (tPSA) to total prostate volume and the total and Gleason grade 4/5 volume of prostate cancer (PCa). J Urol, 2001. 165(Suppl): p. 204-205.

296. Stamey, T.A., Preoperative serum prostate-specific antigen (PSA) below 10 migro/l predicts neither the presence of prostate cancer nor the rate of postoperative PSA failure. Clin Chem, 2001. 47: p. 631-634.

297. Saedi, M.S., T.M. Hill, R.K. Kuus, A. Kumar, J. Payne, S.D. Mikolajczyk, R.L. Wolfert and H.G. Rittenhouse, The precursor form of the human kallikrein 2, a kallikrein homologous to prostate-specific antigen, is present in human sera and is increased in prostate cancer and benign prostatic hyperplasia. Clin Chem, 1998. 44: p. 2115-2119.

298. Wang, T.J., J. Linton, H.G. Rittenhouse, J.A. Finlay, L.J. Sokoll, D.W. Chan, A.W. Partin and D.J. Tindall, The development of dual monoclonal antibody immunoassay for accurate measurement of serum human kallikrein 2 complex (chK2). J Urol, 2000. 163(Suppl): p. 180A.

299. Mikolajczyk, S.D., L.S. Millar, K.M. Marker, H.G. Rittenhouse, R.L. Wolfert, L.S. Marks, M.C. Charlesworth and D.J. Tindall, Identification of a novel complex between human kallikrein 2 and protease inhibitor-6 in prostate cancer tissue. Cancer Res, 1999. 59: p. 3927-3930.

300. Yousef, G.M., C.V. Obiezu, L.Y. Luo, M.H. Black and E.P. Diamandis, Prostase/KLK-L1 is a new member of the human kallikrein gene family, is expressed in prostate and breast tissues, and is hormonally regulated. Cancer Res, 1999. 59: p. 4252-4256.

301. Yoshida, S., M. Taniguchi, T. Suemoto, T. Oka, X. He, S. Shiosaka, S. Yoshida, M. Taniguchi, A. Hirata and S. Shiosaka, cDNA cloning and expression of a novel serine protease, TLSP Sequence analysis and expression of human neuropsin cDNA and gene. Biochim Biophys Acta, 1998. 1399: p. 225-228.

302. Yousef, G.M., A. Magklara and E.P. Diamandis, KLK12 is a novel serine protease and a new member of the human kallikrein gene family-differential expression in breast cancer. Genomics, 2000. 69: p. 331-341.

303. Yousef, G.M., A. Scorilas and E.P. Diamandis, Genomic organization, mapping, tissue expression, and hormonal regulation of trypsin-like serine protease (TLSP PRSS20), a new member of the human Kallikrein gene family. Genomics, 2000. 63: p. 88-96.

304. Yousef, G.M., A. Chang and E.P. Diamandis, Identification and characterization of KLK-L4, a new kallikrein-like gene that appears to be down-regulated in breast cancer tissues. J Biol Chem, 2000. 275: p. 11891-11898.

305. Yousef, G.M., A. Magklara, A. Chang, K. Jung, D. Katsaros and E.P. Diamandis, Cloning of a new member of the human kallikrein gene family, klk14, which is down-regulated in different malignancies. Cancer Res, 2001. 61: p. 3425-3431.

306. Yousef, G.M., A. Scorilas, K. Jung, L.K. Ashworth and E.P. Diamandis, Molecular cloning of the human kallikrein 15 gene (KLK15). Up-regulation in prostate cancer. J Biol Chem, 2001. 276: p. 53-61.

307. Takayama, T.K., C.A. Carter and T. Deng, Activation of prostate-specific antigen precursor (pro-PSA) by prostin, a novel human serine protease identified by degenerate PCR. Biochemistry, 2001. 40: p. 1679-1687.

308. Xu, L.L., B.G. Stackhouse, K. Florence, W. Zhang, N. Shanmugam, I.A. Sesterhenn, Z. Zou, V. Srikantan, M. Augustus, V. Roschke, K. Carter, D.G. McLeod, J.W. Moul, D. Soppett, and S. Srivastava, PSGR, a novel prostate-specific gene with homology to a G protein-coupled receptor, is overexpressed in prostate cancer. Cancer Res, 2000. 60: p. 6568-6572.

309. Tsavaler, L., M.H. Shapero, S. Morkowski and R. Laus, Trp-p8, a novel prostate-specific gene, is up-regulated in prostate cancer and other malignancies and shares high homology with transient receptor potential calcium channel proteins. Cancer Res, 2001. 61: p. 3760-3769.

310. Lin, B., J.T. White, C. Ferguson, R. Bumgarner, C. Friedman, B. Trask, W. Ellis, P. Lange, L. Hood and P.S. Nelson, Part 1: a novel human prostate-specific, androgen-regulated gene that maps to chromosome 5q12. Cancer Res, 2000. 60: p. 858-863.

311. Sidiropoulus, M., A. Chang, K. Jung and E.P. Diamandis, Expression and regulation of prostate androgen regulated transcript-1 (part 1) and identification of differential expression in prostate cancer. Br J Cancer, 2001. 85: p. 393-397.

312. Magee, J.A., T. Araki, S. Patil, T. Ehrig, L. True, P.A. Humphrey, W.J. Catalona, M.A. Watson and J. Milbrandt, Expression profiling reveals hepsin overexpression in prostate cancer. Cancer Res, 2001. 61: p. 5692-5696.

313. Welsh, J.B., L.M. Sapinoso, A.I. Su, S.G. Kern, J. Wang-Rodriguez, C.A. Moskaluk, H.F. Frierson Jr and G.M. Hampton, Analysis of gene expression identifies candidate markers and pharmacological targets in prostate cancer. Cancer Res, 2001. 61: p. 5974-5978.

314. Dhanasekaran, S.M., T.R. Barrette, D. Ghosh, R. Shah, S. Varambally, K. Kurachi, K.J. Pienta, M.A. Rubin and A.M. Chinnaiyan, Delineation of prognostic biomarkers in prostate cancer. Nature, 2001. 412: p. 822-826.

315. Jemal, A., A. Thomas, T. Murray and M. Thun, Cancer Statistics 2002. CA Cancer J Clin, 2002. 52(1): p. 23-47.

316. Merrill, R.M., A.L. Potosky and E.J. Feuer, Changing trends in U.S. prostate cancer incidence rates. J. Natl. Cancer Inst., 1996. 88: p. 1683-1685.

317. Wingo, P.A., L.A. Ries, H.M. Rosenberg, D.S. Miller and B.K. Edwards, Cancer incidence and mortality, 1973-1995: a report card for the U.S. Cancer, 1998. 82: p. 1197-1207.

318. Meyer, F., L. Moore, I. Bairati and Y. Fradet, Downward trend in prostate cancer mortality in Quebec and Canada. J. Urol., 1999. 161: p. 1189-1191.

319. Hoeksema, M.J. and C. Law, Cancer mortality rates fall: a turning point for the nation. J. Natl. Cancer Inst., 1996. 88: p. 1706-1707.

320. Candas, B. and F. Labrie. Unequal decrease of prostate cancer specific death rates through the Province of Quebec between 1991 and 1999. in 14th Int. Symposium J. Steroid Biochem. Mol. Biol. 2000. Quιbec, Canada.

321. Labrie, F., Screening and early hormonal treatment of prostate cancer are accumulating strong evidence and support. Prostate, 2000. 43(3): p. 215-222.

322. Prostate Cancer Triallists' Collaborative Group, Maximum androgen blockade in advanced prostate cancer: an overview of the randomised trials. Lancet, 2000. 355: p. 1491-1498.

323. Labrie, F., B. Candas, L. Cusan, J.L. Gomez, P. Diamond, R. Suburu and M. Lemay, Diagnosis of advanced or noncurable prostate cancer can be practically eliminated by prostate-specific antigen. Urology, 1996. 47: p. 212-217.

324. Candas, B., L. Cusan, J.-L. Gomez, P. Diamond, R.E. Suburu, J. Lιvesque, G. Brousseau, A. Bιlanger and F. Labrie, Evaluation of prostatic specific antigen and digital rectal examination as screening tests for prostate cancer. Prostate, 2000. 45(1): p. 19-35.

325. Schrφder, F.H., P. van der Maas, P. Beemsterboer, A.B. Kruger, R. Hoedemaeker, J. Rietbergen and R. Kranse, Evaluation of the digital rectal examination as a screening test for prostate cancer. J. Natl. Cancer Inst., 1998. 90: p. 1817-1823.

326. Schrφder, F.H., M. Roobol-Bouts, A.N. Vis, T. van der Kwast and R. Kranse, Prostate-specific antigen-based early detection of prostate cancer-validation of screening without rectal examination. Urology, 2001. 57(1): p. 83-90.

327. Labrie, F., A. Dupont, R. Suburu, L. Cusan, M. Tremblay, J.L. Gomez and J. Emond, Serum prostate specific antigen (PSA) as prescreening test for prostate cancer. J. Urol., 1992. 147: p. 846-852.

328. Lee, F., P.J. Littrup, L. Loft-Christensen, B.S. Kelly Jr, T.A. McHugh, D.B. Siders, A.E. Mitchell and J.E. Newby, Predicted prostate specific antigen results using transrectal ultrasound gland volume. Differentiation of benign prostatic hyperplasia and prostate cancer. Cancer, 1992. 70(Suppl.): p. 211-220.

329. Littrup, P.J., C.R. Williams, T.K. Egglin and R.A. Kane, Determination of prostate volume by transrectal US for cancer screening. Part II. Clinical utility of transrectal accuracy of in vivo and in vitro techniques. Radiology, 1991. 179: p. 45-53.

330. Myschetzky, P.S., R.E. Suburu, B.S. Kelly Jr., M.L. Wilson, S.C. Chen and F. Lee, Determination of prostate gland volume by transrectal ultrasound:

REFERENCES

correlation with radical prostatectomy specimens. Scand. J. Urol. Nephrol. Suppl., 1991. 137: p. 107-111.

331. Hodge, K.K., J.E. McNeal, M.F. Terris and T.A. Stamey, Random systematic versus directed ultrasound guided transrectal core biopsies of the prostate. J. Urol., 1989. 142: p. 71-75.

332. Epstein, J.I., P.C. Walsh, M. Carmichael and C.B. Brendler, Pathologic and clinical findings to predict tumor extent of nonpalpable (stage T1c) prostate cancer. JAMA, 1994. 271: p. 368-374.

333. Catalona, W.J., D.S. Smith, T.L. Ratliff, K.M. Dodds, D.E. Coplen, J.J. Yuan, J.A. Petros and G.L. Andriole, Measurement of prostate-specific antigen in serum as a screening test for prostate cancer. N. Engl. J. Med., 1991. 324: p. 1156-1161.

334. Labrie, F., A. Dupont, R. Suburu, L. Cusan, J.L. Gomez, M. Koutsilieris, P. Diamond, J. Emond, M. Lemay and B. Txtu, Optimized strategy for detection of early stage, curable prostate cancer: role of prescreening with prostatic-specific antigen. Clin. Invest. Med., 1993. 16: p. 425-439.

335. Stormont, T.J., G.M. Farrow, R.P. Myers, M.L. Blute, H. Zincke, T.M. Wilson and J.E. Oesterling, Clinical stage B0 or T1c prostate cancer: nonpalpable disease identified by elevated serum prostate-specific antigen concentration. Urology, 1993. 41: p. 3-8.

336. Brawer, M.K. and P.H. Lange, Adjuvant therapy after radical prostatectomy. Probl. Urol., 1990. 4: p. 461-472.

337. Brawer, M.K., M.P. Chetner, J. Beatie, D.M. Buchner, R.L. Vessella and P.H. Lange, Screening for prostatic carcinoma with prostate specific antigen. J. Urol., 1992. 147: p. 841-845.

338. Mettlin, C., Early detection of prostate cancer following repeated examinations by multiple modalities: results of the American Cancer Society National Prostate Cancer Detection Project. Clin. Invest. Med., 1993. 16: p. 440-447.

339. Hugosson, J., G. Aus, C. Becker, S. Carlsson, H. Eriksson, H. Lilja, P. Lodding and G. Tibblin, Would prostate cancer detected by screening with prostate-specific antigen develop into clinical cancer if left undiagnosed? A comparison of two population-based studies in Sweden. BJU Int, 2000. 85(9): p. 1078-84.

340. American Cancer Society, Surveillance Research, cancer facts and figures. CA Cancer J. Clin., 2000: p. 4-9.

341. American Urological Association, Board of Directors Report: Early detection of prostate. American Urological Association, 2001. March.

342. Bolla, M., D. Gonzalez, P. Warde, J.B. Dubois, R.O. Mirimanoff, G. Storme, J. Bernier, A. Kuten, C. Sternberg, T. Gil, L. Collette, and M. Pierart, Improved survival in patients with locally advanced prostate cancer treated with radiotherapy and goserelin. N. Engl. J. Med., 1997. 337: p. 295-300.

343. Pilepich, M.V., R. Caplan, R.W. Byhardt, C.A. Lawton, M.J. Gallagher, J.B. Mesic, G.E. Hanks, C.T. Coughlin, A. Porter, W.U. Shipley, and D. Grignon, Phase III trial of androgen suppression using Goserelin in unfavorable prognosis carcinoma of the prostate treated with definitive radiotherapy: report of Radiation Therapy Oncology Group protocol 85-31. J. Clin. Oncol., 1997. 15: p. 1013-1021.

344. Hanks, G.E., J. Lu, M. Machtay, V. Venkatesan, W. Pinover, R. Byhardt and S.A. Rosenthal. RTOG Protocol 92-02: A Phase III Trial of the Use of Long Term Androgen Suppression Following Neoadjuvant Hormonal Cytoreduction and Radiotherapy in Locally Advanced Carcinoma of the Prostate. in 36th Annual Meeting of the American Society of Clinical Oncology. 2000. New Orleans, LA, USA.

345. Granfors, T., H. Modig, J.E. Damber and R. Tomic, Combined orchiectomy and external radiotherapy versus radiotherapy alone for nonmetastatic prostate cancer with or without pelvic lymph node involvement: a prospective randomized study. J. Urol., 1998. 159(6): p. 2030-2034.

346. Lee, F., S.T. Torp-Pedersen, D.B. Siders, P.J. Littrup and R.D. McLeary, Transrectal ultrasound in the diagnosis and staging of prostatic carcinoma. Radiology, 1989. 170: p. 609-615.

347. The Medical Research Council Prostate Cancer Working Party Investigators Group, Immediate versus deferred treatment for advanced prostatic cancer: initial results of the Medical Research Council trial. Br. J. Urol., 1997. 79: p. 235-246.

348. Labrie, F., L. Cusan, J.L. Gomez, P. Diamond and A. Bılanger, Long-term neoadjuvant and adjuvant combined androgen blockade is needed for efficacy of treatment in localized prostate cancer. Mol. Urol., 1997. 1: p. 253-261.

349. Labrie, F., L. Cusan, J.L. Gomez, A. Belanger and B. Candas, Long-term combined androgen blockade alone for localized prostate cancer. Mol. Urol., 1999. 3(3): p. 217-225.

350. Laverdiere, J., J.L. Gomez, L. Cusan, R. Suburu, P. Diamond, M. Lemay, B. Candas, A. Fortin and F. Labrie, Beneficial effect of combination therapy administered prior and following external beam radiation therapy in localized prostate cancer. Int. J. Radiat. Oncol. Biol. Phys., 1997. 37: p. 247-252.

351. Labrie, F., L. Cusan, J.L. Gomez, P. Diamond, R. Suburu, M. Lemay, B. Tetu, Y. Fradet and B. Candas, Downstaging of early stage prostate cancer before radical prostatectomy: the first randomized trial of neoadjuvant combination therapy with Flutamide and a luteinizing hormone-releasing hormone agonist. Urology, 1994. 44(6A): p. 29-37.

352. Pilepich, M.V., J.M. Krall, M. Al-Saffaf, M.J. John, R.L.S. Dogget, W.T. Sause, C.A. Lawton, R.A. Abrams, M. Rotman, P. Rubin, W.U. Shipley, D. Grignon, R. Caplan, and J.D. Cox, Androgen deprivation with radiation therapy compared with radiation therapy alone for locally advanced prostatic carcinoma: a randomized comparative trial of the Radiation Therapy Oncology Group. Urology, 1995. 45: p. 616-623.

353. Brown, M.L., L. Fintor and P.A. Newman-Horm, The economic burden of cancer. J. Natl. Cancer Inst., 1993. 85: p. 351-353.

354. Labrie, F., Intracrinology and cancer therapy. Science Watch, 1994. 5: p. 3-8.

355. Labrie, F., L. Cusan, J.L. Gomez, P. Diamond and B. Candas, Combination of screening and preoperative endocrine therapy: the potential for an important decrease in prostate cancer mortality. J. Clin. Endocrinol. Metab., 1995. 80: p. 2002-2013.

356. Labrie, F., Combined androgen blockade: its unique efficacy for the treatment of localized prostate cancer, in Cancer: Principle and Practice of Oncology, V.T. De Vita, S. Hellman, and S.A. Rosenberg, Editors. 1999, Lippincott-Raven: Philadelphia. p. 1-9.

357. Labrie, F., A. Dupont, L. Cusan, J.L. Gomez, P. Diamond, M. Koutsilieris, R. Suburu, Y. Fradet, M. Lemay, B. Tʀtu, J. Emond, and B. Candas, Downstaging of localized prostate cancer by neoadjuvant therapy with flutamide and lupron: the first controlled and randomized trial. Clin. Invest. Med., 1993. 16: p. 499-509.

358. Littrup, P.J., R.A. Kane, C.J. Mettlin, G.P. Murphy, F. Lee, A. Toi, R. Badalament and R. Babaian, Cost-effective prostate-cancer detection. Reduction of low-field biopsies. Cancer, 1994. 74: p. 3146-3158.

359. Aus, G., J. Hugosson and L. Norlın, Long-term survival and mortality in prostate cancer treated with noncurative intent. J. Urol., 1995. 154: p. 460-465.

360. Hillner, B.E., D.G. McLeod, E.D. Crawford and C.L. Bennett, Estimating the cost effectiveness of total androgen blockade with flutamide in M1 prostate cancer. Urology, 1995. 45: p. 633-640.

361. Bartsch, G., W. Horninger, H. Klocker, W. Oberaigner, G. Severi, C. Robertson and P. Boyle, Decrease in prostate cancer mortality following introduction of prostate specific antigen (PSA) screening in the federal state of Tyrol, Austria. AUA Annual Meeting. J. Urol., 2000. 163(4): p. P. 88, Abst. 387.

362. Han, M., A.W. Partin, S. Piantadosi, J.I. Epstein and P.C. Walsh, Era specific biochemical recurrence-free survival following radical prostatectomy for clinically localized prostate cancer. J Urol, 2001. 166(2): p. 416-419.

363. Stamey, T.A., Cancer of the Prostate: An analysis of some important contributions and dilemmas. Mono Urol, 1982. 3: p. 67-94.

364. McNeal, J.E., D.G. Bostwick, R.A. Kindrachulk, E.A. Redwine, F.S. Freiha and T.A. Stamey, Patterns of progression in prostate cancer. Lancet, 1986. 1: p. 60-63.

365. Quinlan, D.M., A.W. Partin and P.C. Walsh, Can aggressive prostatic carcinomas be identified and can their natural history be altered by treatment? Urology, 1995. 46(3 Suppl): p. 77-82.

366. Jewett, H.J., The present status of radical prostatectomy for stages A and B prostatic cancer. Urol Clin North Am, 1975. 2(1): p. 105-124.

367. Lee, W.R., G.E. Hanks and A. Halon, Increasing prostate-specific antigen profile following definitive radiation therapy for localized prostate cancer: clinical observations. J Clin Oncol, 1997. 15(1): p. 230-238.

368. Johansson, J.E., H.O. Adami, S.O. Andersson, R. Bergstrom, L. Holmberg and U.B. Krusemo, High

REFERENCES

10-year survival rate in patients with early, untreated prostatic cancer. JAMA, 1992. 267: p. 2191-2196.

369. Krongrad, A., H. Lai and S. Lai, Variation in prostate cancer survival explained by significant prognosis factors. J Urol, 1997. 158(4): p. 1487-1490.

370. Carroll, P.R., J.J. Presti, E. Small and M.R. Roach, Focal therapy for prostate cancer 1996: maximizing outcome. Urology, 1997: p. 84-94.

371. Crawford, E.D., W.R. Fair, G.J. Kellof, M.M. Lieber, G.J. Miller, P.T. Scardaino and E.P. DeAntoni, Chemoprevention of prostate cancer: guidelines for possible intervention strategies. J Cell Biochem, 1992(Suppl 16H): p. 140-145.

372. Kurhanewicz, J., M.G. Swanson, P.J. Wood and D.B. Vigneron, Magnetic resonance imaging and spectroscopic imaging: Improved patient selection and potential for metabolic intermediate endpoints in prostate cancer chemoprevention trials. Urology, 2001. 57(4 Suppl 1): p. 124-128.

373. Yu, K.K. and H. Hricak, Imaging prostate cancer. Radiol Clin North Am, 2000. 38(1): p. 59-85.

374. Kurhanewicz, J., D.B. Vigneron, R.G. Males, M.G. Swanson, K.K. Yu and H. Hricak, The prostate: MR imaging and spectroscopy. Present and future. Radiol Clin North Am, 2000. 38: p. 115-138.

375. Schall, M.D., R.E. Lenkinski, H.M. Pollack, Y. Imai and H.Y. Kressel, Prostate: MR imaging with an endorectal surface coil. Radiology, 1989. 172(2): p. 570-574.

376. Hricak, H., S. White, D. Vigneron, J. Kurhanewicz, A. Kosco, D. Levin, J. Weiss, P. Narayan and P.R. Carroll, Carcinoma of the prostate gland: MR imaging with pelvic phased-array coils versus integrated endorectal — pelvic phased-array coils. Radiology, 1994. 193(3): p. 703-709.

377. Sonnad, S.S., C.P. Langlotz and J.S. Schwartz, Accuracy of MR imaging for staging prostate cancer: a meta-analysis to examine the effect of technologic change. Acad Radiol, 2001. 8(2): p. 149-157.

378. May, F., T. Treumann, P. Dettmar, R. Hartung and J. Breul, Limited value of endorectal magnetic resonance imaging and transrectal ultrasonography in the staging of clinically localized prostate cancer. BJU Int, 2001. 87(1): p. 66-69.

379. Yu, K.K., J. Scheidler, H. Hricak, D.B. Vigneron, C.J. Zaloudek, R.G. Males, S.J. Nelson, P.R. Carroll and J. Kurhanewicz, Prostate cancer: prediction of extracapsular extension with endorectal MR imaging and three-dimensional proton MR spectroscopic imaging. Radiology, 1999. 213(2): p. 481-8.

380. Presti, J.J., R. Hovey, P.R. Carroll and K. Shinohara, Prospective evaluation of prostate specific antigen and prostate specific antigen density in the detection of nonpalpable and state T1C carcinoma of the prostate. U Urol, 1996. 156(5): p. 1685-1690.

381. Presti, J.J., R. Hovey, V. Bhargava, P.R. Carroll and K. Shinohara, Prospective evaluation of prostate specific antigen and prostate specific antigen density in the detection of carcinoma of the prostate: ethnic variations (see comments). J Urol, 1997. 157(3): p. 907-911.

382. Sommer, F.G., H.V. Nghiem, R. Herfkens, J. McNeal and R.N. Low, Determining the volume of prostate carcinoma: value of MR imaging with an external-array coil. AJR, 1993. 161(1): p. 81-86.

383. White, S., H. Hricak, R. Forstner, J. Kurhanewicz, D.B. Vigneron, C.J. Zaloudek, J.M. Weiss, P. Narayan and P.R. Carroll, Prostate cancer: effect of postbiopsy hemorrhage on interpretation of MR images. Radiology, 1995. 195(2): p. 385-390.

384. Hricak, H., The prostate gland. 1991, London England. 311.

385. Scheidler, J., H. Hricak, D.B. Vigneron, K.K. Yu, D.L. Sokolov, L.R. Huang, C.J. Zaloudek, S.J. Nelson, P.R. Carroll and J. Kurhanewicz, Prostate cancer: localization with three-dimensional proton MR spectroscopic imaging—clinicopathologic study. Radiology, 1999. 213(2): p. 473-480.

386. Kurhanewicz, J., D.B. Vigneron, H. Hricak, P. Narayan, P. Carroll and S.J. Nelson, Three-dimensional H-1 MR spectroscopic imaging of the in situ human prostate with high (0.24-0.7-cm3) spatial resolution. Radiology, 1996. 198(3): p. 795-805.

387. Weider, J., G. Schmidts, E. Casola, E. vanSonnenberg, B.F. Stainken and C.L. Parsons, Transrectal Ultrasound-Guided Transperineal Cryoablation in the Treatment of Prostate Carcinoma: Preliminary Results. J Urol, 1995. 154: p. 435-441.

388. Costello, L.C. and R.B. Franklin, Concepts of citrate production and secretion by prostate: 1. Metabolic relationships. Prostate, 1991. 18(1): p. 25-46.

389. Kahn, T., K. Beurrig, B. Schmitz-Dreager, J.S. Lewin, G. Feurst and U. Meodder, Prostatic carcinoma and benign prostatic hyperplasia: MR imaging with histopathologic correlation. Radiology, 1989. 173(3): p. 847-851.

390. Schiebler, M.L., J.E. Tomaszewski, M. Bezzi, H.M. Pollack, H.Y. Kressel, E.K. Cohen, H.G. Altman, W.B. Gefter, A.J. Wein and L. Axel, Prostatic carcinoma and benign hyperplasia: correlation of high-resolution MR and histopathologic findings. Radiology, 1989. 172(1): p. 131-137.

391. Costello, L.C. and R.B. Franklin, Novel role of zinc in the regulation of prostate citrate metabolism and its implications in prostate cancer. Prostate, 1998. 35(4): p. 285-296.

392. Liang, J.Y., Y.Y. Liu, J. Zou, R.B. Franklin, L.C. Costello and P. Feng, Inhibitory effect of zinc on human prostatic carcinoma cell growth. Prostate, 1999. 40(3): p. 200-207.

393. Costello, L.C. and R.B. Franklin, Bioenergetic theory of prostate malignancy. Prostate, 1994. 25(3): p. 162-166.

394. Aboagye, E.O. and Z.M. Bhujwalla, Malignant transformation alters membrane choline phospholipid metabolism of human mammary epithelial cells. Cancer Res, 1999. 59(1): p. 80-84.

395. Daly, P.F., R.C. Lyon, P.J. Faustino and J.S. Cohen, Phospholipid metabolism in cancer cells monitored by 31P NMR spectroscopy. J Biol Chem, 1987. 262(31): p. 14875-14878.

396. Cullis, P.R. and M.J. Hope, Physical properties and functional roles of lipids in membranes. Amsterdam, 1991: p. 1-41.

397. Mountford, C.E. and L.C. Wright, Organization of lipids in the plasma membranes of malignant and stimulated cells: a new model. Trends Biochem Sci, 1988. 13(5): p. 172-177.

398. Kurhanewicz, J., R. Dahiya, J.M. Macdonald, P. Jajodia, L.H. Chang, T.L. James and P. Narayan, Phosphorus metabolite characterization of human prostatic adenocarcinoma in a nude mouse model by 31P magnetic resonance spectroscopy and high pressure liquid chromatography. NMR Biomed, 1992. 5(4): p. 185-192.

399. Kurhanewicz, J., R. Dahiya, J.M. Macdonald, L.H. Chang, T.L. James and P. Narayan, Citrate alterations in primary and metastatic human prostatic adenocarcinomas: 1H magnetic resonance spectroscopy and biochemical study. Magn Reson Med, 1993. 29(2): p. 149-157.

400. Kurhanewicz, J., D.B. Vigneron, S.J. Nelson, H. Hricak, J.M. MacDonald, B. Konety and P. Narayan, Citrate as an in vivo marker to discriminate prostate cancer from benign prostatic hyperplasia and normal prostate peripheral zone: detection via localized proton spectroscopy. Urology, 1995. 45(3): p. 459-466.

401. Fowler, A.H., A.A. Pappas, J.C. Holder, A.E. Finkbeiner, G.V. Dalrymple, M.S. Mullins, J.R. Sprigg and R.A. Komoroski, Differentiation of human prostate cancer from benign hypertrophy by in vitro 1H NMR. Magn Reson Med, 1992. 25(1): p. 140-147.

402. Cornel, E.B., G.A. Smits, G.O. Oosterhof, H.F. Karthaus, F.M. Deburyne, J.A. Schalken and A. Heerschap, Characterization of human prostate cancer, benign prostatic hyperplasia and normal prostate by in vitro 1H and 31P magnetic resonance spectroscopy. J Urol, 1993. 150(6): p. 2019-2024.

403. Cai, H., P. Erhardt, J. Troppmair, M.T. Diaz-Meco, G. Sithanandam, U.R. Rapp, J. Moscat and G.M. Cooper, Hydrolysis of phosphatidylcholine couples Ras to activation of Raf protein kinase during mitogenic signal transduction. Mol Cell Biol, 1993. 13(12): p. 7645-7651.

404. Cuadrado, A., A. Carnero, F. Dolfi, B. Jimenez and J.C. Lacal, Phosphorylcholine: a novel second messenger essential for mitogenic activity of growth factors. Oncogene, 1993. 8(11): p. 2959-2968.

405. Exton, J.H., Phosphatidylcholine breakdown and signal transduction. Biochim Biophys Acta, 1994. 1212(1): p. 26-42.

406. Pelech, S.L. and D.E. Vance, Signal transduction via phosphatidylcholine cycles. Trends Biochem Sci, 1989. 14: p. 28-30.

407. Agris, P.F. and I.D. Campbell, Proton nuclear magnetic resonance of intact Friend leukemia cells: phosphorylcholine increase during differentiation. Science, 1982. 216(4552): p. 1325-1327.

408. Carpinelli, G., F. Podo, V.M. Di, E. Proietti, S. Gessani and F. Belardelli, Modulations of glycerophosphorylcholine and phosphorylcholine in Friend erythroleukemia cells upon in vitro induced erythroid differentiation: a 31P NMR study. Febs Lett, 1984. 176(1): p. 88-92.

409. Galons, J.P., J. Fantini, D.J. Vion, P.J. Cozzone and

P. Canioni, Metabolic changes in undifferentiated and differentiated human colon adenocarcinoma cells studied by multinuclear magnetic resonance spectroscopy. Biochimie, 1989. 71(8): p. 949-961.

410. Kurhanewicz, J., D.B. Vigneron and S.J. Nelson, Three-dimensional magnetic resonance spectroscopic imaging of brain and prostate cancer. Neoplasia, 2000. 2(1-2): p. 166-189.

411. Cheng, L.L., C.L. Wu, M.R. Smith and R.G. Gonzalez, Non-destructive quantitation of spermine in human prostate tissue samples using HRMAS H-1 NMR spectroscopy at 9.4 T. Febs Lett, 2001. 494(1-2): p. 112-116.

412. Schiebler, M.L., K.K. Miyamoto, M. White, S.J. Maygarden and J.L. Mohler, In vitro high resolution 1H-spectroscopy of the human prostate: benign prostatic hyperplasia, normal peripheral zone and adenocarcinoma. Magn Reson Med, 1993. 29(3): p. 285-291.

413. Swanson, M.G., R.G. Males, D.B. Vigneron, J.K. James, I. Cha, P.J. Wood, S.J. Nelson, R.E. Hurd and J. Kurhanewicz, 1H HR-MAS spectroscopic analysis of post-surgical prostate tissue targeted using 3D MRI/MRSI. Proceedings of the International Society for Magnetic Resonance in Medicine, Denver Colorado, 2000. 8: p. 97.

414. van der Graaf, M., R.G. Schipper, G.O. Oosterhof, J.A. Schalken, A.A. Verhofstad and A. Heerschap, Proton MR spectroscopy of prostatic tissue focused on the detection of spermine, a possible biomarker of malignant behavior in prostate cancer. Magma, 2000. 10(3): p. 153-159.

415. Heby, O., Role of polyamines in the control of cell proliferation and differentiation. Differentiation, 1981. 19(1): p. 1-20.

416. Heston, W.D., Prostatic polyamines and polyamine targeting as a new approach to therapy of prostatic cancer. Cancer Surv., 1991. 11: p. 217-238.

417. Swanson, M.G., D.B. Vigneron, T.K. Tran, N. Sailasuta, R.E. Hurd and J. Kurhanewicz, Single-voxel oversampled J-resolved spectroscopy of in vivo human prostate tissue. Magnetic resonance in Medicine, 2001. 45(6): p. 973-980.

418. Yu, K.K., H. Hricak, R. Alagappan, D. Chernoff, P. Bacchetti and C. Zaloudek, Detection of extracapsular extension of prostate carcinoma by endorectal/phased array coil MR imaging: multivariate analysis. Radiology, 1997. 202: p. 697-702.

419. Bostwick, D.G., S.D. Graham Jr, P. Napalkov, P.A. Abrahamsson, P.A. di Sant'agnese, F. Algaba, P.A. Hoisaeter, F. Lee, P. Littrup and F.K. Mostofi, Staging of early prostate cancer: a proposed tumor volume-based pronostic index. Urology, 1993. 41(5): p. 403-411.

420. Stamey, T.A., J.E. McNeal, F.S. Freiha and E. Redwine, Morphometric and clinical studies on 68 consecutive radical prostatectomies. J. Urol., 1988. 139: p. 1235-1241.

421. Wefer, A.E., H. Hricak, D.B. Vigneron, F.V. Coakley, Y. Lu, J. Wefer, U. Mueller-Lisse, P.R. Carroll and J. Kurhanewicz, Sextant localization of prostate cancer: comparison of sextant biopsy, magnetic resonance imaging and magnetic resonance spectroscopic imaging with step section histology (see comments). J Urol, 2000. 164(2): p. 400-404.

422. Wefer, A.E., H. Hricak, W. Okuno, P. Carroll and J. Kurhanewicz. Magnetic Resonance Imaging and Spectroscopy-targeted prostate biopsy. in 95th Meeting of the American Urological Association. 2000. Atlanta, Georgia.

423. Zagars, G.K., Prostate specific antigen as an outcome variable for T1 and T2 prostate cancer treated by radiation therapy. J Urol, 1994. 152(5): p. 1786-1791.

424. Blasko, J.C., K. Wallner, P.D. Grimm and H. Radge, PSA based disease control following ultrasound guided I-125 implantation for stage T1/T2 prostatic carcinoma. J. Urol., 1995. 154: p. 1096-1099.

425. Coakley, F.V., H. Hricak, A.E. Wefer, J.L. Speight, J. Kurhanewicz and M. Roach, Brachytherapy for prostate cancer: endorectal MR imaging of local treatment-related changes. Radiology, 2001. 219(3): p. 817-821.

426. Chen, M., H. Hricak, C.L. Kalbhen, J. Kurhanewicz, D.B. Vigneron, J.M. Weiss and P.R. Carroll, Hormonal ablation of prostatic cancer: effects on prostate morphology, tumor detection, and staging by endorectal coil MR imaging. Ajr Am J Roentgenol, 1996. 166(5): p. 1157-1163.

427. Parivar, F., H. Hricak, K. Shinohara, J. Kurhanewicz, D.B. Vigneron, S.J. Nelson and P.R. Carroll, Detection of locally recurrent prostate cancer after cryosurgery: evaluation by transrectal ultrasound, magnetic resonance imaging, and three-dimensional proton magnetic resonance spectroscopy. Urology, 1996. 48(4): p. 594-599.

428. Parivar, F. and J. Kurhanewicz, Detection of recurrent prostate cancer after Cryosurgery. Current Opinion in Urology, 1998. 8: p. 83-86.
429. Roach, M., 3rd, J. Kurhanewicz and P. Carroll, Spectroscopy in prostate cancer: hope or hype? Oncology (Huntingt), 2001. 15(11): p. 1399-410; discussion 1415-6, 1418.
430. Mueller-Lisse, U.G., D.V. Vigneron, H. Hricak, M.G. Swanson, P. Carroll, A. Bessette, J. Scheidler, A. Srivastava, R.M. Males, I. Cha, and J. Kurhanewicz, Localized Prostate Cancer: Effect of Hormone Deprivation Therapy Measured by Combined Three-dimensional 1H-MR Spectroscopy and MR Imaging: Clinico-Pathologic Case-Control Study. Radiology, 2001. 221: p. 380-390.
431. Mueller-Lisse, U.G., M.G. Swanson, D.B. Vigneron, H. Hricak, A. Bessette, R.G. Males, P.J. Wood, S. Noworolski, S.J. Nelson, I. Barken, P.R. Carroll, and J. Kurhanewicz, Time-dependent effects of hormone-deprivation therapy on prostate metabolism as detected by combined magnetic resonance imaging. Magnetic Resonance in Medicine, 2001. 46(1): p. 49-57.
432. Costello, L.C. and R.B. Franklin, Concepts of citrate production and secretion by prostate: 2. Hormonal relationships in normal and neoplastic prostate. Prostate, 1991. 19(3): p. 181-205.
433. Montironi, R., R. Pomante, L. Diamanti and C. Magi-Galluzzi, Apoptosis in prostatic adenocarcinoma following complete androgen ablation. Urol Int, 1998. 60(Suppl 1): p. 25-29.
434. Pickett, B., E. Vigneault, J. Kurhanewicz, L. Verhey and M. Roach, Static field intensity modulation to treat a dominant intra-prostatic lesion to 90 Gy compared to seven field 3-dimensional radiotherapy. International Journal of Radiation Oncology, Biology and Physics, 1999. 44(4): p. 921-929.
435. Zaider, M., M.J. Zelefsky, E.K. Lee, K.L. Zakian, H.I. Amols, J. Dyke, G. Cohen, Y. Hu, A.K. Endi, C. Chui, and J.A. Koutcher, Treatment planning for prostate implants using magnetic-resonance spectroscopy imaging. International Journal of Radiation Oncology, Biology and Physics, 2000. 47(4): p. 1085-1096.
436. Stamey, T.A. and J.E. McNeal, Adenocarcinoma of the prostate, in Cambell's Urology, P.C. Walsh, et al., Editors. 1992, WB Saunders Co: Philadelphia. p. 1200-1201.
437. Lerner, S.P., C. Seale-Hawkins, C.E. Carlton Jr and P.T. Scardino, The risk of dying of prostate cancer in patients with clinically localized disease. J. Urol., 1991. 146: p. 1040-1045.
438. Pontes, J.E., Z. Wajsman and R.P. Huben, Prognostic factors in localized prostate carcinoma. J Urol, 1985. 134: p. 1137-1139.
439. Rifkin, M.D., E.A. Zertouni and C.A. Gatsonis, Comparison of magnetic resonance imaging and ultrasonography in staging early prostate cancer. New Engl J Med, 1990. 323: p. 621-626.
440. Ennis, R.D. and R.E. Peschel, Radiation therapy for prostate cancer. Cancer, 1993. 72: p. 2644-2650.
441. Gomella, L.G., G.V. Raj and J.G. Moreno, Reverse transcriptase polymerase chain reaction for prostate specific antigen in the management of prostate cancer. J Urol, 1997. 158: p. 326-337.
442. Deguchi, T., M. Yang, S. Ito and Y. Nishino, Detection of micrometastatic prostate cancer cells in the bone marrow of patients with prostate cancer. Br J Cancer, 1997. 75: p. 634-638.
443. Wood Jr, D.P., E.R. Banks and S. Humphrey, Identification of bone metastases in patients with prostate cancer. Cancer, 1994. 74: p. 2533-2540.
444. Cama, C., C.A. Olsson and A.J. Raffo, Molecular staging of prostate cancer, a compariso9n of an enhanced reverse transcriptase polymerase chain reaction assay for prostate specific antigen versus prostate specific membrane antigen. J Urol, 1995. 153: p. 1373-1378.
445. Katz, A.E., G.M. de Vries and M.D. Begg, Enhanced reverse tarnscriptase-polymerase chain reaction as an indicator of true pathologic stage in patients with prostate cancer. Cancer, 1995. 75: p. 1642-1648.
446. Grasso, Y.Z., M.K. Gupta and H.S. Levin, Combined nested rt-PCR assay for prostate specific antigen and prostate specific membrane antigen in prostate cancer patients: correlation with pathologic stage. Cancer Res, 1998. 58: p. 1456-1459.
447. Loric, S., F. Dumas and P. Eschwege, Enhanced detection of hematogenous circulating prostatic cells in patients with prostate adenocarcinoma by using nested reverse transcriptase polymerase chain reaction assay based on prostate specific membrane antigen. Clin Chem, 1995. 41: p. 1698-1704.
448. Melchior, S.W., E. Corey and W.J. Ellis, Early tumor cell dissemination in patients with clinically

localized carcinoma of the prostate. Clin Cancer Res, 1997. 3: p. 249-256.
449. Olsson, C.A., M.C. de Vries and M.C. Benson, The use of rt-PCR for prostate specific antigen assay to predict surgical failures before radical prostatectomy: molecular staging of the prostate cancer. Br J Urol, 1996. 77: p. 411-417.
450. Israeli, R.S., W.H. Miller and S.L. Su, Sensitive reverse transcriptase polymerase chain reaction detection of circulating prostatic tumor cells:comparison of prostate-specific membrane antigen and prostate-specific antigen-based assays. Cancer Res, 1994. 54: p. 6306-6310.
451. Su, S.L., D.W. Heston and M. Perotti, Evaluating neoadjuvant therapy effectiveness on systemic disease: use of a prostate-specific membrane reverse transcriptase polymerase chain reaction. Urology, 1997. 49: p. 95-101.
452. Kantoff, P.W., S. Halabi, D.A. Farmer, D.F. Hayes, N.A. Vogelzang and E.J. Small, Prognostic significance of reverse transcriptase polymerase chain reaction for prostate-specific antigen in men with hormone-refractory prostate cancer. J Clin Oncol, 2001. 19: p. 3025-3028.
453. Koutsilieris, M., P. Lembessis, V. Luu-The and A. Sourla, Repetitive and site-specific molecular staging of prostate cancer using reverse transcriptase polymerase chain reaction for PSA and PSMA. Clin Exp Metastasis, 1999. 17: p. 741-746.
454. Kibel, A.S., K. Krithivas and B. Shamel, Constitutive expression of high levels of prostate specific antigen in the absence of prostate carcinoma. Urology, 1996. 48: p. 741-746.
455. Eschwege, P., F. Dumas and P. Blancet, Heamatogenous dissemination of prostatic epithelial cells during radical prostatetomy. Lancet, 1995. 346: p. 1528-1530.
456. Sourla, A., P. Lembessis, C. Mitsiades, T. Dimopoulos, M. Skouteris, M. Metsinis, A. Ntounis, A. Ioannidis, A. Katsoulis, V. Kyragiannis, T. Lambou, A. Tsintavis, and M. Koutsilieris, Conversion of nested reverse-transcriptase polymerase chain reaction from positive to negative status at peripheral blood during androgen ablation therapy is associated with long progression-free survival in stage D2 prostate cancer patients. Anticancer Res, 2001. 21: p. 3665-3570.
457. Belliveau, R.E. and R.P. Spencer, Incidence and staging of bone lesions detected by 99mTc polyphosphate scans in patients with tumors. Cancer, 1975. 36: p. 65-72.
458. Galasko, C.S., Mechanisms of bone destruction in the development of skeletal metastases. Nature, 1976. 263: p. 507-508.
459. Koutsilieris, M., Skeletal metastases in advanced prostate cancer: cell biology and therapy. Crit. Rev. Oncol. Hematol., 1995. 18: p. 51-64.
460. Koutsilieris, M., Osteoblastic metastasis in advanced prostate cancer. Anticancer Res, 1993. 13: p. 443-449.
461. Guise, T.A. and G.R. Mundy, Cancer and bone. Endocr Rev, 1998. 19: p. 18-54.
462. Galasko, C.S., Mechanism of lytic and blastic metastatic disease of bone. Clin Orth, 1982. 12: p. 20-27.
463. Mundy, G.R., Mechanisms of bone metastasis. Cancer, 1997. 80: p. 1546-1556.
464. Koutsilieris, M., N. Faure, G. Tolis, B. Laroche, G. Robert and C.F. Ackman, Objective response and disease outcome in 59 patients with stage D2 prostatic cancer treated with either Buserelin or orchiectomy. Disease aggressivity and its association with response and outcome. Urology, 1986. 27: p. 221-228.
465. Koutsilieris, M., B. Laroche, M. Thabet and Y. Fradet, The assessment of disease aggressivity in stage D2 prostate cancer patients. Anticancer Res, 1990. 10: p. 333-336.
466. Crawford, E.D., M.A. Eisenberger, D.G. McLeod, J.T. Spaulding, R. Benson, F.A. Dorr, B.A. Blumenstein, M.A. Davis and P.J. Goodman, A controlled trial of leuprolide with and without flutamide in prostatic carcinoma. N. Engl. J. Med., 1989. 321(7): p. 419-424.
467. Mitsiades, C. and M. Koutsilieris, Molecular biology and cellular physiology of refractoriness to androgen ablation therapy in advanced prostate cancer. Exper Opin Investig Drugs, 2001. 6: p. 1099-1115.
468. Koutsilieris, M., C. Mitsiades and A. Sourla, Insulin-like growth factor I and urikonase-type plasminogen activator bioregulation system as a survival mechanism of prostate cancer cells in osteoblastic metastases: development of antisurvival factor therapy for hormone-refractory prostate cancer. Mol Med, 2000. 6: p. 251-267.

469. Koutsilieris, M., S.A. Rabbani and D. Goltzman, Selective osteoblast mitogen can be extracted from prostatic tissue. Prostate, 1986. 9: p. 109-115.
470. Reyes-Moreno, C., A. Sourla, I. Choki, C. Doillon and M. Koutsilieris, Osteoblast-derived survival factors protect PC-3 human prostate cancer cell from adriamycin apoptosis. Urology, 1998. 52: p. 341-347.
471. Koutsilieris, M., C. Mitsiades, T. Dimopoulos, A. Ioannidis, A. Ntounis and T. Lambou, A combination therapy of dexamethasone and somatostatin analog reintroduces objective clinical responses to LHRH analog in androgen ablation-refractory prostate cancer patients. J Clin Endocrinol Metab, 2001. 86: p. 5729-5736.
472. Koutsilieris, M., M.A. Dimopoulos, C. Doillon, A. Sourla, C. Reyes-Moreno and I. Choki, The molecular concept of prostate cancer. Cancer J., 1996. 9: p. 89-94.
473. Berenson, J.R., R. Vescio and K. Henick, A phase I, open label, dose ranging trial of intravenous bolus zolendronic acid, a novel bisphosphonate, in cancer patients with metastatic bone disease. Cancer, 2001. 91: p. 144-154.
474. Labrie, F., A. Dupont and A. Bılanger, Complete androgen blockade for the treatment of prostate cancer, in Important Advances in Oncology, V.T. de Vita, S. Hellman, and S.A. Rosenberg, Editors. 1985, J.B. Lippincott: Philadelphia. p. 193-217.
475. Labrie, F., A. Bılanger, L. Cusan, J. Simard, V. Luu-The, C. Labrie, J.L. Gomez, P. Diamond and B. Candas, History of LHRH agonists and combination therapy in prostate cancer. Endocrine-Related Cancer, 1996. 3: p. 243-278.
476. Koutsilieris, M. and C.S. Mitsiades, Combination of dexamethasone and of a somatostatin analogue in the treatment of advanced prostate cancer. Expert Opin Invest Drugs, 2002. 11(2): p. 283-293.
477. Labrie, F., A. Dupont, A. Bélanger, L. Cusan, M. Giguère, N. Bergeron, W. Wegrzycki, M. Brochu, E. Turina, S. Pinault, Y. Lacourcière, and J. Emond, Antihormone treatment in stage D2 prostate cancer patients relapsing under treatment with Flutamide and castration: addition of aminoglutethimide and low dose hydrocortisone to combination therapy. Brit. J. Urol., 1989. 63: p. 634-638.
478. Labrie, F., Intracrinology. Mol. Cell. Endocrinol., 1991. 78: p. C113-C118.
479. Garnick, M.B., Prostate cancer: screening, diagnosis, and management. Ann. Int. Med., 1993. 118: p. 804-818.
480. Dupont, A., J.L. Gomez, L. Cusan, M. Koutsilieris and F. Labrie, Response to Flutamide withdrawal in advanced prostate cancer in progression under combination therapy. J. Urol., 1993. 150: p. 908-913.
481. Kelly, W.K., S. Slovin and H.I. Scher, Steroid hormone withdrawal syndromes. Pathophysiology and clinical significance. Urol Clin North Am, 1997. 24: p. 421-431.
482. Small, E.J. and N.J. Vogelzang, Second-line therapy for advanced prostate cancer: a shifting paradigm. J Clin Oncol, 1997. 15: p. 382-388.
483. Tannock, I.F., Is there evicence that chemotherapy is of benefit to patients with carcinoma of the prostate? J Clin Oncol, 1985. 3: p. 1013-1021.
484. Hudes, G.R., R. Greenberg and R.L. Krigel, Phase II study of estramustine and vinblastine, two microtubule inhibitors, in hormone-refractory prostate cancer. J Clin Oncol, 1992. 10: p. 1754-1761.
485. Oh, W.K., Chemotherapy for patients with advanced prostate carcinoma. Cancer, 2000. 88: p. 3015-3021.
486. Small, E.J., P. Fratesi and D.M. Reese, Immunotherapy of hormone-refractory prostate cancer with antigen-loaded dendritic cells. J Clin Oncol, 2000. 18: p. 3894-3903.
487. Eisenberger, M.A., R. Simon, P.J. O'Dwyer, R.E. Wittes and M.A. Friedman, A reevaluation of non-hormonal cytotoxic chemotherapy in the treatment of prostatic carcinoma. J Clin Oncol, 1985. 3: p. 827-841.
488. Dowling, A.J. and I.F. Tannock, Systemic treatment for prostate cancer. Cancer Treat Rev, 1998. 24: p. 283-301.
489. Borst, P., R. Evers, M. Kool and J. Wijnhlds, A family of drug transporters: the multidrug resistance-associated proteins. J Natl Cancer Inst, 2000. 92: p. 1295-1302.
490. Bertino, J.R., E. Goker, R. Gorlick, W.W. Li and D. Banerjee, Resistance mechanisms to methotrexate in tumors. Stem Cells, 1996. 14: p. 5-9.
491. Nicholson, D.W., From bench to clnic with apoptosis-based therapeutic agents. Nature, 2000. 407: p. 810-816.

REFERENCES

492. Mitsiades, C.S., M. Koutsilieris, A. Sourla, C. Doillon and T. Lembessis, Three-dimensional type I collagen co-culture systems for the study of cell-cell interactions and treatment response in bone metastases. J Musculoskel Neuron Interact, 2000. 1: p. 153-155.

493. Shain, K.H., T.H. Landowski and W.S. Dalton, The tumor microenvironment as a determinant of cancer cell survival: a possible mechanism for de novo drug resistance. Curr Opin Oncol, 2000. 12: p. 557-563.

494. Osborne, C.K., Steroid hormone receptors in breast cancer management. Breast Cancer Res Treat, 1998. 51: p. 227-238.

495. Quigley, C.A., A. De Bellis, K.B. Marschke, M.K. el-Awady, E.M. Wilson and F.S. French, Androgen receptor defects: historical, clinical and molecular perspectives (published erratum appears in Endocr Rev 1995 Aug; 16(4):546). Endocr Rev, 1995. 16: p. 271-321.

496. van der Kwast, T.H., J. Schalken and J.A. Ruizeveld de Winter, Androgen receptors in endocrine-therapy-resistant human prostate cncer. Int J Cancer, 1991. 48: p. 189-193.

497. Lopez-Otin, C. and E.P. Diamandis, Breast and prostate cancer: an analysis of common epidemiological, genetic and biochemical features. Endocr Rev, 1998. 19: p. 365-396.

498. Hobisch, A., Z. Culig, C. Radmayr, G. Bartsch, H. Klocker and A. HIttmair, Distant metastases from prostatic carcinoma express receptor protein. Cancer Res, 1995. 55: p. 3068-3072.

499. Eder, I.E., Z. Culig and R. Ramoner, Inhibition of LncaP prostate cancer cells by means of androgen receptor antisense oligonucleotides. Cancer Gene Ther, 2000. 7: p. 997-1007.

500. Taplin, M.E., G.J. Bubley, T.D. Shuster and e. al., Mutation of the androgen-receptor gene in metastatic androgen-independent prostate cancer. N. Engl. J. Med., 1996. 332: p. 1393-1398.

501. Veldscholte, J., C. Ris-Stalpers, G.G. Kuiper, G. Jenster, C. Berrevoets, E. Claassen, H.C. van Rooij, J. Trapman, A.O. Brinkmann and E. Mulder, A mutation in the ligand binding domain of the androgen receptor of human LNCaP cells affects steroid binding characteristics and response to anti-androgens. Biochem. Biophys. Res. Commun., 1990. 173: p. 534-540.

502. Suzuki, H., K. Akakura, A. Komiya, S. Aida, S. Akimoto and J. Shimazaki, Codon 877 mutation in the androgen receptor gene in advanced prostate cancer: relation to antiandrogen withdrawal syndrome. Prostate, 1996. 29: p. 153-158.

503. Culig, Z., H. Klocker and J. Eberle, DNA sequence of the androgen receptor in prostatic tumor cell lines and tissue specimens assessed by means of the polymerase chain reaction. Prostate, 1993. 22: p. 11-22.

504. Viskorpi, T., E. Hyytinen and P. Koivisto, In vivo amplification of the androgen receptor gene and prostate progression of human prostate cancer. Nat. Genet., 1996. 9: p. 401-406.

505. Koivisto, P., J. Kononen, C. Palmberg, T. Tammela, E. Hyytinen, J. Isola, J. Trapman, C. Cleutjens, A. Noordzij, T. Visakorpi, and O.P. Kallioniemi, Androgen receptor gene amplification: a possible molecular mechanism for androgen deprivation therapy failure in prostate cancer. Cancer Res., 1997. 57: p. 314-319.

506. Gottlieb, B., H. Lehvaslaiho, L.K. Beitel, R. Lumbroso, L. Pinsky and M. Trifiro, The androgen receptor gene mutations Database. Nucleic Acids Res, 1998. 26: p. 234-238.

507. Ruijter, E., C. van de Kaa, G. Miller, D. Ruiter, F. Debruyne and J. Schalken, Molecular genetics and epidemiology of prostate carcinoma. Endocr Rev, 1999. 20: p. 22-45.

508. Suzuki, H., N. Sato, Y. Watabe, M. Masai, S. Seino and J. Shimazaki, Androgen receptor gene mutations in human prostate cancer. J Steroid Biochem Mol Biol, 1993. 46: p. 759-765.

509. Castagnaro, M., D.W. Yandell, B. Dockhorn-Dworniczak, H.J. Wolfe and C. Poremba, Androgen receptor gene mutations and p53 gene analysis in advanced prostate cancer. Verh Dtsch Ges Pathol, 1993. 77: p. 119-123.

510. Evans, B.A., M.E. Harper and C.E. Daniells, Low incidence of androgen receptor gene mutations in human prostatic tumors using single strand conformation polymorphism analysis. Prostate, 1996. 28: p. 162-171.

511. Elo, J.P., L. Kvist and K. Leinonen, Mutated human androgen receptor gene detected in a prostatic cancer patient is also activated by estradiol. J Clin Endocrinol Metab, 1995. 80: p. 3494-3500.

512. Peterziel, H., Z. Culig and J. Stober, Mutant andro-

gen receptors in prostatic tumors distinguish between amino-acid-sequence requirements for transactivation and ligand binding. Int J Cancer, 1995. 63: p. 544-550.
513. Tilley, W.D., G. Buchanan, T.E. Hickey and J.M. Bentel, Mutations in the androgen receptor gene are associated with progession of human prostate cancer to androgen independence. Clin. Cancer Res., 1996. 2: p. 277-285.
514. Crocitto, L.E., B.E. Henderson and G.A. Coetzee, Identification of two germline point mutations in the 5'UTR of the androgen receptor gene in men with prostate cancer. J Urol, 1997. 158(1599-1601).
515. Koivisto, P., M. Kolmer, T. Visakorpi and O.P. Kallioniemi, Androgen receptor gene and hormonal therapy failure of prostate cancer. Am J Pathol, 1998. 152: p. 1-9.
516. Bubendorf, L., M. Kolmer and J. Kononen, Hormone therapy failure in human prostate cancer: analysis by complementary DNA and tissue microarrays. J Natl Cancer Inst, 1999. 91: p. 1758-1764.
517. Jacobs, S.C., D. Pinka and R. Lawson, Prostatic osteoblast factor. Invest Urol, 1988. 17: p. 195-199.
518. Koutsilieris, M., S.A. Rabbani and D. Goltzman, Effects of human prostatic mitogens on rat bone cells and fibroblasts. J Endocrinol, 1987. 115: p. 447-454.
519. Polychronakos, C., U. Janthly, J.G. Lehoux and M. Koutsilieris, Mitogenic effects of insulin and insulin-like growth factors on PA-III rat prostate adenocarcinoma cells: characterization of the receptors involved. Prostate, 1991. 19: p. 313-321.
520. Koutsilieris, M., Prostate-derived growth factors for bone cells: implications for bone physiology and pathophysiology: review. In Vivo, 1988. 2: p. 377-383.
521. Matuo, Y., N. Nishi, S. Matsui, A.A. Sandberg, J.T. Isaacs and F. Wada, Heparin binding affinity of rat prostatic growth factor in normal and cancerous prostates: partial purification and characterization of rat prostatic growth factor in the Dunning tumor. Cancer Res, 1987. 47: p. 188-192.
522. Nishikawa, K., Y. Yoshitake, M. Minemura, K. Yamada and Y. Matuo, Localization of basic fibroblast growth factor (bFGF) in a metastatic cell line (AT-3) established from the Dunning prostatic carcinoma of rat: application of a specific monoclonal antibody. Adv Exp Med Biol, 1992. 324: p. 131-139.
523. Mansson, P.E., P. Adams, M. Kan and W.L. McKeehan, Heparin-binding growth factor gene expression and receptor characteristics in normal rat prostate and two transplantable rat prostate tumors. Cancer Res, 1989. 49: p. 2485-2494.
524. Steiner, M.S. and E.R. Barrack, Transforming growth factor-beta 1 overproduction in prostate cancer: effects on growth in vivo and in vitro. Mol Endocrinol, 1992. 6: p. 15-25.
525. Chen, D., J.Q. Feng and M. Feng, Sequence and expression of bone morphogenetic protein 3 mRNA in prolonged cultures of fetal rat calvarial osteoblasts and in rat prostate adenocarcinoma PA III cells. DNA Cell Biol, 1995. 14: p. 235-239.
526. Harris, S.E., M.A. Harris, P. Mahy, J. Wozney, J.Q. Feng and G.R. Mundy, Expression of bone morphogenetic protein messenger RNAs by normal rat and human prostate and prostate cancer cells. Prostate, 1994. 24: p. 204-211.
527. Lagenstroer, P., R. Tang, E. Shapiro, B. Divish, T. Opgenorth and H. Lepor, Endothelin-1 in the human prostate: tissue levels, source of produciton and isometric tension studies. J Urol, 1993. 150: p. 495-499.
528. Nelson, J.B., S.P. Hedican and D.J. George, Identification of entothelin-1 in the pathophysiology of metastatic adenocarcinoma of the prostate. Nat Med, 1995. 1: p. 944-949.
529. Koutsilieris, M., S.A. Rabbani, H.P. Bennett and D. Goltzman, Characteristics of prostate-derived growth factors for cells of the osteoblast phenotype. J Clin Invest, 1987. 80: p. 941-946.
530. Simpson, E., J. Harrod, G. Eilon, J.W. Jacobs and G.R. Mundy, Identification of a messenger ribonucleic acid fraction in human prostatic cancer cells coding for a novel oestoblast-stimulating factor. Endocrinology, 1985. 117: p. 1615-1620.
531. Koutsilieris, M., G. Frenette, C. Lazure, J.G. Lehoux, M.V. Govindan and C. Polychronakos, Urokinase-type plasminogen activator: a paracrine factor regulating the bioavailability of IGFs in PA-III cell-induced osteoblastic metastases. Anticancer Res, 1993. 13: p. 481-486.
532. Frenette, G., R.R. Tremblay, C. Lazure and J.Y. Dubι, Prostatic kallikrein hK2, but not prostate-specific antigen (hK3), activates single-chain uroki-

REFERENCES

nase-type plasminogen activator. Int J Cancer, 1997. 71: p. 897-899.

533. Wun, T.C., L. Ossowski and E. Reich, A proenzyme form of human urokinase. J Biol Chem, 1982. 257: p. 7262-7268.

534. Reyes-Moreno, C. and M. Koutsilieris, Glucocorticoid receptor function possibly modulates cell-cell interactions in osteoblastic metastases on rat skeleton. Clin Exp Metastasis, 1997. 15: p. 205-217.

535. Webber, M.M. and A. Waghray, Urokinase-mediated extracellular matrix degradation by human prostatic carcinoma cells and its inhibition by retinoic acid. Clin Cancer Res, 1995. 1: p. 755-761.

536. Mizukami, I.F., B.A. Garni-Wagner and L.M. DeAngelo, Immunologic detection of the cellular receptor for urokinase plasminogen activator. Clin Immunol Immunopathol, 1994. 71(96-104).

537. Crowley, C.W., R.L. Cohen, B.K. Lucas, G. Liu, M.A. Shuman and A.D. Levinson, Prevention of metastasis by inhibition of the urokinase receptor. Proc Natl Acad Sci USA, 1993. 90: p. 5021-5025.

538. Quax, P.H., A.C. de Bart, J.A. Schalken and J.H. Verheijen, Plasminogen activator and matrix metalloproteinase production and extracellular matrix degradation by rat prostate cancer cells in vitro: correlation with metastatic behavior in vivo. Prostate, 1997. 32: p. 196-204.

539. Achbarou, A., S. Kaiser and G. Tremblay, Urokinase overproduction results in increased skeletal metastasis by prostate cancer cells in vivo. Cancer Res, 1994. 54: p. 2372-2377.

540. Jankun, J., R.W. Keck, E. Skrzypczak-Jankun and R. Swiercz, Inhibitors of urokinase reduce size of prostate cancer xenografts in severe combined immunodeficient mice (published erratum appears in Cancer Res 1998 Jan 1;58(1):179). Cancer Res, 1997. 57: p. 559-563.

541. Hienert, G., J.C. Kirchheimer, G. Christ, H. Pfluger and B.R. Binder, Plasma urokinase-type plasminogen activator correlates to bone scintigraphy in prostatic carcinoma. Eur Urol, 1988. 15: p. 256-258.

542. Rabbani, S.A., J. Desjardins and A.W. Bell, An amino-terminal fragment of urokinase isolated from a prostate cancer cell line (PC-3) is mitogenic for osteoblast-like cells. Biochem Biophys Res Commun, 1990. 173: p. 1058-1064.

543. Rabbani, S.A., A.P. Mazar and S.M. Bernier, Structural requirements for the growth factor activity of the amino-terminal domain of urokinase. J Biol Chem, 1992. 267: p. 14151-14156.

544. Rabbani, S.A., J. Gladu, A.P. Mazar, J. Henkin and D. Goltzman, Induction in human osteoblastic cells (SaOS2) of the early response genes fos, jun, and myc by the amino terminal fragment (ATF) of urokinase. J Cell Physiol, 1997. 172: p. 137-145.

545. Koutsilieris, M. and C. Polychronakos, Proteinolytic activity against IGF-binding proteins involved in the paracrine interactions between prostate adenocarcinoma cells and osteoblasts. Anticancer Res, 1992. 12: p. 905-910.

546. Reyes-Moreno, C., G. Frenette, J. Boulanger, E. Lavergne, M.V. Govindan and M. Koutsilieris, Mediation of glucocorticoid receptor function by transforming growth factor beta 1 (TGFb1) expression in PC-3 human prostate cancer cells. Prostate, 1995. 26: p. 260-269.

547. Boulanger, J., C. Reyes-Moreno and M. Koutsilieris, Mediation of glucocorticoid receptor function by the activation of latent transforming growth factor beta 1 in MG-63 human osteosarcoma cell. Int J Cancer, 1995. 61: p. 692-697.

548. Rajah, R., B. Valentinis and P. Cohen, Insulin-like growth factor (IGF)-binding protein-3 induces apoptosis and mediates the effects of transforming growth factor-beta1 on programmed cell death through a p53- and IGF-independent mechanism. J Biol Chem, 1997. 272: p. 12181-12188.

549. Behrakis, P. and M. Koutsilieris, Pulmonary Metastases in metastatic prostate cancer: host tissue-tumor cell interactions and response to hormone therapy. Anticancer Res, 1997. 17(1517-1518).

550. Landstrom, M., J.E. Damber and A. Bergh, Prostatic tumor regrowth after initially successful castration therapy may be related to a decreased apoptotic cell death rate. Cancer Res, 1994. 54: p. 4281-4224.

551. Koutsilieris, M., C. Reyes-Moreno, I. Choki, A. Sourla, C. Doillon and N. Pavlidis, Chemotherapy cytotoxicity of human MCF-7 and MDA-MB 231 breast cancer cells is altered by osteoblast-derived growth factors. Mol Med, 1999. 5: p. 86-97.

552. Choki, I., A. Sourla, C. Reyes-Moreno and M. Koutsilieris, Osteoblast-derived growth factors enhance adriamycin-cytostasis of MCF-7 human

breast cancer cells. Anticancer Res, 1998. 18: p. 4213-4224.

553. Koutsilieris, M., A. Sourla, G. Pelletier and C.J. Doillon, Three-dimensional type I collagen gel system for the study of osteoblastic metastases produced by metastatic prostate cancer. J. Bone Miner. Res., 1994. 9(Novembre): p. 1823-1832.

554. Sourla, A., C. Doillon and M. Koutsilieris, Three-dimensional type I collagen gel system containing MG-63 osteoblasts-like cells as a model for studying local bone reaction caused by metastatic cancer cells. Anticancer Res, 1996. 16: p. 2773-2780.

555. Mantzoros, C.S., A. Tzonou, L.B. Signorello, M. Stampfer, D. Trochopoulos and H.O. Adami, Insulin-like growth factor 1 in relation to prostate cancer and benign prostatic hyperplasia. Br J Cancer, 1997. 76: p. 1115-1118.

556. Chan, J.M., M.J. Stampfer and E. Giovannucci, Plasma insulin-like growth factor-I and prostate cancer risk: a prospective study. Science, 1998. 279: p. 563-566.

557. Delany, A.M. and E. Canalis, Transcriptional repression of insulin-like growth factor I by glucocorticoids in rat bone cells. Endocrinology, 1995. 136: p. 4776-4781.

558. Koutsilieris, M., PA-III rat prostate adenocarcinoma cells (review). In Vivo, 1992. 6: p. 199-203.

559. Chen, T.L., J.B. Mallory and R.L. Hintz, Dexamethasone and 1,25(OH)2 vitamin D3 modulate the synthesis of insulin-like growth factor-I osteoblast-like cells. Calcif Tissue Int, 1991. 48: p. 278-282.

560. Koutsilieris, M., C. Reyes-Moreno, A. Sourla, V. Dimitriadou and I. Choki, Growth factors mediate glucocorticoid receptor function and dexamethasone-induced regression of osteoblastic lesions in hormone refractory prostate cancer. Anticancer Res, 1997. 17: p. 1461-1465.

561. Villafuerte, B.C., S. Goldstein, D.G. Robertson, C.I. Pao, L.J. Murphy and L.S. Phillips, Nutrition and somatomedin XXIX. Molecular regulation of IGFBP-1 in hepatocyte primary culture. Diabetes, 1992. 41: p. 835-842.

562. Giustina, A. and J.D. Veldhuis, Pathophysiology of the neuroregulation of growth hormone secretion in experimental animals and the human. Endocr Rev, 1998. 19: p. 717-719.

563. Davies, P.H., S.E. Stewart, L. Lancranjan, M.C. Sheppard and P.M. Stewart, Long-term therapy with long-acting octreotide (Sandostatin-LAR) for the management of acromegaly. Clin Endocrinol (Oxf), 1998. 48: p. 311-316.

564. Ezzat, S., S.G. Ren, G.D. Braunstein and S. Melmed, Octreotide stimulates insulin-like growth factor-binding protein-1: a potential pituitary-independent mechanism for drug action. J Clin Endocrinol Metab, 1992. 75: p. 1459-1463.

565. Koutsilieris, M., M. Tzanela and T. Dimopoulos, Novel concept of antisurvival factor (ASF) therapy produces an objective clinical response in four patients with hormone-refractory prostate cancer: case report. Prostate, 1999. 38: p. 313-316.

566. Soloway, M.S., S.W. Hardeman and D. Hickey, Stratification of patients with metastatic prostate cancer based on extent of disease on initial bone scan. Cancer, 1988. 61: p. 195-202.

567. Elomaa, I., T. Taube, C. Blomqvist, P. Rissanen, S. Rannikko and O. Alfthan, Aminoglutethimide for advanced prostatic cancer resistant to conventional hormonal therapy. Eur Urol, 1988. 14: p. 104-106.

568. Ponder, B.A., R.J. Shearer and R.D. Pocock, Response to aminoglutethimide and cortisone acetate in advanced prostatic cancer. Br J Cancer, 1984. 50: p. 757-763.

569. Plowman, P.N., L.A. Perry and T. Chard, Androgen suppression by hydrocortisone without aminoglutethimide in orchiectomised men with prostatic cancer. Br J Urol, 1987. 59: p. 255-257.

570. Manni, A., R.J. Santen and A.E. Boucher, Androgen depletion and repletion as a means of potentiating the effect of cytotoxic chemotherapy in advanced prostate cancer. J Steroid Biochem, 1987. 27: p. 551-556.

571. Enomoto, Y., H. Fukuhara and S. Kurimoto, A case of hormone-refractory prostate cancer responsive to low-dose prednisolone therapy. Nippon Hinyokika Gakkai Zasshi, 1997. 88: p. 636-639.

572. Kelly, W.K., H.I. Scher and M. Mazumdar, Suramin and hydrocortisone: determining drug efficacy in androgen-independent prostate cancer. J Clin Oncol, 1995. 13: p. 2214-2222.

573. Figg, W.D., G. Kroog and P. Duray, Flutamide withdrawal plus hydrocortisone resulted in clinical complete response in a patient with prostate carcinoma. Cancer, 1997. 79: p. 1964-1968.

574. Small, E.J., A. Baron and R. Bok, Simultaneous

antiandrogen withdrawal and treatment with ketoconazole and hydrocortisone in patients with advanced prostate carcinoma. Cancer, 1997. 80: p. 1755-1759.
575. Hellmann, K., R.H. Phillips and M. Goold, High dose dexamethasone and base of brain irradiation for hormone refractory metastatic carcinoma of the prostate. Clin Exp Metastasis, 1993. 11: p. 227-229.
576. Sinisi, A.A., A. Bellastella and D. Prezioso, Different expression patterns of somatostatin receptor subtypes in cultured epithelial cells from human normal prostate and prostate cancer. J Clin Endocrinol Metab, 1997. 82: p. 2566-2569.
577. Brevini, T.A., R. Bianchi and M. Motta, Direct inhibitory effect of somatostatin on the growth of the human prostatic cancer cell line LNCaP: possible mechanism of action. J Clin Endocrinol Metab, 1993. 77: p. 626-631.
578. Koppan, M., A. Nagy, A.V. Schally, J.M. Arencibia, A. Plonowski and G. Halmos, Targeted cytotoxic analogue of somatostatin AN-238 inhibits growth of androgen-dependent Dunning R-3327-AT-1 prostate cancer in rats at nontoxic doses. Cancer Res, 1998. 58: p. 4132-4137.
579. Nagy, A., A.V. Schally and G. Halmos, Synthesis and biological evaluation of cytotoxic analogs of somatostatin containing doxorubicin or its intensely potent derivative, 2-pyrrolinodoxorubicin. Proc Natl Acad Sci USA, 1998. 95: p. 1794-1799.
580. Figg, W.D., A. Thibault and M.R. Cooper, A phase I study of the somatostatin analogue somatuline in patients with metastatic hormone-refractory prostate cancer. Cancer, 1995. 75: p. 2159-2164.
581. Maulard, C., P. Richaud, J.P. Droz, D. Jessueld, F. Dufour-Esquerre and M. Housset, Phase I-II study of the somatostatin analogue lanreotide in hormone-refractory prostate cancer. Cancer Chemother Pharmacol, 1995. 36: p. 259-262.
582. Vainas, G., V. Pasaitou and G. Galaktidou, The role of somatostatin analogues in complete antiandrogen treatment in patients with prostatic carcinoma. J Exp Clin Cancer Res, 1997. 16: p. 199-126.
583. Caligaris-Cappio, F., L. Bergui and M.G. Gregoretti, Role of bone marrow stromal cells in the growth of human multiple myeloma. Blood, 1991. 77: p. 2688-2693.
584. Treon, S.P. and K.C. Anderson, Interleukin-6 in multiple myeloma and related plasma cell dyscrasias. Curr Opin Hematol, 1998. 5: p. 42-48.
585. Bataille, R., D. Chappard and C. Marcelli, Recruitement of new osteoblasts and osteoclasts is the earliest critical event in the pathogenesis of human multiple myeloma. J Clin Invest, 2992. 88: p. 62-66.
586. Caligaris-Cappio, F., M.G. Gregoretti, P. Ghia and L. Bergui, In vitro growth of human multiple myeloma: implications for biology and therapy. Hematol Oncol Clin North Am, 1992. 6: p. 257-271.
587. Borsellino, N., A. Belldegrun and B. Bonavida, Endogenous interleukin 6 is a resistance factor for cis-diamminedichloroplatinum and etoposide-mediated cytotoxicity of human prostate carcinoma cell lines. Cancer Res, 1995. 55: p. 4633-4639.
588. Drachenberg, D.E., A.A. Elgamal, R. Rowbotham, M. Peterson and G.P. Murphy, Circulating levels of interleukin-6 in patients with hormone refractory prostate cancer. Prostate, 1999. 41: p. 127-133.
589. Manolagas, S.C., The role of IL-6 type cytokines and their receptors in bone. Ann N Y Acad Sci, 1998. 840: p. 194-204.
590. Swolin-Eide, D. and C. Ohlsson, Effects of cortisol on the expression of interleukin-6 and interleukin-1 beta in human osteoblast-like cells. J Endocrinol, 1998. 156: p. 107-114.
591. Hierl, T., I. Borcsok, U. Sommer, R. Ziegler and C. Kasperk, Regulation of interleukin-6 expression in human osteoblastic cells in vitro. Exp Clin Endocrinol Diabetes, 1998. 106: p. 324-333.
592. Song, S., M.G. Wientjes, Y. Gan and J.L. Au, Fibroblast growth factors: an epigenetic mechanism of broad spectrum resistance to anticancer drugs. Proc Natl Acad Sci USA, 2000. 97: p. 8658-8663.
593. Meyer, G.E., E. Yu, J.A. Siegal, J.C. Petteway, B.A. Blumenstein and M.K. Brawer, Serum basic fibroblast growth factor in men with and without prostate carcinoma. Cancer, 1995. 76: p. 2304-2311.
594. Cronauer, M.V., A. Hittmair and I.E. Eder, Basic fibroblast growth factor levels in cancer cells and in sera of patients suffering from proliferative disorders of the prostate. Prostate, 1997. 31: p. 223-233.
595. Di Raimondo, F., M.P. Azzaro and G. Palumbo, Angiogenic factors in multiple myeloma: higher levels in bone marrow than in peripheral blood. Hematologica, 2000. 85: p. 800-805.
596. Cleutjens, C.B., K. Steketee, C.C. van Eekelen, J.A.

vander Korput, A.O. Brinkmann and J. Trapman, Both androgen receptor and glucocorticoid receptor are able to induce prostate-specific antigen expression, but differ in their growth-stimulating properties of LNCaP cells. Endocrinology, 1997. 138: p. 5293-5300.

597. Shan, J.D., K. Porvari and M. Ruokonen, Steroid-involved transcriptional regulation of human genes encoding prostatic acid phosphatase, prostate-specific antigen, and prostate-specific glandular kallikrein. Endocrinology, 1997. 138: p. 3764-3770.

598. Young, C.Y., B.T. Montgomery, P.E. Andrews, S.D. Qiu, D.L. Bilhartz and D.J. Tindall, Hormonal regulation of prostate-specific antigen messenger RNA in human prostatic adenocarcinoma cell line LNCaP. Cancer Res., 1991. 51: p. 3748-3752.

599. Montgomery, B.T., C.Y. Young and D.L. Bilhartz, Hormonal regulation of prostate specific antigen (PSA) glycoprotein in the human prostatic adenocarcinoma cell line, LNCaP. Prostate, 1992. 21: p. 63-73.

600. Revilla, M., I. Arribas, M. Sanchez-Chapado, L.F. Villa, F. Bethencourt and H. Rico, Total and regional bone mass and biochemical markers of bone remodeling in metastatic prostate cancer. Prostate, 1998. 35: p. 243-247.

601. Akimoto, S., Y. Furuya, K. Akakura and H. Ito, Comparison of markers of bone formation and resorption in prostate cancer patients to predict bone metastasis. Endocr J, 1998. 45: p. 97-104.

602. Takeuchi, S., K. Arai, H. Saitoh, K. Yoshida and M. Miura, Urinary pyridinoline and deoxypyridinoline as potential markers of bone metastasis in patients with prostate cancer. J Urol, 1996. 156: p. 1691-1695.

603. Charhon, S.A., M.C. Chapuy, E.E. Delvin, A. Valentin-Opran, C.M. Edouard and P.J. Meunier, Histomorphometric analysis of sclerotic bone metastases from prostatic carcinoma special reference to osteomalacia. Cancer, 1983. 51: p. 918-924.

604. Urwin, G.H., R.C. Percival, S. Harris, M.N. Beneton, J.L. Williams and J.A. Kanis, Generalised increase in bone resorption in carcinoma of the prostate. Br J Urol, 1985. 57: p. 721-723.

605. Clarke, N.W., J. McClure and N.J. George, Disodium pamidronate identifies differential osteoclastic bone resorption in metastatic prostate cancer. Br J Urol, 1992. 69: p. 64-70.

606. Zhang, J., J. Dai and Y. Qi, Osteoprotegerin inhibits prostate cancer-induced osteoclastogenesis and prevents prostate tumor growth in the bone. J Clin Invest, 2001. 107: p. 1235-1244.

607. Berenson, J.R., A. Lichtenstein and L. Porter, Efficacy of pamidronate in reducing skeletal events in patients with advanced multiple myeloma. Myeloma Aredia Study Group, 1996. N Engl J Med(334).

608. Diel, I.J., E.F. Solomayer and S.D. Costa, Reduction in new metastases in breast cancer with adjuvant clodronate treatment. N Engl J Med, 1998. 339: p. 357-363.

609. Liedholm, H. and A.B. Linne, Alendronate in postmenopausal osteoporosis. N Engl J Med, 1996. 334: p. 733-734.

610. McGrath Jr, H., Alendronate in postmenopausal osteoporosis. N Engl J Med, 1996. 334: p. 734-735.

611. Disla, E., B. Tamayo and A. Fahmy, Intermittent etodronate and corticosteroid-induced osteoporosis. N Engl J Med, 1997. 337: p. 1921.

612. Saag, K.G., R. Emkey and T.J. Schnitzer, Alendronate for the prevention and treatment of glucocorticoid-induced osteoporosis. Glucocorticoid - induced osteoporosis intervention study group, 1998. N Engl J Med(339).

613. Smith, M.R., F.J. McGovern and A.L. Zietman, Pamidronate to prevent bone loss during androgen-deprivation therapy for prostate cancer. N Engl J Med, 2001. 345: p. 948-955.

614. Lee, M.V., E.M. Fong, F.R. Singer and R.S. Guenette, Bisophosphonate treatment inhibits the growth of prostate cancer cells. Cancer Res, 2001. 61: p. 2602-2608.

615. Senaratne, S.G., G. Pirianov, J.L. Mansi, T.R. Arnett and K.W. Colston, Bisphosphonates induce apoptosis in human breast cancer cell lines. Br J Cancer, 2000. 82: p. 1459-1468.

616. Aaronson, N., J. Seidenfeld and D.J. Samson, Relative effectiveness and cost-effectiveness of methods of androgen suppression in the treatment of advanced prostatic cancer., in Summary, Evidence-Report/Technology Assessment. 1999, Blue Cross/Blue Shield Association: Rockville, Maryland.

617. Beland, G., M. Elhilali, Y. Fradet, B. Laroche, E.W. Ramsey, J. Trachtenberg, P.M. Venner and H.D. Tewari, A controlled trial of castration with and

REFERENCES

without nilutamide in metastatic prostatic carcinoma. Cancer, 1990. 66(5 Suppl): p. 1074-9.

618. Boccardo, F., M. Pace, A. Rubagotti, D. Guarneri, A. Decensi, F. Oneto, G. Martorana, L. Giuliani, F. Selvaggi, M. Battaglia, and et al., Goserelin acetate with or without flutamide in the treatment of patients with locally advanced or metastatic prostate cancer. The Italian Prostatic Cancer Project (PONCAP) Study Group. Eur J Cancer, 1993. 29A(8): p. 1088-93.

619. Bono, A.V., F. DiSilverio, G. Robustelli della Cuna, C. Benvenuti, M. Brausi, P. Ferrari, A. Gibba and L. Galli, Complete androgen blockade versus chemical castration in advanced prostatic cancer: analysis of an Italian multicentre study. Italian Leuprorelin Group. Urol Int, 1998. 60 Suppl 1: p. 18-24.

620. Brisset, J.M., L. Boccon Gibod, H. Botto, M. Camey, G. Cariou, J.M. Duclos, F. Duval, D. Gonties, R. Jorest, L. Lamy, and et al., Anandron (RU 23908) associated to surgical castration in previously untreated stage D prostate cancer: a multicenter comparative study of two doses of the drug and of a placebo. Prog. Clin. Biol. Res., 1987: p. 411-422.

621. Crawford, E.D., B.S. Kasmis, D. Gandara, J.A. Smith, M.S. Soloway, P.H. Lange, D.F. Lynch, A. Al-Juburi, R.B. Bracken, H.A. Wise, N. Heyden, and C. Bertagna, A randomized, controlled clinical trial of leupoprolide and anandron (LA) versus leuproprolide and placebo (LP) for advanced prostate cancer (D2CaP). Proceedings American Society of Clinical Oncology, 1990. 9(135): p. 523.

622. Denis, L., J. Carnelro de Moura, A. Bono, R. Sylvester, P. Whelan, D. Newling and M. Depauw, Goserelin acetate and flutamide vs bilateral orchiectomy: a phase III EORTC trial (30853). EORTC GU Group and EORTC Data Center. Urology, 1993. 42: p. 119-129.

623. Dijkman, G.A., R.A. Janknegt, T.M. Dereijke and F.M.J. Debruyne, Long-term efficacy and safety of nilutamide plus castration in advanced prostate-cancer, and the significance of early prostate specific antigen normalization. J. Urol., 1997. 158: p. 160-163.

624. Eisenberger, M.A., B.A. Blumenstein, E.D. Crawford, G. Miller, D.G. McLeod, P.J. Loehrer, G. Wilding, K. Sears, D.J. Culkin, I.M. Thompson, A.J. Bueschen, and B.A. Lowe, Bilateral orchiectomy with or without flutamide for metastatic prostate cancer. N. Engl. J. Med., 1998. 339: p. 1036-1042.

625. Ferrari, P., G. Castagnetti, G. Ferrari, B. Baisi and A. Dotti, Combination treatment versus LHRH alone in advanced prostatic cancer. Urol Int, 1996. 56 Suppl 1: p. 13-7.

626. Fourcade, R.O., P. Colombel and M. Mangin. Zoladex plus flutamide versus zoladex plus placebo in advanced prostatic carcinoma: extended follow-up of the French multi-center study. in Third International Symposium on Recent Advances in Urological Cancer: diagnosis and treatment. 1992. Paris, France.

627. Iversen, P., F. Rasmussen, P. Klarskov and I.J. Christensen, Long-term results of Danish Prostatic Cancer Group trial 86. Goserelin acetate plus flutamide versus orchiectomy in advanced prostate cancer. Cancer, 1993. 72(12): p. 3851-3854.

628. Knonagel, H., J.F. Bolle, F. Hering, E. Senn, T. Hodel, H. Neuenschwander and C. Biedermann, [Therapy of metastatic prostatic cancer by orchiectomy plus Anandron versus orchiectomy plus placebo. Initial results of a randomized multicenter study]. Helv Chir Acta, 1989. 56(3): p. 343-5.

629. Namer, M., J. Toubol, A. Caty, J.E. Couette, J. Douchez, P. Kerbrat and J.P. Droz, A randomized double-blind study evaluating Anandron associated with orchiectomy in stage D prostate cancer. J Steroid Biochem Mol Biol, 1990. 37(6): p. 909-15.

630. Navratil, H., Double-blind study of Anandron versus Placebo in stage D2 prostate cancer patients receiving Buserelin. Results on 49 cases from a multicenter study. Prog. Clin. Biol. Res., 1987. 243A: p. 401-410.

631. Periti, P., M. Rizzo, T. Mazzei and M. E., Depot leuprorelin acetate alone or with nilutamide in the treatment of metastatic prostate carcinoma: interim report of a multicenter, double-blind, placebo-controlled study (Meeting abstract). Can J Infect, 1995. 6(Suppl. C): p. 292C.

632. Schulze, H., H. Kaldenhoff and T. Senge, Evaluation of total versus partial androgen blockade in the treatment of advanced prostatic cancer. Urol Int, 1988. 43(4): p. 193-7.

633. Tyrrell, C.J., J.E. Altwein, F. Klippel, E. Varenhorst, G. Lunglmayr, F. Boccardo, I.M.

Holdaway, J.M. Haefliger and J.P. Jordaan, A multicenter randomized trial comparing the luteinizing hormone-releasing hormone analogue goserelin acetate alone and with flutamide in the treatment of advanced prostate cancer. The International Prostate Cancer Study Group. J Urol, 1991. 146(5): p. 1321-1326.

634. Zalcberg, J.R., D. Raghaven, V. Marshall and P.J. Thompson, Bilateral orchidectomy and flutamide versus orchidectomy alone in newly diagnosed patients with metastatic carcinoma of the prostate—an Australian multicentre trial. Br J Urol, 1996. 77(6): p. 865-9.

635. Moinpour, C.M., M.J. Savage, A. Troxel, L.C. Lovato, M. Eisenberger, R.W. Veith, B. Higgins, R. Skeel, M. Yee, B.A. Blumenstein, E.D. Crawford, and F.L. Meyskens, Quality of life in advanced prostate cancer: results of a randomized therapeutic trial. J. Natl. Cancer Inst., 1998. 90(20): p. 1537-1544.

636. Schmitt, B., C. Bennett, J. Seidenfeld, D. Samson and T. Wilt, Maximal androgen blockade for advanced prostate cancer. Cochrane Database Syst Rev, 2000(2): p. CD001526.

637. Prostate Cancer Triallists' Collaborative Group, Maximum androgen blockade in advanced prostate cancer: an overview of 22 randomized trials with 3283 deaths in 5710 patients. Lancet, 1995. 346: p. 265-269.

638. Reese, D.M., Choice of hormonal therapy for prostate cancer [In Process Citation]. Lancet, 2000. 355(9214): p. 1474-1475.

639. Laufer, M., S.R. Denmeade, V.J. Sinibaldi, M.A. Carducci and M.A. Eisenberger, Complete androgen blockade for prostate cancer: what went wrong? J Urol, 2000. 164(1): p. 3-9.

640. Schellhammer, P., R. Sharifi, N. Block, M. Soloway, P. Venner, A.L. Patterson, M. Sarosdy, N. Vogelzang, J. Jones and G. Kolvenbag, A controlled trial of bicalutamide versus flutamide, each in combination with luteinizing hormone-releasing hormone analogue therapy, in patients with advanced prostate cancer. Urology, 1995. 45: p. 745-752.

641. Denis, L., EORTC 30853. Cancer, 1993. 71: p. 1050-1058.

642. McLeod, D.G., Tolerability of Nonsteroidal Antiandrogens in the Treatment of Advanced Prostate Cancer. Oncologist, 1997. 2(1): p. 18-27.

643. Kolvenbag, G.J.C.M. and G.R.P. Blackledge, Worldwide activity and safety of bicalutamide: a summary review. Urology, 1996. 47(Suppl 1A): p. 70-79.

644. Delaere, K.P. and E.L. Van Thillo, Flutamide monotherapy as primary treatment in advanced prostatic carcinoma. Semin Oncol, 1991. 18(5 Suppl 6): p. 13-18.

645. Lundgren, R., Flutamide as primary treatment for metastatic prostatic cancer. Br J Urol, 1987. 59(2): p. 156-8.

646. Chodak, G.W., Bicalutamide-associated fulminant hepatic failure. Urology, 1997. 50(6): p. 1027.

647. FDA, Recent prescription approvals, changes, and safety information. Oncology Spectrums, 2001. 3(7): p. 487.

648. Decensi, A.U., F. Boccardo, D. Guarneri, N. Positano, M.C. Paoletti, M. Costantini, G. Martorana and L. Giuliani, Monotherapy with nilutamide, a pure nonsteroidal antiandrogen, in untreated patients with metastatic carcinoma of the prostate. The Italian Prostatic Cancer Project. J Urol, 1991. 146(2): p. 377-81.

649. Chatelain, C., V. Rousseau and J. Cosaert, French multicentre trial comparing Casodex (ICI 176,334) monotherapy with castration plus nilutamide in metastatic prostate cancer: a preliminary report. Eur Urol, 1994. 26 Suppl 1: p. 10-4.

650. Wong, P.W., N. Macris, L. DiFabrizio and N.S. Seriff, Eosinophilic lung disease induced by bicalutamide: a case report and review of the medical literature. Chest, 1998. 113(2): p. 548-50.

651. Azuma, T., S. Kurimoto, K. Mikami and M. Oshi, Interstitial pneumonitis related to leuprorelin acetate and flutamide. J Urol, 1999. 161(1): p. 221.

652. Kim, S.P., E.M. Moran and E.D. Bowes, The antiandrogen transfer. Prostate, 2000. 2: p. 88-93.

653. Fair, W.R., A. Aprikian and V. Reuter, Neoadjuvant hormonal manipulation. A strategy for chemoprevention trials. J. Cell. Biochem., 1992. 16H(Suppl.): p. 118-121.

654. Scott, W.W., M. Menon and P.L. Walsh, Hormonal therapy of prostatic cancer. Cancer, 1980. 45: p. 1929-1936.

655. Vaillancourt, L., B. Tҳtu, Y. Fradet, A. Dupont, J. Gomez, L. Cusan, E.R. Suburu, P. Diamond, B. Candas and F. Labrie, Effect of neoadjuvant

endocrine therapy (combined androgen blockade) on normal prostate and prostatic carcinoma. Am. J. Surg. Pathol., 1996. 20: p. 86-93.

656. Têtu, B., J.R. Srigley, J.C. Boivin, A. Dupont, G. Monfette, S. Pinault and F. Labrie, Effect of combination endocrine therapy (LHRH agonist and Flutamide) on normal prostate and prostatic adenocarcinoma: A histopathologic and immunohistochemical study. Am. J. Surg. Pathol., 1991. 15: p. 111-120.

657. van der Kwast, T.H., B. Tetu, Y. Fradet, A. Dupont, J. Gomez, L. Cusan, P. Diamond and F. Labrie, Androgen receptor modulation in benign human prostatic tissue and prostatic adenocarcinoma during neoadjuvant endocrine combination therapy. Prostate, 1996. 28: p. 227-231.

658. van der Kwast, T.H., B. Txtu, E.R. Suburu, J. Gomez, M. Lemay and F. Labrie, Cycling activity of benign prostatic epithelial cells during long-term androgen blockade: evidence for self-renewal of luminal cells. J Pathol, 1998. 186: p. 406-409.

659. van der Kwast, T.H., B. Txtu, B. Candas, J.L. Gomez, L. Cusan and F. Labrie, Prolongued neoadjuvant combined androgen blockade leads to a further reduction of prostatic tumor volume: three versus six months of endocrine therapy. Urology, 1999. 53: p. 523-529.

660. Civantos, F., M.A. Marcial, E.R. Banks, C.K. Ho, V.O. Speights, P.A. Drew, W.M. Murphy and M.S. Soloway, Pathology of androgen deprivation therapy in prostate carcinoma. A comparative study of 173 patients. Cancer, 1995. 75(7): p. 1634-1641.

661. Murphy, W.M., M.S. Soloway and G.H. Barrows, Pathologic changes associated with androgen deprivation therapy for prostate cancer. Cancer, 1991. 68: p. 821-828.

662. Hellstrom, M., P. Ranepall, K. Wester, S. Brandsted and C. Busch, Effects of androgen deprivation on epithelial and mesenchymal tissue components in localized prostate cancer. Br. J. Urol., 1997. 79: p. 421-426.

663. Witjes, W.P., C.C. Schulman, F.M.J. Debruyne and members of the EORTC Study Group on Neoadjuvant Treatment of Prostate Cancer, Preliminary results of a prospective randomized study comparing radical prostatectomy versus radical prostatectomy versus radical prostatectomy associated with neoadjuvant hormonal combination therapy in T2-3 N0 M0 prostatic carcinoma. Urology, 1997. 49: p. 65-69.

664. Bono, A.V., F. Pagano, R. Montironi, F. Zattoni, A. Manganelli, F.P. Selvaggi, G. Comeri, G. Fiiaccavento, S. Guazzieri, C. Selli, A. Lembo, S. Cosciani-Cunico, D. Potenzoni, G. Muto, L. Diamanti, A. Santinelli, R. Mazzucchelli, and T. Prayer-Galletti, Effect of complete androgen blockade on pathologic stage and resection margin status of prostate cancer: progress pathology report of the Italian PROSIT study. Urology, 2001. 57: p. 117-121.

665. Labrie, F., L. Cusan, J. Gomez, P. Diamond, E.R. Suburu, M. Lemay, B. Txtu, Y. Fradet, A. Bulanger and B. Candas, Neoadjuvant hormonal therapy: the Canadian Experience. Urology, 1997(56-64).

666. Fair, W.R., M.S. Cookson, N. Stroumbakis, D. Cohen, A.G. Aprikian, Y. Wang, P. Russo, S.M. Soloway, P. Sogani, J. Sheinfeld, H. Herr, G. Dalgabni, C.B. Begg, W.D. Heston, and V.E. Reuter, The indications, rationale, and results of neoadjuvant androgen deprivation in the treatment of prostate cancer: memorial sloan-kettering cancer center results. Urology, 1997. 49: p. 46-55.

667. Amling, C.L., M.L. Blute, E.J. Bergstralh, J.M. Slezak, S.K. Martin and H. Zincke, Preoperative androgen-deprivation therapy for clinical sage T3 prostate cancer. Semin Urol Oncol, 1997. 15: p. 222-229.

668. Gleave, M.E., S.L. Goldenberg, E.C. Jones, N. Bruchovsky and L.D. Sullivan, Biochemical and pathological effects of 8 months of neoadjuvant androgen withdrawal therapy before radical prostatectomy in patients with clinically confined prostate cancer. J. Urol., 1996. 155: p. 213-219.

669. Soloway, M.S., R. Sharifi, Z. Wajsman, D. McLeod, D.P. Wood Jr and A. Puras-Baez, Randomized prospective study comparing radical prostatectomy alone versus radical prostatectomy preceded by androgen blockade in clinical stage B2 (T2bNxM0) prostate cancer. J. Urol., 1995. 154: p. 424-428.

670. Zheng, W., M. Bazinet, L.R. Bigin, A. Aprikian, P.I. Karakiewicz and M.M. Elhilali, Histological changes induced by neoadjuvant androgen ablation may result in the underdetection of positive surgical margins and capsular involvement by prostate cancer. J Urol, 1996. 155(Suppl): p. 554A.

671. Gleave, M.E., S.L. Goldenberg, J. Warner, J. Chin,

L. Klotz, M. Jewett, M. Chetner, V. Kassabian, J. Zadra and C.U.-O. Group, Randomized comparative study of 3 vs 8 months of neoadjuvant hormonal therapy prior to radical prostatetomy: biochemical & pathological effects. J Urol, 1999. 161: p. 154.

672. Armas, O.A., A.G. Aprikian, J. Melamed, C. Cordon Cardo, D.W. Cohen, R. Erlandson, W.R. Fair and V.E. Reuter, Clinical and pathobiological effects of neoadjuvant total androgen ablation therapy on clinically localized prostatic adenocarcinoma. Am. J. Surg. Pathol., 1994. 18: p. 971-991.

673. Têtu, B., Morphologic changes induced by neoadjuvant combination hormone therapy on prostatic tissue and prostate cancer. Endocrine Related Cancer, 1996. 3: p. 165-170.

674. Ohori, M., T.M. Wheeler, M.W. Kattan, Y. Goto and P.T. Scardino, Prognostic significance of positive surgical margins in radical prostatectomy specimens. J. Urol., 1995. 154(5): p. 1818-1824.

675. Epstein, J.I., G. Pizov and K. Webster, Correlation of pathologic findings with progression after radical retropubic prostatectomy. Cancer, 1993. 71: p. 3582-3593.

676. Catalona, W.J. and L.V. Avioli, Diagnosis, staging, and surgical treatment of prostatic carcinoma. Arch. Intern. Med., 1987. 147: p. 361-363.

677. Meyer, F., I. Bairati, C. Bedard, L. Lacombe, B. Tetu and Y. Fradet, Duration of neoadjuvant androgen deprivation therapy before radical prostatectomy and disease-free survival in men with prostate cancer. Urology, 2001. 58(2 Suppl 1): p. 71-7.

678. Sarosdy, M.F., P.F. Schellhammer, R. Johnson, K. Carroll and G.J. Kolvenbag, Does prolonged combined androgen blockade have survival benefits over short-term combined androgen blockade therapy? Urology, 2000. 55: p. 391-395.

679. Tran, T.A., T.A. Jennings, J.S. Ross and T. Nazeer, Pseudomyxoma ovariilike posttherapeutic alteration in prostatic adenocarcinoma: a distinctive pattern in patients receiving neoadjuvant androgen ablation therapy. Am J Surg Pathol, 1998. 22: p. 347-354.

680. Smith, D.M. and W.M. Murphy, Histologic changes in prostatic carcinomas treated with leuprolide (luteinizing hormone-releasing hormone effect): Distinction from poor tumor differentiation. Cancer, 1994. 73: p. 1472-1477.

681. Hellstrom, M., M. Haggman, S. Brandstedt, M. de la Torre, K. Pedersen, I. Jarlsfeldt, H. Wijkstrom and C. Busch, Histopathological changes in androgen-deprived localized prostatic cancer - a study in total prostatectomy specimens. Eur. Urol., 1993. 24: p. 461-465.

682. Kaltz-Wittmer, C., U. Klenk, A. Glaessgen, D.E. Aust, J. Diebold, U. Lohrs and G.B. Baretton, FISH analysis of gene aberrations (MYC, CCND1, ERBB2, RB and AR) in advanced prostatic carcinomas before and after androgen deprivation therapy. Lab Invest, 2000. 80: p. 1455-1464.

683. Osman, I., H.I. Scher, M. Drobnjak, D. Verbel, M. Morris, D. Agus, J.S. Ross and C. Cordon-Cardo, HER02/neu (p185neu) protein expression in the natural or treated history of prostate cancer. Clin Cancer Res, 2001. 7: p. 2643-2647.

684. Shi, Y., F.H. Brands, S. Chatterjee, A.C. Feng, S. Groshen, J. Schewe, G. Lieskovsky and R.J. Cote, Her-2/neu expression in prostate cancer: high level of expression associated with exposure to hormone therapy and androgen independent disease. J Urol, 2001. 166: p. 1514-1519.

685. Signoretti, S., R. Montironi, J. Manola, A. Altimari, C. Tam, G. Bubley, S. Balk, G. Thomas, I. Kaplan, L. Hlatky, P. Hahnfeldt, P. Kantoff, and M. Loda, Her-2-neu expression and progression toward androgen independence in human prostate cancer. J Natl Cancer Inst, 2000. 92: p. 1918-1925.

686. Kubota, Y., K. Fujinami, H. Uemura, Y. Dobashi, H. Miyamoto, Y. Iwasaki, H. Kitamura and T. Shuin, Retinoblastoma gene mutations in primary human prostate cancer. Prostate, 1995. 27: p. 314-320.

687. Montironi, R., C. Magi-Galluzzi, G. Muzzonigro, E. Prete, M. Polito and F. Fabris, Effects of combination endocrine treatment on normal prostate, prostatic intraepithelial neoplasia, and prostatic adenocarcinoma. J Clin Pathol, 1994. 47: p. 906-913.

688. Montironi, R., C. Magi-Galluzzi and G. Fabris, Apoptotic bodies in prostatic intraepithelial neoplasia and prostatic adenocarcinoma following total androgen ablation. Pathol Res Pract, 1995. 191: p. 873-880.

689. Van de Voorde, W.M., A.A. Elgamal, H. van Poppel, E.K. Verbeken, L.V. Baert and J.M. Lauweryns, Morphologic and immunohistochemi-

REFERENCES

cal changes in prostate cancer after preoperative hormonal therapy. Cancer, 1994. 74: p. 3164-3175.

690. Kruithof-Dekker, I.G., B. Tӿtu, P. Janssen and T.H. van der Kwast, Elevated estrogen receptor expression in human prostatic stromal cells by androgen ablation therapy. J Urol, 1996. 156: p. 1194-1197.

691. Ferguson, F., H. Zincke, E. Ellison, E. Bergstrahl and D.G. Bostwick, Decrease of prostatic intraepithelial neoplasia following androgen deprivation therapy in patients with stage T3 carcinoma treated by radical prostatectomy. Urology, 1994. 44: p. 91-95.

692. Montie, J.E., Follow-up after radical prostatectomy or radiation therapy for prostate cancer. Urol. Clin. North Am., 1994. 21: p. 673-676.

693. van der Kwast, T.H., F. Labrie and B. Tӿtu, Persistence of high-grade prostatic intra-epithelial neplasia under combined androgen blockade therapy. Hum Pathol, 1999. 30: p. 1503-1507.

694. Grignon, D. and M. Troster, Changes in immunohistochemical staining in prostatic adenocarcinoma following diethylstillbestrol therapy. Prostate, 1985. 7: p. 195-202.

695. Helpap, B., Treated prostatic carcinoma. Histological, immunohistochemical and cell kinetic studies. Appl Pathol, 1985. 3: p. 230-241.

696. van Poppel, H., D. De Ridder, A.A. Elgamal, W. van de Voorde, P. Werbrouck, K. Ackaert, R. Oyen, G. Pittomvils, L. Baert and M.o.t.B.u.-o.s. group, Neoadjuvant hormonal therapy before radical prostatectomy decreases the number of positive surgical margins in stage T2 prostate cancer: interim results of a prospective randomized trial. J Urol, 1995. 154: p. 429-434.

697. Dhom, G. and S. Degro, Therapy of prostatic cancer and histophathologic follow-up. Prostate, 1982. 3: p. 531-542.

698. Dalkin, B.L., F.R. Ahmann, R. Nagle and C.S. Johnson, Randomized study of neoadjuvant testicular androgen ablation therapy before radical prostatectomy in men with clinically localized prostate cancer. J Urol, 1996. 155: p. 1357-1360.

699. Goldenberg, S.L., L.H. Klotz, J.R. Srigley, M.A.S. Jewett, D. Mador, Y. Fradet, J. Barkin, J. Chin, J.M. Paquin, M.J. Bullock, S. Laplante, and C.U.O. Group, Controlled Study Comparing Radical Prostatectomy Alone and Neoadjuvant Androgen Withdrawal in the Treatment of Localized Prostate Cancer. J Urol, 1996. 156: p. 873-877.

700. Yang, X.J., K. Lecksell, K. Short, J. Gottesman, L. Peterson, J. Bannow, P.F. Schellhammer, W.P. Fitch, G.B. Hodge, R. Parra, S. Rouse, J. Waldstreicher, and J.I. Epstein, Does long-term finasteride therapy effect the histologic features of benign prostatic tissue and prostate cancer on needle biopsy? Urology, 1999. 53: p. 696-700.

701. Kolata, G., Prostate cancer consensus hampered by lack of data. Science, 1987. 236: p. 1626-1627.

702. Middleton, R.G., I.M. Thompson, M.S. Austenfeld, W.H. Cooner, R.J. Correa, R.P. Gibbons, H.C. Miller, J.E. Oesterling, M.I. Resnick, S.R. Smalley, and et al., Prostate Cancer Clinical Guidelines Panel Summary report on the management of clinically localized prostate cancer. The American Urological Association. J. Urol., 1995. 154: p. 2144-2148.

703. Labrie, F. and B. Candas, The Quebec study shows a 69% decrease in prostate cancer death [Letter to the Editor: Reply by the authors]. Prostate, 1999. 40: p. 137.

704. Shröder, F.H., P.V.D. Maas, P. Beemsterboer, A.B. Kruger, R. Hoedemaeker and J. Rietbergen, Evaluation of the digital rectal examination as a screening test for prostate cancer. J Natl Cancer Inst, 1998: p. 1817-1823.

705. Shröder, F.H., M. Roobol-Bouts, A.N. Vis, T.V.D. Kwast and R. Kranse, Prostate-specific antigen-based early detection of prostate cancer-validation of screening without rectal examination. Urology, 2001. 57(1): p. 83-90.

706. Labrie F., Candas B., Cusan L., Gomez J.L., Lévesque J., Chevrette E., and Brousseau G., Chapter 4, in Prostate cancer: understanding the pathophysiology and re-designing a therapeutic approach, F. Labrie and M. Koutsilieris, Editors. 2002, Paschalidis Medical Publications: Athens, Greece. p. 67-78.

707. Labrie, F., A. Bélanger, L. Cusan, C. Sıguin, G. Pelletier, P.A. Kelly, J.J. Reeves, F.A. Lefebvre, A. Lemay and J.P. Raynaud, Antifertility effects of LHRH agonists in the male. J. Androl., 1980. 1: p. 209-228.

708. Faure, N., F. Labrie, A. Lemay, A. Bélanger, Y. Gourdeau, B. Laroche and G. Robert, Inhibition of serum androgen levels by chronic intranasal and subcutaneous administration of a potent luteinizing hormone-releasing hormone (GNRH) agonist in adult men. Fertil. Steril., 1982. 37: p. 416-424.

709. Labrie, F., A. Dupont, A. Bélanger, L. Cusan, Y. Lacourcière, G. Monfette, J.G. Laberge, J. Emond, A.T. Fazekas, J.P. Raynaud, and J.M. Husson, New hormonal therapy in prostatic carcinoma: combined treatment with an LHRH agonist and an antiandrogen. Clin. Invest. Med., 1982. 5: p. 267-275.

710. Tolis, G., D. Ackman, A. Stellos, A. Mehta, F. Labrie, A.T.A. Fazekas, A.M. Comaru-Schally and A.V. Schally, Tumor growth inhibition in patients with prostatic carcinoma treated with LHRH agonists. Proc. Natl. Acad. Sci., 1982. 79: p. 1658-1662.

711. VACURG, Treatment and survival of patients with cancer of the prostate. Surg. Gynecol. Obstet., 1967. 124: p. 1011-1017.

712. Robinson, M.R. and B.S. Thomas, Effect of hormone therapy on plasma testosterone levels in prostatic cancer. Br. Med. J., 1971. 4: p. 391-394.

713. Peeling, W.B., Phase III studies to compare goserelin (Zoladex) with orchiectomy and with diethylstilbestrol in treatment of prostatic carcinoma. Urology, 1989. 33: p. 45-52.

714. Labrie, C., A. Bélanger and F. Labrie, Androgenic activity of dehydroepiandrosterone and androstenedione in the rat ventral prostate. Endocrinology, 1988. 123: p. 1412-1417.

715. Bennett, C.L., T.D. Tosteson, B. Schmitt, P.D. Weinberg, M.S. Ernstoff and S.D. Ross, Maximum androgen-blockade with medical or surgical castration in advanced prostate cancer: a meta-analysis of nine published randomized controlled trials and 4128 patients using Flutamide. Prostate Cancer and Prostatic Diseases, 1999. 2: p. 4-8.

716. Janknegt, R.A., C.C. Abbou, R. Bartoletti, L. Bernstein-Hahn, B. Bracken, J.M. Brisset, F.C. Da Silva, G. Chisholm, E.D. Crawford, F.M.J. Debruyne, G.D. Dijkman, J. Frick, L. Goedhals, H. Knφnagel, and P.M. Venner, Orchiectomy and Nilutamide or placebo as treatment of metastatic prostatic cancer in a multinational double-blind randomized trial. J. Urol., 1993. 149: p. 77-83.

717. Caubet, J.F., T.D. Tosteson, E.W. Dong, E.M. Naylon, G.W. Whiting, M.S. Ernstoff and S.D. Ross, Maximum androgen blockade in advanced prostate cancer: a meta-analysis of published randomized controlled trials using nonsteroidal antiandrogens. Urology, 1997. 49: p. 71-78.

718. Denis, L.J., F. Keuppens, P.H. Smith, P. Whelan, J.L. Carneiro de Moura, D. Newling, A. Bono and R. Sylvester, Maximal androgen blockade: final analysis of EORTC Phase III trial 30853. Eur. Urol., 1998. 33: p. 144-151.

719. Brawer, M.K., E.D. Crawford, F. Labrie, A. Mendoza-Valdez, P.D. Miller and D.P. Petrylak, Advanced disease. Reviews in Urology, 2001: p. in press.

720. Labrie, F., B. Candas, J.L. Gomez and L. Cusan, Can combined androgen blockade provide long-term control or possible cure of localized prostate cancer? Urology, 2002. 60(1): p. 115-9.

721. Wirth, M., C. Tyrrell, M. Wallace, K.P. Delaere, M. Sanchez-Chapado, J. Ramon, J. Hetherington, F. Pina, C.F. Heynes, T.M. Borchers, T. Morris, and A. Stone, Bicalutamide (Casodex) 150 mg as immediate therapy in patients with localized or locally advanced prostate cancer significantly reduces the risk of disease progression. Urology, 2001. 58(2): p. 146-51.

722. Brawer, M.K., T.A. Stamey, J. Fowler, M. Droller, E. Messing and W.R. Fair, Perspectives on prostate cancer diagnosis and treatment: a roundtable. Urology, 2001. 58(2): p. 135-40.

723. Kelloff, G.J., R. Lieberman, V.E. Steele, C.W. Boone, R.A. Lubet, L. Kopelovich, W.A. Malone, J.A. Crowell, H.R. Higley and C.C. Sigman, Agents, biomarkers, and cohorts for chemopreventive agent development in prostate cancer. Urology, 2001. 57(4 Suppl 1): p. 46-51.

724. Kelloff, G.J., R. Lieberman, V.E. Steele, C.W. Boone, R.A. Lubet, L. Kopelovitch, W.A. Malone, J.A. Crowell and C.C. Sigman, Chemoprevention of prostate cancer: concepts and strategies. Eur Urol, 1999. 35(5-6): p. 342-50.

725. Kelloff, G.J., R. Lieberman, M.K. Brawer, E.D. Crawford, F. Labrie and G.J. Miller, Strategies for chemoprevention of prostate cancer. Prostate Cancer and Prostatic Diseases, 1999. 2: p. 27-33.

726. Kelloff, G.J., J.A. Crowell, V.E. Steele, R.A. Lubet, C.W. Boone, W.A. Malone, E.T. Hawk, R. Lieberman, J.A. Lawrence, L. Kopelovich, I. Ali, J.L. Viner, and C.C. Sigman, Progress in cancer chemoprevention. Ann N Y Acad Sci, 1999. 889: p. 1-13.

727. Lieberman, R., Androgen deprivation therapy for prostate cancer chemoprevention: current status and future directions for agent development. Urology, 2001. 58(2 Suppl 1): p. 83-90.

REFERENCES

728. Messina, M. and S. Barnes, The role of soy products in reducing risk of cancer. J Natl Cancer Inst, 1991. 83(8): p. 541-6.

729. Keloff, G.J., J.A. Crowell, E.T. Hawk, V.E. Steele, R.A. Lubet, C.W. Boone, J.M. Covey, L.A. Doody, G.S. Omenn, P. Greenwald, W.K. Hong, D.R. Parkinson, D. Bagheri, G.T. Baxter, M. Blunden, M.K. Doeltz, K.M. Eisenhauer, K. Johnson, K. Longfellow, D.G. Longfellow, G.G. Knapp, W.F. Malone, S.G. Nayfeild, H.E. Seifried, L.M. Swall, and C.C. Sigman, Clinical development plan: genistein. J Cell Biochem Supp, 1996. 26: p. 114-126.

730. Tabary, O., S. Escotte, J.P. Couetil, D. Hubert, D. Dusser, E. Puchelle and J. Jacquot, Genistein inhibits constitutive and inducible NFkappaB activation and decreases IL-8 production by human cystic fibrosis bronchial gland cells. Am J Pathol, 1999. 155(2): p. 473-81.

731. Adlercreutz, H., K. Hockerstedt, C. Bannwart, S. Bloigu, E. Hamalainen, T. Fotsis and A. Ollus, Effect of dietary components, including lignans and phytoestrogens, on enterohepatic circulation and liver metabolism of estrogens and on sex hormone binding globulin (SHBG). J Steroid Biochem, 1987. 27(4-6): p. 1135-44.

732. Adlercreutz, H., T. Fotsist, L. Schweigerert, M. Pepper, H. Attalla, Y. Zhang, K. Wahala, R. Montesano, P.P. Nawroth and T. Hase, Isoflavonoids and 2-methoxyestradiol: inhibitors of tumor cell growth and angiogenesis. Proc Ann Meeting Am Assoc Cancer Res, 1994. 35: p. 693-694.

733. Giovannucci, E., A. Ascherio, E.B. Rimm, M.J. Stampfer, G.A. Colditz and W.C. Willett, Intake of carotenoids and retinol in relation to risk of prostate cancer. J Natl Cancer Inst, 1995. 87(23): p. 1767-76.

734. Gann, P.H., J. Ma, E. Giovannucci, W. Willett, F.M. Sacks, C.H. Hennekens and M.J. Stampfer, Lower prostate cancer risk in men with elevated plasma lycopene levels: results of a prospective analysis. Cancer Res, 1999. 59(6): p. 1225-30.

735. Di Mascio, P., S. Kaiser and H. Sies, Lycopene as the most efficient biological carotenoid singlet oxygen quencher. Arch Biochem Biophys, 1989. 274: p. 532-538.

736. Sharoni, Y., E. Giron, M. Rise and J. Levy, Effects of lycopene-enriched tomato oleoresin on 7,12-dimethylbenz(a)anthracene-induced rat mammary tumors. Cancer Detect Prev, 1997. 21: p. 118-123.

737. Narisawa, T., Y. Fukaura, M. Hasebe, S. Nomura, S. Oshima, H. Sakamoto, T. Inakuma, Y. Ishiguro, J. Takayasu and H. Nishino, Prevention of N-methylnitrosourea-induced colon carcinogenesis in F344 rats by lycopene and tomato juice rich in lycopene. Jpn J Cancer Res, 1998. 89: p. 1003-1008.

738. Okajima, E., M. Tsutsumi, S. Ozono, H. Akai, A. Denda, H. Nishino, S. Oshima, H. Sakamoto and Y. Konishi, Inhibitory effect of tomato juice on rat urinary bladder carcinogenesis after N-butyl-N-(4-hydroxybutyl)nitrosamine initiation. Jpn J Cancer Res, 1998. 89: p. 22-26.

739. Ross, R.K., M.C. Pike, G.A. Coetzee, J.K.V. Reichardt, M.C. Yu, H. Feigelson, F.Z. Stanczyk, L.N. Kolonel and B.E. Henderson, Androgen metabolism and prostate cancer: Establishing a model of genetic susceptibility. Cancer Res, 1998. 58: p. 4497-4504.

740. Lieberman, R., W.G. Nelson, W.A. Sakr, F.L. Meyskens, E.A. Klein, G. Wilding, A.W. Partin, J.J. Lee and S.M. Lippman, Executive summary of the National Cancer Institute workshop (on prostate cancer prevention). Urology, 2001. 57(Suppl 4A): p. 4-27.

741. van der Kwast, T.H., F. Labrie and B. Tetu, Prostatic intrepithelial neoplasia and endocrine manipulation. Eur Urol, 1999. 35: p. 508-510.

742. Nevalainen, M.T., P.L. Harkonen, E.M. Valve, W. Ping, M. Nurmi and P.M. Martikainen, Hormone regulation of human prostate in organ culture. Cancer Res, 1993. 53: p. 5199-5207.

743. Lucia, M.S., M.A. Anzano, M.V. Slayter, M.R. Anver, D.M. Green, M.W. Shrader, D.L. Logsdon, C.L. Driver, C.C. Brown, C.W. Peer, A.B. Roberts, and M.B. Sporn, Chemopreventive activity of tamoxifen, N-(4-hydroxyphenyl)retinamide, and the vitamin D analogue Ro24-5531 for androgen-promoted carcinomas of the rat seminal vesicle and prostate. Cancer Res, 1995. 55: p. 5621-5627.

744. Sato, M., C.H. Turner, T. Wang, M.D. Adrian, E. Rowley and H.U. Bryant, LY353381.HCl: a novel raloxifene analog with improved SERM potency and efficacy in vivo. J Pharmacol Exp Ther, 1998. 287: p. 1-7.

745. Hoque, A., D. Albanes, S.M. Lippman, M.R. Spitz, P.R. Taylor, E.A. Klein, I.M. Thompson, P.

Goodman, J.L. Stanford, J.J. Crowley, C.A. Coltman, and R.M. Santella, Cancer Causes. Control, 2000. 12: p. 627-633.

746. Bosland, M.C., Use of animal models in defining efficacy of chemopreventive agents against prostate cancer. Eur Urol, 1999. 35: p. 459-463.

747. Maroukalou, I.G., M. Anver, L. Garret and J.E. Green, Prostate and mammary adenocarcinoma in transgenic mice carrying a rat C3(1) simian virus 40 large tumor antigen fusion gene. Proc Natl Acad Sci USA, 1994. 91: p. 11236-11240.

748. Foster, B.A., J.R. Gingrich, E.D. Kwon, C. Madias and N.M. Greenberg, Characterization of prostatic epithelial lines derived from transgenic adenocarcinoma of the mouse prostate (TRAMP) model. Cancer Res, 1997. 57: p. 3325-3330.

749. Kadmon, D., Chemoprevention in prostate cancer: The role of difluoromethylornithine (DFMO). J Cell Biochem, 1992. 16H: p. 122-127.

750. Gupta, S., N. Ahmad, S.R. Marengo, G.T. MacLenna, N.M. Greenberg and H. Mukhtar, Chemoprevention of prostate carcinogenesis by alpha-difluoromethylornithine in TRAMP mice. Cancer Res, 2000. 60: p. 5125-5133.

751. McCormick, D.L., K.V.N. Rao, V.E. Steele, R.A. Lubet, G.J. Kelloff and M.C. Bosland, Chemoprevention of rat prostate carcinogenesis by 9-cis-retinoic acid. Cancer Res, 1999. 59: p. 521-524.

752. Schwartz, G.G., T.A. Oeler, M.R. Uskokovic and R.R. Bahnson, Human prostate cancer cells: Inhibition of proliferation by vitamin D analogues. Anticancer Res, 1994. 14: p. 1077-1081.

753. Getzenberg, R.H., B.W. Light, P.E. Lapco, B.R. Konety, A.K. Nangia, J.S. Ancierno, R. Dhir, Z. Shurin, R.S. Day, D.L. Trump, and C.S. Johnson, Vitamin D inhibition of prostate adenocarcinoma growth and metastasis in the Dunning rat prostate model system. Urology, 1997. 50: p. 999-1006.

754. Gupta, S., N. Ahmad and H. Mukhtar, Prostate cancer chemoprevention by green tea. Semin Urol Oncol, 1999. 17: p. 70-76.

755. Gupta, S., N. Ahmad, R.R. Mohan, M.M. Husain and H. Mukhtar, Prostate cancer chemoprevention by green tea: in vitro and in vivo inhibition of testosterone-mediated induction of ornithine decarboxylase. Cancer Res, 1999. 59: p. 2115-2120.

756. Paganini-Hill, A., A. Chao, R.K. Ross and B.E. Henderson, Aspirin use and chronic diseases: a cohort study of the elderly. Br Med J, 1989. 299: p. 1247-1250.

757. Thun, M.J., M.M. Namboodiri, E.E. Calle, W.D. Flanders and C.W. Heath Jr, Aspirin use and risk of fatal cancer. Cancer Res, 1993. 53: p. 1322-1327.

758. Schreinemachers, D.M. and R.B. Everson, Aspirin use and lung, colon and breast cancer incidence in a prospective study. Epidemiology, 1994. 5: p. 138-146.

759. Norrish, A.E., R.T. Jackson and C.U. McRae, Non-steroidal anti-inflammatory drugs and prostate cancer progression. Int J Cancer, 1998. 77: p. 511-515.

760. Rose, P. and J.M. Connolly, Effects of fatty acids and eisocsanoid synthesis inhibitors on the growth of two human prostate cancer cell lines. Prostate, 1991. 18: p. 243-254.

761. Chaudry, A.A., K.W.J. Wahle, S. McClinton and L.E.F. Moffat, Arachidonic acid metatolism in benign and malignant prostatic tissue in vitro: effects of fatty acids and cyclooxygenase inhibitors. Int J Cancer, 1994. 57: p. 176-180.

762. Viljoen, T.C., C.H. van Aswegen and D.J. du Plessis, Influence of acetylsalicylic acid and metabolites on DU-145 prostatic cancer cell proliferation. Oncology, 1995. 52: p. 465-469.

763. Tjandrawinata, R.R., R. Dahiya and M. Hughes-Fulford, Induction of cyclo-oxygenase-2 mRNA by prostaglandin E2 in human prostatic carcinoma cells. Br J Cancer, 1997. 75: p. 1111-1118.

764. Liu, X.H., S. Yao, A. Kirschenbaum and A.C. Levine, NS398, a selective cyclooxygenase-2 inhibitor, induces apoptosis and down-regulates bcl-2 expression in LNCaP cells. Cancer Res, 1998. 58: p. 245-249.

765. Hsu, A.L., T.T. Ching, D.S. Wang, X. Song, V.M. Rangnekar and C.S. Chen, The cyclooxygenase-2 inhibitor celecoxib induces apoptosis by blocking Akt activation in human prostate cancer cells independently of bcl-2. J Biol Chem, 2000. 275: p. 11397-11403.

766. Goluboff, E.T., D. Prager, D. Rukstalis, B. Giantonio, M. Madorsky, I. Barken, I.B. Weinstein, A.W. Partin and C.A. Olsson, Safety and efficacy of exisulind for treatment of recurrent prostate cancer after radical prostatectomy. J Urol, 2001. 166: p. 882-886.

767. Wechter, W.J., D.D. Leipold, E.D. Murray Jr, D. Quiggle, J.D. McCracken, R.S. Barrios and N.M.

Greenberg, E-7869 (R-flubiprofen) inhibits progression of prostate cancer in the TRAMP mouse. Cancer Res, 2000. 60: p. 2203-2208.
768. Bostwick, D.G. and J. Qian, Effect of androgen deprivation therapy on prostatic intraepithelial neoplasia. Urology, 2001. 58(Suppl 2A): p. 91-93.
769. Kelloff, G.J., C.W. Boone, W.F. Malone, V.E. Steele and L.A. Doody, Introductory remarks: development of chemopreventive agents for prostate cancer. J Cell Biochem, 1992. 16H: p. 1-8.
770. Landis, S.H., T. Murray, S. Bolden and P.A. Wingo, Cancer Statistics, 1999. CA Cancer J. Clin., 1999. 49: p. 8-31.
771. Cookson, M.S., V.E. Reuter, I. Linkov and W.R. Fair, Glutathione S-transferase PI (GST-pi) class expression by immunohistochemistry in benign and malignant prostate tissue. J Urol, 1997. 157: p. 673-676.
772. Xie, W., Y.C. Wong and S.W. Tsao, Correlation of increased apoptosis and proliferation with development of prostatic intraepithelial neoplasia (PIN) in ventral prostate of the Noble rat. Prostate, 2000. 44: p. 31-39.
773. Sakr, W.A. and A.W. Partin, Histologic markers of risk and role of high-grade prostatic intraepithelial neoplasia. Urology, 2001. 57(Suppl 4): p. 115-120.
774. Bostwick, D.G., R. Montironi and I.A. Sesterhenn, Diagnosis of prostatic intraepithelial neoplasia: Prostate Working Group/consensus report. Scand J Urol Nephrol Suppl, 2000. 205: p. 3-10.
775. Bull, J.H., G. Ellison, A. Patel, M. Walker, M. Underwood, F. Khan and L. Paskins, Identification of potential diagnostic markers of prostate cancer and prostatic intraepithelial neoplasia using cDNA microarray. Br J Cancer, 2001. 84: p. 1512-1519.
776. D'Amico, A.V., M. Schnall, R. Whittington, S.B. Malkowicz, D. Schultz, J.E. Tomaszewski and A. Wein, Endorectal coil magnetic resonance imaging identifies locally advanced prostate cancer in select patients with clinically localized disease. Urology, 1998. 51: p. 449-454.
777. Barentsz, J.O., M. Engelbrecht, G.J. Jager, J.A. Witjes, J. de LaRosette, B.P. van der Sanden, H.J. Huisman and A. Heerschap, Fast dynamic gadolinium-enhanced MR imaging of urinary bladder and prostate cancer. J Magn Reson Imaging, 1999. 10: p. 295-304.
778. Cote, R.J., E.C. Skinner, C.E. Salem, S.J. Mertes, F.Z. Stanczyk, B.E. Henderson, M.C. Pike and R.K. Ross, The effect of finasteride on the prostate gland in men with elevated serum prostate-specific antigen levels. Br J Cancer, 1998. 78: p. 413-418.
779. Bostwick, D.G., R.J. Neumann, J. Qian and L. Cheng, Reversibility of prostatic intraepithelial neoplasia: implications for chemoprevention. Eur Urol, 1999. 35: p. 492-495.
780. Feigelson, H.S., R.K. Ross, M.C. Yu, G.A. Coetzee, J.K.V. Reichardt and B.E. Henderson, Genetic susceptibility to cancer from exogenous and endogenous exposures. J Cell Biochem, 1996. 25: p. 15-22.
781. Powell, I.J. and F.L. Meyskens, African American men and hereditary/familial prostate cancer: Intermediate-risk populations for chemoprevention trials. Urology, 2001. 57(Suppl 4): p. 178-181.
782. Tindall, D.J. and P.T. Scardino, Defeating prostate cancer: crucial directions for research - Excerpt from the report of the Prostate Cancer Progress Review Group. Prostate, 1999. 38: p. 166-171.
783. Irvine, R.A., M.C. Yu, R.K. Ross and G.A. Coetzee, The CAG and GGC microsatellites of the androgen receptor gene are in linkage disequilibrium in men with prostate cancer. Cancer Res, 1995. 55(9): p. 1937-40.
784. Giovannucci, E., M.J. Stampfer, K. Krithivas, M. Brown, D. Dahl, A. Brufsky, J. Talcott, C.H. Hennekens and P.W. Kantoff, The CAG repeat within the androgen receptor gene and its relationship to prostate cancer. Proc Natl Acad Sci U S A, 1997. 94(7): p. 3320-3.
785. Hakimi, J.M., M.P. Schoenberg, R.H. Rondinelli, S. Piantadosi and E.R. Barrack, Androgen receptor variants with short glutamine or glycine repeats may identify unique subpopulations of men with prostate cancer. Clin Cancer Res, 1997. 3(9): p. 1599-608.
786. Ingles, S.A., R.K. Ross, M.C. Yu, R.A. Irvine, G. La Pera, R.W. Haile and G.A. Coetzee, Association of prostate cancer risk with genetic polymorphisms in vitamin D receptor and androgen receptor. J Natl Cancer Inst, 1997. 89(2): p. 166-70.
787. Platz, E.A., E. Giovannucci, D.M. Dahl, K. Krithivas, C.H. Hennekens, M. Brown, M.J. Stampfer and P.W. Kantoff, The androgen receptor gene GGN microsatellite and prostate cancer risk. Cancer Epidemiol Biomarkers Prev, 1998. 7(5): p. 379-84.

788. Bratt, O., A. Borg, U. Kristoffersson, R. Lundgren, Q.X. Zhang and H. Olsson, CAG repeat length in the androgen receptor gene is related to age at diagnosis of prostate cancer and response to endocrine therapy, but not to prostate cancer risk. Br J Cancer, 1999. 81(4): p. 672-6.
789. Correa-Cerro, L., G. Wohr, J. Haussler, P. Berthon, E. Drelon, P. Mangin, G. Fournier, O. Cussenot, P. Kraus, W. Just, T. Paiss, J.M. Cantu, and W. Vogel, (CAG)nCAA and GGN repeats in the human androgen receptor gene are not associated with prostate cancer in a French-German population. Eur J Hum Genet, 1999. 7(3): p. 357-62.
790. Edwards, S.M., M.D. Badzioch, R. Minter, R. Hamoudi, N. Collins, A. Ardern-Jones, A. Dowe, S. Osborne, J. Kelly, R. Shearer, D.F. Easton, G.F. Saunders, D.P. Dearnaley, and R.A. Eeles, Androgen receptor polymorphisms: association with prostate cancer risk, relapse and overall survival. Int J Cancer, 1999. 84(5): p. 458-65.
791. Ekman, P., Genetic and environmental factors in prostate cancer genesis: identifying high-risk cohorts. Eur Urol, 1999. 35(5-6): p. 362-9.
792. Lange, E.M., H. Chen, K. Brierley, H. Livermore, K.J. Wojno, C.D. Langefeld, K. Lange and K.A. Cooney, The polymorphic exon 1 androgen receptor CAG repeat in men with a potential inherited predisposition to prostate cancer. Cancer Epidemiol Biomarkers Prev, 2000. 9(4): p. 439-42.
793. Beilin, J., L. Harewood, M. Frydenberg, H. Mameghan, R.F. Martyres, S.J. Farish, C. Yue, D.R. Deam, K.A. Byron and J.D. Zajac, A case-control study of the androgen receptor gene CAG repeat polymorphism in Australian prostate carcinoma subjects. Cancer, 2001. 92(4): p. 941-9.
794. Latil, A.G., R. Azzouzi, G.S. Cancel, E.C. Guillaume, B. Cochan-Priollet, P.L. Berthon and O. Cussenot, Prostate carcinoma risk and allelic variants of genes involved in androgen biosynthesis and metabolism pathways. Cancer, 2001. 92(5): p. 1130-7.
795. Chang, B.L., S.L. Zheng, G.A. Hawkins, S.D. Isaacs, K.E. Wiley, A. Turner, J.D. Carpten, E.R. Bleecker, P.C. Walsh, J.M. Trent, D.A. Meyers, W.B. Isaacs, and J. Xu, Polymorphic GGC repeats in the androgen receptor gene are associated with hereditary and sporadic prostate cancer risk. Hum Genet, 2002. 110(2): p. 122-9.
796. Xue, W., R.A. Irvine, M.C. Yu, R.K. Ross, G.A. Coetzee and S.A. Ingles, Susceptibility to prostate cancer: interaction between genotypes at the androgen receptor and prostate-specific antigen loci. Cancer Res, 2000. 60(4): p. 839-41.